W9-BVF-887

HOLISTIC MEDICINE

Published by arrangement with
Robert Briggs Associates, San Francisco.

Books by Kenneth R. Pelletier

Mind as Healer, Mind as Slayer

Toward a Science of Consciousness

Holistic Medicine

Co-author of
Consciousness: East and West

Kenneth R. Pelletier

HOLISTIC

From Stress

A Merloyd Lawrence Book

MEDICINE

to Optimum Health

DELACORTE PRESS / SEYMOUR LAWRENCE

A MERLOYD LAWRENCE BOOK
Published by
Delacorte Press / Seymour Lawrence
1 Dag Hammarskjold Plaza
New York, N.Y. 10017

ACKNOWLEDGMENTS

Grateful acknowledgment is made for permission to reprint the following material:

Questionnaire in Chapter II adapted by permission of Alfred A. Knopf, Inc., from TYPE A BEHAVIOR AND YOUR HEART by Meyer Friedman, M.D. and Ray H. Roseman, M.D. Copyright © 1974 by Meyer Friedman. Published in Great Britain by Wildwood House Ltd., London.

"Health Hazard Appraisal" reprinted by permission of Methodist Hospital, Indianapolis, Indiana, and Dr. Jack Hall.

Nutrition Chart in Chapter VI from *Body Forum Magazine*. Used by permission.

Vitamin Chart from A GUIDE TO GOOD NUTRITION by Michael Volen, M.D., and David Bresler, Ph.D., © 1976 by Center for Integral Medicine, P.O. Box 967, Pacific Palisades, California, 90272. Used by permission.

List of Dietary Goals from *Nutrition: How Much Can Government Help?* used by permission of Concern, Inc., Washington, D.C.

List of Exercise Testing Facilities reprinted from *The Jogger* with permission of the National Jogging Association, Washington, D.C.

Nutrition, Health and Activity Profile used by permission of Pacific Research Systems, Los Angeles, California.

Copyright © 1979 by Kenneth R. Pelletier
Introduction copyright © 1979 by Norman Cousins
All rights reserved. No part of this book may be reproduced or transmitted in any form or by any means, electronic or mechanical, including photocopying, recording or by any information storage and retrieval system, without the written permission of the Publisher, except where permitted by law.
Manufactured in the United States of America
First printing

Designed by Laura Bernay

Library of Congress Cataloging in Publication Data

Pelletier, Kenneth R.
Holistic medicine.

"A Merloyd Lawrence book."
Bibliography: p.262
Includes index.
1. Holistic medicine. 2. Medicine—Philosophy.
3. Medicine, Preventive. 4. Health. I. Title.
R723.P382   610   79-9509
ISBN 0-440-05288-2

TO ELIZABETH ANNE BERRYHILL
who already knew the path of the heart

Acknowledgments

Many friends and colleagues contributed a great deal to make this book a reality. Most of all I am indebted to R. James Yandell, M.D., Ph.D., and Norman S. Tresser, M.D., because we have worked together as friends to create a clinic from a dream. During these last three years, two remarkable men, Hans Selye, M.D., Ph.D., and Gregory Bateson, have given their sustaining support. Knowing them has been an inspiration to me.

For many years now, I have been fortunate to know Robert Briggs as a friend who has consistently given sage advice and counsel. Through him, I came to know Seymour Lawrence and Merloyd Lawrence, who encouraged me to write and to explore. For this I am very thankful.

A true Renaissance is taking place and a prolific sharing of ideas and visions is occurring among extraordinary people. To be a part of this time and place with these friends and colleagues is a unique gift and I am sincerely grateful to: Robert O. Becker, M.D., Harold H. Bloomfield, M.D., David E. Bresler, Ph.D., James R. Brown, M.D., Rick J. Carlson, J.D., Norman Cousins, Leonard J. Duhl, M.D., Daniel Goleman, Ph.D., James S. Gordon, M.D., Ram Dass, John W. Travis, M.D., O. Carl Simonton, M.D., C. Norman Shealy, M.D., Ph.D., Richard Strohman, Ph.D., and two very special friends, Arthur M. Young and Ruth Forbes Young. From these people and their work, I have learned so much and I am greatly indebted to them.

Finally, the research, preparation, and preliminary editing of this book was only possible through the efforts of Antoinette A. Gattozzi, Lee Peake, Joan Lynne Schleicher, Frances Wilcox, and Celia Zaentz. Each of these people, in a unique manner, personifies the gift of standing on the earth and reaching toward the heavens.

KENNETH R. PELLETIER
San Francisco, California
April 1979

Contents

Introduction

The more the human species pushes back the frontiers of space and the more its capacity for awe is stretched as a result, the more certain it is that the most mysterious and wondrous object in the entire universe is human life itself. Our scientific research serves mainly to enlarge our respect for what remains to be learned about life. Perhaps it is just as well that humans have yet to comprehend fully the wonder of their own beings; otherwise, they would probably spend all their time in the celebration of life and have no time for anything else.

We may not be able to unravel the ultimate mystery of life, but one thing is certainly within our capacity: We can do a better job of caring for human life than we are now doing. It is in this respect that science and common sense converge. For the ultimate mission of human intelligence is the potentiation of self. This process is not confined to the full development of human abilities. It involves in equal measure the way human beings ward off breakdown and cope with it when it occurs. It has to do with the will to live and the physiological benefits of creativity and of the positive emotions.

Medical science is coming to understand that the human mind is not walled off from the supposedly involuntary activities of the autonomic nervous system. At the School of Medicine at Stanford University; at the Menninger Foundation in Topeka, Kansas; at the Brain

Research Institute of the University of California, Los Angeles, and at least a dozen other places medical scientists are dealing with evidence that the brain is an advanced apothecary, producing or ordering the endocrine system to produce the changes in the body's chemistry. In this way, the mind can govern the ability of the body not just to overcome pain but to regulate such functions as respiration, digestion, circulation, and even the way cells reproduce.

These findings undergird the basic concept of holistic health, which holds that the human being is a fully coherent and integrated life-support system with built-in mechanisms of balance and control. In this sense, the mind is regarded not just as a biological switchboard but a center for total management. And it is recognized that the mind must not be bypassed or underestimated in any effort to deal with breakdowns, whether from stress or pathological organisms.

The widespread interest in holistic health is a recent development in the United States and elsewhere, but the central philosophy is as old as medicine itself. Great medical teachers have always impressed upon their students the need to make a careful assessment of everything that may interact in the cause and course of a disease. Hippocrates, the first major historical name in medicine, was both a theoretician and a practitioner. He tried to close existing gaps between the understanding of disease and its treatment. He was quintessentially holistic when he insisted that it is natural for the human body to heal itself, and that this process can generally take place even without the intervention of a physician *(vis medicatrix naturae)*. He believed that the essential function of the physician— here again Hippocrates was being nothing if not holistic—was to avoid any treatment that might interfere with the healing process or that might do harm *(primum non nocere)*.

This holistic principle has been restated many times as a basic guideline for sound medical practice. A half-century ago, Arturo Castiglioni, in his *History of Medicine,* wrote that "the physician above all should keep in mind the welfare of the patient, his constantly changing state, not only in the visible signs of his illness but also in his state of mind, which must necessarily be an important factor in the success of the treatment. One would be blind not to recognize that before and after the advent of modern scientific medicine there were great and able healers of the sick who were not men of science, but who had the ability to reassure the patient and thus favorably to influence the course of the illness. It is also obvious that there have been excellent scientists who were very mediocre practitioners. Thus history teaches that any division of the science and art of medicine is necessarily harmful to practice."

If holistic concepts are not new, how are we to account for the extraordinary new popular interest and their development into a national and indeed a worldwide movement? Several factors are involved:

1. Medication

Ever since the dangers of thalidomide for pregnant women were discovered, many thousands of people have become aware that modern drugs are not to be regarded solely in a life-saving role; they can be powerfully dangerous, even when taken as directed by the physician. Antibiotics made their appearance as miracle drugs; they were able to destroy potent microorganisms beyond the reach of other medications. But bacteria became inured and resistant to antibiotics, requiring ever more powerful strains of antibiotic killers. This in turn made the human body increasingly vulnerable to the harmful effects of the antibiotics. The chain reaction was costly and destructive. So the physician had to weigh carefully the relative dangers and benefits. The same was true of steroid drugs. The dramatic and almost instantaneous improvements brought about by the cortisones had to be balanced off against disturbances to the endocrine system.

There were other new drugs, more effective than ever before in preventing or combatting hypertension, or in regulating the human heartbeat, or in restoring sluggish organs, or in combatting unusual growths — all of them powerfully effective but each imposing penalties or risks. These dangers were often as great as, and sometimes greater than, the benefits; their use was therefore brought into serious question.

The public's awareness of these dangers rose very sharply in the 1960s and 1970s as consumer consciousness expanded into the health field. The result was a growing distrust not just of the highly sophisticated new drugs but of almost all medications in general. People became attracted to the emphasis of holistic medicine on eliminating basic causes of breakdown and illness rather than on the use of hazardous drugs. It was felt that doctors had a tendency to overmedicate and to fail to maintain the necessary vigilance over patients who continued to take potent drugs long past the point where their use was indicated—often resulting in health problems even more severe than the ones for which the medication was originally prescribed. People tended to forget that much of the pressure on doctors to prescribe the exotic new drugs came from the public itself.

In any case, the reaction against drugs became an important part of the appeal of holistic medicine.

2. Nutrition

Inevitably, distrust of powerful medication figured in the surging new emphasis on proper nutrition, which was seen both as a precondition of good health and as a substitute for drugs in the treatment of many illnesses. Books on nutrition found an eager audience. The public became more aware, as the result of the White House Conference on Nutrition in 1965, and through the growing literature of protest against drugs, that medical schools failed to teach nutrition or at least to accord it the same importance in their curriculum as physiology, pathology, pharmacology, anatomy, or biochemistry. Actually, nutrition was not being ignored or bypassed but taught as an integral part of other subjects. Even so, the fact that it has no standing of its own in most medical schools ran counter to the public's conviction that nutrition was at the very top of factors affecting health. And the more some doctors tried to combat this view—generally by asserting that the average food market shopping basket provided everything needed for a balanced diet—the more convinced people became that doctors were opposed to them on nutritional matters. The fact that so few doctors questioned their patients in detail about their food habits provided yet additional evidence on this point.

3. Over-specialization and Technology

The reasons behind the massive trend to specialization were logical enough. The general practitioner had no way of keeping up with the fast-developing new knowledge, let alone the vast array of new technology and techniques. Even as they made allowances for these facts, however, the public felt uncomfortable about the extent to which specialization was changing medical practice. People saw a contradiction between the traditional view of the doctor as a reassuring father figure who took care of all their medical needs and the pluralization of the doctor-patient relationship brought about by specialists who presided over separate parts of their anatomy. Holistic medicine has tried to counteract this trend by putting emphasis on the integrating factors.

Patients found it difficult to accept this new impersonalization produced by the new technology. Moreover, the machines pronounced verdicts with a finality that seemed to run counter to one of the oldest rules of medical diagnosis: Always allow for the fact that certain individuals may have all the symptoms of a particular disease yet be atypical or even completely free of that disease. In any case, holistic medicine puts its emphasis on human contact and human warmth, regarding medical technology as generally cold and unappealing.

4. Growing Sophistication of the Public

The rapid rise in the educational level of Americans was reflected in the ability of many people to inform themselves to a far greater extent than ever before about health matters. Many millions of Americans got into the habit of following medical developments. In their own relationships with physicians they no longer were disposed to accept medical decisions unquestioningly. They tended to evaluate doctors according to the willingness of the physician to enter into a dialogue with them based on mutual respect.

5. New Interest in the Powers of the Mind

Enough verifiable data have appeared about the ability of the human mind to play a major role in overcoming illness to make this entire field enormously attractive to laymen. It is manifestly true that interest in these matters outruns systematic knowledge; even so, many people eagerly snatch at new findings or speculations having to do with the reach of the mind. And they are disappointed when they discover that their doctors are not equally well informed or excited about such developments and prospects. With each new popular book on the potentialities of the human mind or on its influence over the autonomic nervous system, the gap has widened between the public and the medical profession. Not all doctors, of course, are disdainful of the new trends. The biochemical manifestations of mental powers are being well documented. But systematic scrutiny of such phenomena, however, has lagged behind popular interest, the result being that the entire field has been somewhat colored by guesswork and extraordinary claims. Out of it all, however, has emerged the undeniable evidence that the human mind can be trained to play an important part both in preventing disease and in overcoming it when it occurs. The entire biofeedback movement has gained in stature as the result of such new research. In any case, many thousands of Americans are pressing for greater emphasis—by the medical profession—on mind-body interactions and the attack on illness.

To be sure, these are not the only elements involved in the burgeoning growth of the holistic health movement. But they constitute both the main structural props and the rallying points for the growing interest of the educated public. Underlying these ideas, of course, are the traditional essentials of health that have always had a strong place in medical canons—adequate exercise, enough sleep, good air, moderation in personal habits, and so forth.

One of the most knowledgeable figures in the development of the holistic health movement has been Kenneth Pelletier. Through his writings and his talks across the country, he has served as a bridge between public and physician. He has a wide understanding of the nature of the public's concerns, and he is able to articulate for the layman the nature of scientific data bearing on their interest in holistic health. His book *Mind as Healer, Mind as Slayer* was a superb examination of psychosomatic phenomena. Now, in his new book, he has systematically brought together for comprehensive and comprehensible scrutiny all the elements involved in the development of the holistic health philosophy and movement. I know of no aspect of holistic health that is not authoritatively presented in this book. He has performed an important service in bringing proportion and perspective to an area that has grown so fast that at times it seems overloaded and confused. This work is both a handbook and an analytical guide. It comes at just the right time.

NORMAN COUSINS
Department of Psychiatry and Behavioral Sciences
University of California, Los Angeles

Those who dream by night in the dusty recesses of their minds wake in the day to find that it was vanity; but the dreamers of the day are dangerous men, for they may act their dreams with open eyes, to make it possible.

T. E. Lawrence
From the suppressed/introductory chapter of
Seven Pillars of Wisdom

I

Physician Heal Thyself

Each century has its own afflictions. Prior to the industrial revolution, epidemics and plagues were the major cause of disease and death. At the turn of the century, cholera, tuberculosis, dysentery, and typhoid were beginning to abate but not because of increased medical efficacy. Improvements in agriculture, housing, sanitation, nutrition, water purification, and sociopolitical equality played the decisive role in improving the general health of the population and increasing longevity (Dubos, 1961; McKeown, 1976; Powles, 1973). Research focusing upon disease trends has consistently demonstrated that the quality of the environment has been the primary determinant of the general health of any population (McKeown & Record, 1962). In contrast to these environmental changes, specific medical interventions have rarely been demonstrated to be significantly related to a decline in the incidence of disease or to increased life expectancy. A frequently cited exception is the development of antibiotics and vaccines, largely between 1935 and 1955, which led to the further control of infectious disease such as pneumonia and polio.

As the threat of infectious disease receded, however, there appeared to be a commensurate increase in the "afflictions of civilization," including cardiovascular disease; cancer; arthritis; respiratory disorders, including emphysema and bronchitis; and the pervasive incidence of depression. These psychosomatic or stress-related dis-

1

orders have shown little decline in incidence since the turn of the century despite concerted efforts of medical research and treatment. Measurable advances in these areas have been very slow or negligible. Causes of these disorders appear to reside in genetic predispositions, environmental contamination, and especially life-style.

Technological management of these disorders has improved but at enormous cost, with staggering complexity, and with relatively little success overall. For instance, the slight decline in heart disease mortality which began in 1968 has been attributed to changes in adult smoking habits and other preventive measures rather than to increased spending on medical care (Kristein, 1977). Each of these disorders has been explored in *Mind as Healer, Mind as Slayer* (Pelletier, 1977) in terms of their etiology, that is, a maladaptation to psychosocial and environmental stressors. In order to alleviate these modern plagues, a marked transformation of the premises of present-day medical care will be necessary. Just as the decrease in incidence of plagues required major alterations in external environmental factors, the alleviation of these contemporary disorders requires an equally profound alteration of man's internal environment. Clearly there is a pressing need to continue to improve environmental conditions, but it is equally pressing to work toward renewed internal environments.

At the present time there is no comprehensive system of truly preventive care in existence. The analysis and conclusions which follow are a modest beginning, suggestions rather than a definitive statement. There is a pressing need for further research and public policy formulation concerning the fundamental etiology of health and disease. Emphasis in health care must shift toward prevention and health maintenance rather than the crisis care of pathology. Our goals need to focus upon health rather than its absence. This reorientation is the major challenge to all health care delivery systems and practitioners. In an anthology of essays entitled *Doing Better and Feeling Worse* (1977), John H. Knowles, the late president of the Rockefeller Foundation, gathered twenty eminent individuals to focus upon the present crisis in medical care. Overall, the essays acknowledge unequivocally that the effectiveness of medicine is limited, with its greatest efficacy in diagnosis rather than treatment, and that health care is largely a matter of individual initiative. Throughout the book are various recommendations for improving the situation, none of which move much beyond speculation into implementation. Perhaps the most cogent observation is that of Ernest W. Saward, Associate Dean of the University of Rochester School of

Medicine, who emphasized that a substantial improvement in the nation's health depends upon a major change in life-styles. He adds, however, "How this is to occur in American society short of an apocalypse is unclear." The purpose of this book is to document the substantial alternatives which are already emerging to make these major changes possible.

At the outset it is necessary to emphasize that none of these alternatives are antithetical or antagonistic to traditional medical treatment. Scathing diatribes directed at medicine are usually based upon misinformation or distortion. Undoubtedly, there is a trend toward progressive dehumanization and mechanization of patient care as documented in *The Unkindest Cut* (1977), by Marcia Millman from the University of California at Santa Cruz. Moreover, political lobbying by pharmaceutical companies and medical societies renders much of contemporary medicine immune to reform. All this is well documented in *The End of Medicine* (1975), by Rick J. Carlson, which demonstrates how even the present level of highly limited benefits of organized medicine to public health will decrease further over the next twenty-five years. Ivan Illich's *Medical Nemesis* (1976) presented the most cogent and precise analysis of the shortcomings of contemporary medicine but again proved to be long on polemics and short on constructive vision. Actually the word "nemesis" chosen for the title points to the instability at the heart of contemporary medicine. In Greek mythology, Zeus gave Prometheus the task of fashioning men from clay. However, Prometheus acted out of hubris, or overwhelming pride, and stole fire from heaven as his own gift to man. For that act, Nemesis engineered the revenge of chaining Prometheus to a rock in eternal bondage. According to physician Raymond N. F. Killen, "Thus Nemesis has demanded retribution from every nation of the ancient and modern worlds when hubris exceeds humility" (1976), and that is perhaps the greatest indictment of contemporary medicine. When the problem is examined in depth, it becomes evident that the consumers of medical care bear a very substantial responsibility for the creation of the very medical care system which they condemn. Our present system reflects our society's values, beliefs, and symbols.

Another aspect of the problem is unrealistic expectations. Consumers have demanded a medical system based upon expectations of miraculous medical intervention and then become indignant and hostile when these expectations are left unfulfilled. According to Lewis Thomas, president of Memorial Sloan-Kettering Cancer Cen-

ter and author of *The Lives of a Cell,* this attitude is based on mis-
guided notions of health and disease:

> The general belief these days seems to be that the body is
> fundamentally flawed, subject to disintegration at any moment,
> always on the verge of mortal disease, always in need of contin-
> ual monitoring and support by health-care professionals. . . .
> There is a public preoccupation with disease that is assuming
> the dimension of a national obsession. . . . Every mail brings
> word of the imminent perils posed by multiple perils posed by
> multiple sclerosis, kidney disease, cancer, heart disease, cystic
> fibrosis, asthma, muscular dystrophy, and the rest. . . . There is,
> regrettably, no discernible counter propaganda. No agencies
> exist for the celebration of the plain fact that most people are,
> in real life, abundantly healthy (Thomas, 1977).

When people experience themselves as ill and the assumption is
that medicine produces health, the "logical" conclusion is that
there is not enough medicine (Chapman, 1974). This, in turn,
leads to a proliferation of medical schools and paramedical training, and clamor for mechanized procedures such as computer diagnosis, resulting in a further escalation of unrealistic expectations
and no appreciable increase in the realization of health. Many
clinicians and researchers have encouraged the image of an om-
nipotent healer, creating a reciprocal spiraling of unrealistic expectations. Both doctors and laymen are laboring under many
false assumptions concerning who is responsible for alleviating the
modern plagues. It is evident that there are no villains, only mis-
placed efforts.

At present there are two basic approaches to health care, with
numerous overlapping areas and points of mutual enrichment. One
orientation emphasizes the increasing sophistication of biomedical technology such as coronary bypass surgery, kidney dialysis,
and prosthetic joints. Such a system is consistent with widespread
indulgence in self-destructive behavior, for medicine is expected
to repair the resultant damages. The other approach is more "ecological" in orientation and acknowledges that there are finite resources available to the individual to expend just as there are finite
resources of the planet. Changes in self-destructive life-styles are
seen as necessary to prevent the occurrence of severe disorders, as
well as a decrease in our dependency upon more sophisticated biomedical technology. At the interface of these two approaches are

innovations such as biofeedback with its emphasis upon technology, coupled with individual responsibility and humanistic values.

The thrust of this book is in keeping with the most recent evaluation of the national health care system by the Department of Health, Education, and Welfare in 1975 entitled *Forward Plan for Health:* "Further expansion in the nation's health system is likely to produce only marginal increases in the overall health status of the American people. . . . The greatest benefits are likely to accrue from efforts to improve the health habits of all Americans and the environment in which they live and work" (U.S. Department of Health, Education, and Welfare, 1975). From this statement and many other supporting research and clinical reports, it is evident that traditional medicine is one small part of a much larger issue, which is health care and maintenance. Medicine per se is the "diagnosis and treatment of disease" with an emphasis upon pathology or disorders of structure and function. There is virtually no mandate or training in medicine for practitioners to be skilled in health care. One physician, John S. Chapman, noted in a recent editorial in the *Archives of Environmental Health* (1974) that "if the aim is health, as proclaimed, people will strive in vain as long as they try to achieve that goal by proliferation of medical personnel or facilities. . . . Medicine has indeed very little knowledge of or techniques for production of health as a positive activity." As long as doctors and patients labor under the misconception that health can be created by pharmaceuticals or surgery, then bitter resentments toward the medical profession will continue to increase. As long as medical care consumers maintain a "Volkswagen attitude" that they can run themselves as hard as they wish to the breaking point and then medicine will repair the damage by replacing the parts, the present crisis will continue unabated. We are a credit-fixated culture that has a pervasive ethic of buy now and pay later. Organ transplants and renal dialysis epitomize this direction in medicine. Such approaches are clearly limited to a specific population while the alternative approach with an emphasis upon prevention is far more encompassing. This book attempts to define both the scope and limitations of medicine and clarify the more comprehensive sources from which a genuine system of health maintenance can spring.

Future directions in health must involve the positive modification of the conditions which lead to disease rather than simple intervention in the mechanism of a disorder after it has occurred. Health is not the absence of disease but a state of optimum functioning about which we have very little information. Medicine focuses narrowly upon the particular area of acute illness and traumatic injury, but most disorders and health issues far exceed that narrow range of inquiry. As pathology is examined with ever-increasing specialization, the major crises in contemporary medicine are completely overlooked. There is no need to search obscure journals for a constructive critique of this situation, since some of the most articulate spokesmen on the limits of modern medicine are within the system itself. An article by F. J. Ingelfinger, former editor of *The New England Journal of Medicine,* underlines these limits:

> Let us assume that 80 percent of patients have either self-limited disorders or conditions not improvable, even by modern medicine. The physician's actions, unless harmful, will therefore not affect the basic course of such conditions. In slightly over 10 percent of cases, however, medical intervention is dramatically successful, whether the surgeon repairs bones or removes stones, the internist uses antibiotics or palliative measures (e.g., insulin, vitamin B_{12}) appropriately, or the pediatrician eliminates a food that an enzyme-deficient infant cannot absorb or metabolize. But, alas, in the final 9 percent, give or take a point or two, the doctor may diagnose or treat inadequately, or he may just have bad luck. Whatever the reason, the patient ends up with iatrogenic problems. So the balance of accounts ends up marginally on the positive side of zero (Ingelfinger, 1977).

It is more than evident that health never has been and never will be the sole responsibility of doctors but increasingly that of the consumer working in concert with medical, psychological, and environmental counselors. Within this revised context, the role of the physician will change substantially. Such change has been anticipated in a new publication entitled *The Harvard Medical School Health Letter,* which is an excellent general source of health information for the layperson. A statement by Robert H. Moser in *The New England Journal of Medicine* summarizes the motivation behind the *Health Letter:* "It is time we descended from Olympus and began to address the people—to educate them about the realities of health and disease, to teach them what they can do to help themselves, and what we cannot do. They must be taught about the marvelous capabilities and the serious limitations of medicine" (Moser, 1977). Such an orientation can certainly have the effect of changing the present dismal status quo, from marginally positive health toward a level of optimum health.

Ultimately, the solution to the present crisis in health care involves individual responsibility. Secondary to this is the necessity of social and political responsibility through public education and legislation. There is a definite tendency in our culture toward self-destructive behavior and living the "good life" despite dire consequences. A revised medical care system would literally change the way in which most people live their lives. This does not mean that they would "drop out," but rather change many of the self-destructive patterns of their life-styles. Sources of these life-styles are many. Television advertising is one example. A commercial first elicits a certain neurotic concern such as lack of companionship, insufficient achievement, and so on. Then it proceeds to "diagnose" this condition as due to "bad breath," "yellow teeth," "dandruff"; and to "prescribe" the "cure," which is the sponsor's product. The situation is then happily resolved. Among other deceptions, this perpetuates a destructive and pervasive myth that fulfillment resides outside the individual in an object or product. Such a pervasive model advocating the abdication of individual responsibility makes it difficult to change people's attitudes. John H. Knowles has suggested further factors contributing to self-destructive behavior even in the presence of clear information as to its consequences.

> The reasons for this peculiar behavior may include: (1) a denial of death and disease coupled with the demand for instant gratification and the orientation of most people in most cultures to living day by day; (2) the feeling that nature, including death and disease, can be conquered through scientific and technologic advance or overcome by personal will; (3) the dispiriting conditions of old people leads to a decision by some that they don't want infirmities and unhappiness and would just as soon die early; (4) chronic depression in some individuals to the extent that they wish to take care of themselves; (5) the disinterest of the one person to whom we ascribe the ultimate wisdom about health—the physician (Knowles, 1977).

Among the destructive habits in question are overeating, smoking, dependency upon medication, reckless driving, lack of exercise, excess alcohol consumption, and on and on. No one is advocating a new Puritan ethic, but rather that the individuals in our society who engage in inherently destructive life-styles assume responsibility for the outcome rather than turning to medicine as a panacea. This means recognizing their neurotic condition as primary and finding the means of achieving an internal resolution. Such a change from an external to an internal orientation is a pressing need, paralleled by the recognition of our environmental limitations. The psychological and biological resources of man are also limited and need to be utilized with a heightened consciousness.

An effective system of preventive medicine must be based entirely upon each individual's voluntary efforts to practice such measures as the identification and alleviation of stress, conscientious dietary practices, regular exercise, medical and dental screenings, as well as a number of other specific measures. John H. Knowles has stated that each person has "an individual moral obligation to preserve one's own health—a public duty if you will" (Knowles, 1977). Despite the fact that stress management, dietary considerations, exercise implementation, and environmental safeguards are not necessarily an exciting panacea, they have been demonstrated to be central to any holistic system of preventive medicine.

In 1974, Marc Lalonde, Canada's Minister of National Health and Welfare, published the results of an exhaustive study concerning the future direction of the health care system for all of Canada: *A New Perspective of the Health of Canadians* (1975). Each of the above measures was considered basic to both individual and political reform in the Canadian health system. Although the document by Lalonde and his colleagues emphasized individual responsibility, it is equally clear that institutions of medicine and government cannot abdicate their responsibility. Recently, physician Eugene Vayda, who is Chairman of the Department of Medicine at the University of Toronto, has underscored the necessity of truly shared responsibility by noting: "Public health requires collective as well as individual action, and a government sensitive to the needs of its people should not attempt to shirk this responsibility" (1978). Specifically, Vayda cites the fact that government needs to enact and enforce appropriate environmental protection measures, to reorganize the present system both to make it more efficient, as well as to free funding for innovative programs in holistic medicine, and to conduct basic research concerning "why people behave the way they do, as well as an evaluation of the best methods for altering unhealthy forms of behavior" (Vayda, 1978). Critics of the Canadian document have noted that it fails to address itself adequately to these issues and emphasizes individual responsibility while exonerating existing medical and governmental establishments. Although the emphasis here is upon individual approaches to optimum health, it is incumbent upon government to implement active reforms in all of the above areas of concern.

Individual education in preventive care has been and will be a major force in social reform tantamount to any previous evolution in technology as a result of *Sputnik* or in individual rights deriving from the civil rights movement. Eminent health economist Victor Fuchs noted in *Who Shall Live* that ". . . the greatest current potential for improving the health of the American people is to be found in what they do and don't do to and for themselves. Individual decisions about diet, exercise, and smoking are of critical importance, and collective decisions affecting pollution and other aspects of environment are also relevant" (Fuchs, 1974). Clearly, there needs to be an extension and revision of our health care system. This book is intended to provide the means for individuals, practitioners, and government agencies to implement and evaluate a preventive program.

At the present time, it is widely recognized by the general public that the major causes of death and disability in the United States are cardiovascular disease, cancer, and strokes. Because these occur prematurely most of the time, i.e., in middle age, this is an indication that they are potentially preventable. It is also widely accepted that alleviation of these conditions depends directly upon modification of an individual's behavior and habits of living. If the problem is so clear and the resolution at hand, then there must be a major block to its implementation. That impediment appears to be the difficulty of persuading individuals to initiate and sustain new behavior which is not dramatic in its short-term effects. Programs of life-style change are far less appealing and compelling than the programs of massive inoculation, or the exotic drama of coronary bypass surgery. Prevention is both simple and subtle, which is its greatest asset as well as its most severe liability.

Research by Lester Breslow and N. B. Belloc, of the University of California, Los Angeles School of Medicine, has focused upon the positive health behaviors of over 7,000 adults who were studied for a period of five and a half years. From their research, it is evident that seven factors are significantly related to life expectancy and health: "(1) three meals a day at regular times and no snacking; (2) breakfast every day; (3) moderate exercise two or three times a week; (4) adequate sleep (seven or eight hours a night); (5) no smoking; (6) moderate weight; (7) no alcohol or only in moderation" (Belloc & Breslow, 1972, 1973). Results of this study indicated that forty-year-old men who practiced at least six of these seven positive life-style behaviors lived an average of eleven years longer than those who practiced only two or three. Each of these factors will be explored more precisely in later chapters; the main point here is that though the concept of prevention is relatively easy, its implementation is problematic. Changing an individual's behavior requires a sustained intelligible message which is reinforced by peer pressure and results in clearly perceived rewards in a relatively short period of time (Farquhar et al., 1977). If any message is not sustained, a subsequent change in behavior will not be sustained. Advertising agencies realize this all too well.

Drawing upon both governmental and clinical statistics makes it possible to define clearly the major problem areas which would have to be addressed by an effective preventive care program. Each of these is considered at length in later chapters. Among the most pressing problem areas are the incidence of the two most prevalent causes of death and disability in the United States, those of cardiovascular disease and cancer. Based on recent findings it is estimated that up to eighty percent of deaths due to cardiovascular disease are "premature" since they occur in relatively young individuals and are clearly related to negative life-style behavior such as smoking, diet, exercise, and undetected hypertension (Knowles, 1977). Also the incidence of cancer has also been termed "premature" since many of its most prevalent forms appear to be related to self-destructive behavior patterns. Among the observations are the link between smoking to oral, lung, and bladder cancer; correlations between diets laden with excess fats, refined foods low in residue, and artificial additives with the incidence of gastrointestinal, prostate, and breast cancer. In any case, a substantial number of cases of death and disability from both these disorders is premature and could be averted by preventive measures. Such measures have already been instituted and have been demonstrated to have impact. According to the most recent publication of the National Center for Health Statistics, death rates in 1976 moved from an estimated average of 9.1 deaths per thousand in 1975 to 8.9 per thousand in 1976. Declines in the incidence of stroke were particularly dramatic since the average figure of 102.1 deaths per thousand was virtually constant from 1962 to 1973. That figure has steadily declined since 1975 to a low of 88.2 in 1976. According to the National Center, some of the major reasons for this decline are "advances in lowering blood pressure, a reduction in fat intake by many citizens, more vigorous exercise programs, and the development of coronary care units and better emergency care in many hospitals" (*Behavior Today,* 1977). All but the last measure can be implemented by the individual.

Stress and its manifestation in psychosomatic disorders is the most evident single factor contributing to the "afflictions of civilization."

It is increasingly clear that there are distinct stages in the etiology of a stress disorder initiated by chronically elevated physiological responses to environmental stressors (Selye, 1956, 1974; Pelletier, 1977). Second, these excess levels appear to be precipitated by an excess of adaptation to change in too brief a period of time. Research supporting this concept indicates that up to eighty percent of serious illness develops in an identifiable population (Holmes & Rahe, 1967) and also that approximately seventy percent of physical illness develops at periods of time when individuals feel helpless or hopeless (Seligman, 1975). The incidence of disorder in the year following divorces is twelve times higher than the norm and even the death rate for widowers is ten times higher than average in the first year of bereavement. A third and last factor in this etiology are personality factors which channel these excess levels of reactivity, once precipitated by excess adjustment levels, into a specific disorder. Extensive research has focused upon prospective studies of behavioral factors in cardiovascular disease (Friedman & Rosenman, 1974) and the carcinogenic personality indices associated with cancer (Fox, 1976). Evidently it is inadequate simply to prescribe global guidelines for individuals to assess and alleviate stress factors in their ongoing daily activity. Chapter IV contains a computer-scored assessment system showing the toll that excess stress exacts from an individual's life expectancy. Effective preventive measures by which individuals can recognize and alleviate excess stress reactivity, appear to be the single highest priority cited in virtually all approaches to a holistic, preventive medicine.

A third major area which we will examine is the dietary factor in the etiology of the modern plagues. Diet plays a major role in cardiovascular disease and cancer as well as a primary role in many other disorders. Forty percent of our current population, or eighty million people, are twenty pounds or more above the ideal weight for their height, sex, and age. It is clear that the major variable appears to be fat content or cholesterol consumption. One such study leading to this conclusion is the classic Framingham Study which was initiated in 1959 by the United States Public Health Service. Over 5,000 men and women in Framingham, Massachusetts, volunteered to take part in research concerning cardiovascular disease. Each volunteer was given a thorough physical and an examination every two years. No dietary measures were prescribed but when heart disease was evidenced, the researchers looked for causes in the records of the individual's life pattern. From this research, it became evident that elevated serum cholesterol was a major contributing factor to cardiovascular disease. Among the innumerable conclusions based on the study was the observation that men whose blood cholesterol level was elevated fifty percent above the recommended value suffered nearly twice the incidence of cardiovascular disease and that a ten percent weight reduction for men between thirty-five and fifty-five would result in a twenty percent decrease in incidence of cardiovascular disease (U.S. Government Printing Office, 1968). Despite the precision of the Framingham study, more recent research has modified these findings considerably and has recognized lack of exercise to be another contributing factor. Specifics of this more recent research are elaborated in Chapter VII. Although the precise mechanism has yet to be determined, it is clear that dietary factors, particularly excess fat intake, predispose individuals to cancer and cardiovascular disease as well as diabetes, liver and gall bladder disorders, degenerative arthritis, and numerous other disorders (Knowles, 1973, 1977). Consideration of dietary factors in holistic medicine is fraught with controversy and misconception. It is difficult for an individual to decipher the information adequately and devise a pragmatic dietary practice. Chapter VI presents a conservative approach to a healthy diet and Appendix A provides a computer-based assessment system as an initial means to individualize the complexities of dietary factors in health care.

A fourth major impediment to improved national health is the self-destructive behavior pervasive in our culture. Among the most striking manifestations of such behavior are lack of exercise, cigarette smoking, and excessive use of alcohol. Despite the general knowledge that cigarette smoking is injurious to health, the per capita consumption of cigarettes has increased, beginning in 1975. This increase followed a relatively stable period from 1963 to 1965 immediately following the publication of research results by the Surgeon General. The effect of public education appears to be short-lived. Excessive use of alcohol is comparable to cigarette smoking in terms of the pervasive knowledge that it is conducive to disease. Alcohol excess is directly linked to cirrhosis and cancer of the liver, vitamin deficiency, and is a highly ranked "risk factor" in cancer of the mouth and internal neck area including the larnyx and esophogus. Indirectly, intoxication is linked with estimates ranging from fifty to seventy-five percent of all deaths and injuries due to automobile accidents. Alcohol abuse is one more symptom of widespread self-destructive behavior. Establishment of preventive health care in such a climate is clearly a multifaceted problem far beyond the province of medicine. Collectively, the four major problem areas discussed above demonstrate the necessity of individual responsibility.

Undoubtedly, there are numerous other factors which affect health, especially environmental ones: asbestos from automobile brake linings, radiation, geographic variables, hazardous occupations, drinking water, etc. (Page et al., 1976). It is simply not possible to consider all of these factors here, but they all confirm the central thesis of this book, which is the need for a fundamental heightening of the health consciousness of each individual in our culture. Once again, John H. Knowles has made the issue clear: "A successful long-term strategy for improving and maintaining health must place equal responsibility on individual producers and individual consumers—a substantial change in the behavior of both will be required before health is improved measurably in the United States" (Knowles, 1977). Virtually every individual is appalled by the rapidly escalating costs of medical care but few people clearly see the connection between this rise and the fact that the greatest portion of the national expenditure for medical care is for premature, i.e., preventable, disorders. Until this connection is acknowledged, railing against the plight of contemporary medicine is a hollow protest. If each individual is willing to participate in private and public efforts to reduce health hazards in his or her behavior and environment, then the afflictions of civilization can be reduced. If not, then we need to stop complaining about the disproportionate share of the Gross National Product that is consumed under our present medical care system. Whatever advances there will be in the health of the entire culture will be determined by what each of us is willing to do for himself and others.

An orientation has emerged in health care which has been termed holistic medicine, derived from the Greek *holos* meaning "whole." Fundamental to holistic medicine is the recognition that each state of health and disease requires a consideration of all contributing factors: psychological, psychosocial, environmental, and spiritual. Such an approach is obviously inimical to reductionistic ones seeking cause-and-effect relationships, whether based upon unconscious conflicts or aberrant molecular structures. Despite this more comprehensive orientation, the holistic approach is still within the scientific tradition, as will be explored more fully in the next chapter. Critics of such an approach are always eager to point out that there is inadequate research evidence to support its effectiveness. Of course, research is inherently limited at this point because it was started only a few years ago. However, there are already substantial clinical research trials where a holistic approach to preventive care has been evaluated, such as a diabetes management program at the University of Southern California, patient education programs undertaken at the University of Southern California, and the Kaiser Permanente Hospital in Santa Clara (Harrington et al., 1977), and a cardiovascular disease program operated by Stanford University (Farquhar et al., 1977). Each has been demonstrably effective in reducing incidence of disease through preventive education.

Another criticism of holistic approaches is that they are prone to mismanage a medical problem by treating it through psychosocial methods. This would be true if holistic approaches were an alternative to medical care rather than an extension and modification of our present medical model. Crisis intervention medicine and holistic medicine need to work together for the enrichment of both. Citing the need for this mutual cooperation, Hoyle Leigh and Morton F. Reiser from the Department of Psychiatry at Yale University have noted, "Neglect of the psychosocial dimension often results in ineffective or short-sighted medical treatment such as simply treating the vital signs in a patient with an overdose with suicidal intent, and then discharging the patient without follow-up, or on the other extreme, treating a patient with depression associated with the carcinoma of the tail of the pancreas, with psychotherapy alone" (Leigh & Reiser, 1977). Cooperation, not competition, is required.

Another less frequent criticism is that there are few empirical means of preventing disease. This may be partly valid but there are studies which indicate great promise for such an approach and none which clearly indicate negative effects. Empirical evaluation of preventive care would ultimately involve a double-blind study, where neither the researchers nor subjects would know who received treatment and who did not until the evaluation was completed, with matched control populations over a minimum thirty-year time period. Not only is such research extremely costly but it might require several trials to be conclusive, and it is clear that thirty years is simply too long to wait, given the present crisis in health care. A major reason why there is a relative paucity of research to support such an approach is that there has been virtually no funding allocated for that purpose. Of the annual national expenditure, over 130 billion dollars per year for health care, more than $590 for each person in our society, it is appalling that less than 2.5 percent is spent on prevention and the even lower figure of .5 percent for health education (U.S. Government Printing Office, 1975). Without research funding it is hardly likely that preventive measures can be adequately evaluated. An alternative form of evaluation is the more simple one of patient outcome. Virtually every patient acknowledges that stress has either induced or aggravated his or her condition and is quite capable of acknowledging when a procedure aids him in recovery and health maintenance. Whether these variables can be quantified and empirically validated is a quite different issue from whether or not it is effective. Actually, if the *Physician's Desk Reference (PDR)* (Baker et al., 1978), which is a compendium of all pharmaceuticals and their effects, is scanned to determine the effects of a specific pharmaceutical, the potentially adverse side effects frequently outweigh the primary effect and although such procedures are empirical they may not necessarily be therapeutic. Another instance is the application of acupuncture anaesthesia, which has been demonstrated clinically, but not until recent research demonstrated its empirical base in the biochemistry of the endorphins (Arehart-Treichel, 1977; Marx, 1977; Snyder, 1976) did it achieve validity. Caution needs to be exercised in evaluating any clinical procedure, but it is equally important not to discard positive clinical outcome because it does not appear compatible with the prevailing scientific paradigm.

Above all else, a holistic approach to preventive care places emphasis upon positive states of health rather than the absence of pathology. Concepts of health as a positive state with unique attributes date back at least as far as 1947, when the World Health Organization defined health as "physical, mental, and social well-being, not merely the absence of disease or infirmity" (World Health Organization, 1958). Although this definition has been widely criticized for its abstractness and simplicity (Goldsmith, 1972), it has proved to be one of the only enduring definitions of health as a positive state. Recently, Lester Breslow undertook a quantitative approach to this definition and qualified it along three axes of physical, mental, and social well-being (Breslow, 1972). Prior to 1940, indicators of health were based on such data as decreased mortality due to infectious diseases, infant mortality, and life expectancy. However, as the epidemic diseases began to abate and the modern plagues were increasingly evident, such variables become anachronistic. Most recently, emphasis has shifted away from negative, deficiency-oriented definitions of health and toward an attempt at a positive statement. Progress has been extremely slow due to the inadequacy of methods for assessing the quality of life, but most of all due to the lack of a comprehensive overview which integrates the disparate information concerning health (Sorochan, 1968; Patrich, Bush, & Chen, 1973; Parsons, 1972). Now is the time to redirect the priority in health care away from actuarial data and toward an explication of the highest attributes of human behavior. Despite recent attempts to determine health, an observation by the Philadelphia physician Jesse F. Williams in 1930 still stands as a major innovation:

> It is of value to think of health as that condition of the individual that makes possible the highest enjoyment of life, the greatest constructive work, and that shows itself in the best service to the modern world. . . . Health as a freedom from disease is a standard of mediocrity; health as a quality of life is a standard of inspiration and increasing achievement (Williams, 1934).

More recently, Ivan Illich has suggested another definition in *Medical Nemesis:* "Health levels will be at their optimum when the environment brings out autonomous, personal, responsible, coping behavior" (1976).

The final chapter of this book focuses entirely upon the creation of a framework for inquiry into optimal states of functioning, emphasizing the quality of life. At the present time, if an individual is deemed normal by medical or psychological examination, that means he is likely to become ill or die along with everyone else of comparable age, weight, and sex. This is certainly a dismal prognosis. When clinical specialists reflect on their training, they realize that virtually all of their education was spent recognizing and treating disease with no emphasis upon the recognition of optimum health. From such a perspective, the mental image of a patient is an individual who is potentially susceptible to every conceivable physiological and psychological disorder. By contrast it is equally important to begin to create a data base to outline the optimum that can be expected of human performance. Limiting such an inquiry is the fact that optimum levels of health are, unfortunately, not abundant. According to research by Scott Williamson and Innes H. Pearse (1947) in the Peckham Experiment (1971), an intensive study of the town of Peckham in England, the distribution of illness in a population is twenty to thirty percent; sixty to seventy percent of the people, whom the authors term "survivors," have signs and symptoms; and only ten percent or less could be considered healthy. This observation is supported by numerous other studies such as the Manhattan Mental Health and the Australian government studies of epidemiology which indicate that, despite different criteria, virtually all studies determine that only ten percent or less of the people in any given population are healthy. Despite this limitation, the relative rarity of health makes it precious and increasingly important to explore its determinants.

Among the sources which will be explored in the concluding chapter is research on certain individuals who demonstrate an optimal ability to adapt to stress (Audy, 1973; Pelletier & Peper, 1977). From such research it is evident that health is inherently a dynamic, ongoing process. Though it is more than the absence of pathology, it does not necessarily preclude illness. Optimum health is not mutually exclusive of periods of severe disease. For centuries, it has been observed that individuals emerge from periods of profound psychological (Perry, 1962) and physical pathology to function at higher levels of health than their previous norm. Among the most striking examples are those who undergo a "spontaneous remission," where ostensibly terminal cancer is halted in its progress or disappears completely. *Spontaneous Regression of Cancer* by Tilden C. Everson and Warren H. Cole (1956) is a classic study of 176 well-documented cases of a wide variety of cancers which remitted without treatment. Conclusions by the authors indicate that this occurrence was due to hormonal influences or immune mechanisms with absolutely no consideration of psychosocial influences in the patient's life. A later book of the same title by William Boyd (1966) also overlooks any psychosomatic or psychosocial variables in the observed outcome. More recent clinical work by oncologists O. Carl Simonton and Stephanie Matthews-Simonton (1975), indicates that such factors may be the initial factors which induce the immunological system to move toward remission.

Such instances indicate that periods of illness can be a precondition for a profound means for a transformation of the afflicted individual. Hypotheses such as these are even applicable to individuals who have attempted to commit suicide. Psychiatrist David H. Rosen of the University of California School of Medicine in San Francisco conducted interviews with seven of ten known survivors of suicide attempts from the Golden Gate or San Francisco–Oakland Bay Bridge. None of the survivors experienced their lives or distant memories being reviewed but all experienced a sense of tranquility, peace, and transcendence. Each of the survivors reported experiences of "spiritual rebirth" and a renewed "will to live" which altered their lives in a positive direction after their suicide attempts (Rosen, 1975). Inherent to a holistic concept of health is that it contains an attitude of positive volition even in the midst of severe or terminal disorders. At present, illness is inevitable but there is a vast range of reactions to illness which run the gamut from depression and resignation to optimism and active movement toward health.

Moving away from a purely biological perspective on health, there is a great deal of evidence that optimum levels of performance are dependent upon identifiable psychosocial factors. Numerous longevity studies have been conducted which point up common factors associated with subjective well-being and longevity. One example is the research by Erdman Palmore of Duke University. Based on a longitudinal study of 268 volunteers ranging in age from sixty to ninety-four, Palmore noted that four relatively simple factors were noted among these people who enjoyed a functional, long life: "(1) maintain a useful and satisfying role in society; (2) maintain a positive view of life; (3) maintain good physical functioning; and (4) avoid smoking" (Palmore, 1969). Other longevity studies cite more complex and subtle factors but generally cite cultural, vocational, dietary, and physical involvement with satisfaction as the primary requisite. Psychological, subjective states are as important correlates of optimum health as physiological indicators. Interestingly, most research concerning health indicates that it is dependent upon deceptively simple factors. It is far too easy to dismiss such simple guidelines. Their difficulty does not reside in their comprehension but in their practice. As intriguing as the results of longevity research are, the final data are inevitably static in that they cannot indicate the process by which an individual or group attained states of health. They only demonstrate that certain people are more or less at risk than others. Throughout the book this needs to be considered, since the focus is not upon a theoretical description of health but rather upon pragmatic implementation of an individual program of holistic, preventive health.

One of the most intriguing sources of information concerning optimum health is in the form of athletic performance records over the last century. Despite the fact that there has been little change in the anatomy and physiology of man over the last ten thousand years, there has been a remarkable change in athletic performance (Dubos, 1965). Looking through the *Guinness Book of World Records,* spanning the years from 1951 to 1977, there is a clear trend which suggests an enhanced capacity for human performance. Between 1951 and 1977, fourteen seconds has been cut off the mile, high jumpers clear barriers one foot higher, swimmers have reduced the elapsed time in the 100-meter freestyle, etc. Undoubtedly, this trend is predictable and is due in part to more sophisticated training techniques and equipment, improved nutrition, and superior facilities (Astrand & Rodahl, 1970). For whatever reasons, this continued escalation of the upper limits of human performance suggests some of the parameters which need to be considered in plotting optimum states of health. This is not to suggest that athletes or athletics represents an ideal of optimum health, as is a prevalent misconception. Much of athletic training has focused exclusively on the creation of an efficient biological machine with little or no attention to the psychological or emotional attributes of the athlete. One result of such an overly competitive thrust has been numerous injuries, and innumerable surgical procedures, resulting in chronic, premature disability. Such an approach can hardly be termed holistic, nor can it be conducted under the rubric of preventive care.

Levels of fitness characteristic of competitive athletics are not synonymous with optimum health and might actually be destructive. Consideration of this distinction is contained in Chapter VII. "Chronic exercise may be viewed as a type of 'stress'; its profound effects on adrenocortical function are of particular interest in view of the effects of adrenocortical steroids on antibody levels" (Polednak, 1976). Actually, data for several studies have indicated that major athletes die significantly more often from cancer than nonathletes. Anthony P. Polednak of the Center of Human Radiobiology in Illinois conducted a survey of 8,393 college men and his data "suggest that excess risk among major athletes is greatest in cancer of the prostate and of the digestive tract excluding the colon" (1976). Observations such as these can only be adequately comprehended in the context of recent innovative research in psychophysiology and neuroimmunology, which is discussed in later sections. At this point it is sufficient to note that optimum health is a qualitative, not a quantitative, aspect of physical exercise.

Fortunately there are increasing numbers of athletes and books with a holistic approach, acknowledging mind and body integration as a fundamental property of health. Among these are *The Inner Game of Tennis* by Timothy Gallwey, *Golf in the Kingdom* by Michael Murphy, *Beyond Jogging* by Mike Spino, and *The Ultimate Athlete* by George Leonard. Common to each of these books is a turn away from obsessive competition to enjoyment, fulfillment, and personal insight on the part of the athletic participant.

The pioneering work of Abraham Maslow, with its emphasis upon "self-actualizers" (Maslow, 1968), began to open a broader dimension in the understanding of the healthy individual. Maslow suggested a hierarchy of developmental processes in which, once the primary, biological ones were satisfied, individuals evolved toward more humanitarian ideas. Analogous to Maslow's model, is the assumption in holistic medicine that individuals are capable of moving toward an increasingly positive state of health and the fulfillment of personal potential. Individual responsibility is again at the core of this process. In patient-doctor participation, such a progression also exists. At one extreme is virtually total passivity on the part of the patient, as in surgery; at the other are preventive, early-intervention approaches, in which the patient is essentially active and the doctor acts as trained consultant. The former instance involves high risk and invasive techniques, with inherent danger to the patient and the threat of malpractice for the surgeon and anaesthesiologist. At the latter extreme is a minimized risk system which can maximize the individual's participation in an approach of shared responsibility.

Many patients who have no discernible physical disorder are often depressed, bored, anxious, and involved in self-destructive behavior which would eventually lead to overt symptoms of physical disease. Inherent to such states is an agitated state of consciousness which can be quieted and focused through meditative practices (Trungpa, 1975). Ultimately the possibility of holistic health care is dependent upon each individual being willing to undertake the eternal quest of inner harmony. For over 2,000 years, this has been advocated by every system of meditation as the singular means for individual and cultural evolution (Suzuki, 1964; Tulku, 1977). Again, it seems that the most simple solutions are those which are so easily overlooked rather than practiced. Equally unfortunate has been the tendency of individuals in our culture to create an infinite array of movements and cults, many of which insist that any given system of meditation is the only means to attain inner harmony. Meditative disciplines are a mirror to elicit and reflect an individual's inner state and Zen practitioners admonish initiates not to mistake the finger for that to which it points. Far too many individuals have reified the guru or the system as though it were the source rather than the occasion for insight and evolution. Meditation is not inherently holistic and can become as specialized, dogmatic, and narrow as the very systems its practitioners seek to rectify. Clinical biofeedback, too, can also overemphasize the instruments instead of seeing itself simply as one means of treatment in a holistic approach to patient care.

Far before there was a plethora of meditative and biofeedback systems, William James clearly foresaw the necessity for people in the United States to seek out such approaches to psychosomatic health. For a decade, he had decried the increasing sense of "breathlessness and tension . . . lack of inner harmony . . . and absurd feelings of hurry" (James, 1899) that he detected at the turn of the century, when the standard of living rose as its quality deteriorated. Addressing a graduating university class in 1899, James noted:

> Though it is no small thing to inoculate seventy millions of people with new standards, yet, if there is to be any relief, that will have to be done. We must change ourselves from a race that admires jerk and snap for their own sakes, and looks down upon low voices and quiet ways as dull, to one that, on the contrary, has calm for its ideal, and for their own sakes loves harmony, dignity, and ease (James, 1899).

Toward this end he advocated "the ideal of the well-trained and vigorous body maintained neck by neck with that of the well-trained and vigorous mind as the two coequal halves of the higher education for men and women alike." These observations are as prophetic now as they were at the turn of the century and have as yet to be implemented. Even when such concepts are applied, there is a tendency for individuals to enter into a new age of Puritanism with an undying resolve to become strenuously healthy no matter what the cost. Paradoxical as it may seem, optimum health appears to occur only when an individual is no longer fixated upon whether it is present or not. Between the extremes of self-destructive behavior and hypochondriasis resides an ongoing, dynamic process of spontaneous participation in each moment of life. Such an orientation is not the exclusive province of any one discipline. Actually one of the most succinct descriptions of total participation is found in a book by Tristan Jones, who holds nine world records in sailing. In this recent autobiography of one sailing venture entitled *The Incredible Voyage,* he describes that heightened awareness as he considers the possibility of imminent death in a squall:

> Let them peer, eyes aching with want of sleep, into the darkness in a heaving, crazy, thundering hall in God's vastness; let them strain their ears away from the roaring wind and try to pick out the sound of surf on the deadly reefs. Then they can look down their noses, if they like. But don't let them tell me they were not afraid up to a certain point. I say a certain point, because there comes a time when, without any dimunition of the dangers, you get beyond fear. You come to realize that it interferes with logical thought and isn't solving anything. You've done all you can do to avoid disaster, now you are in the

hands of God. When this moment comes, man feels the greatest peace of mind that is possible for him to ever experience. At that moment he realizes that death is not terribly important, even though it is inevitable, and that he has lived his life as well as he could in his own way. If this is the end, then fair enough, he has lived this life, now for the next. Then some regret; not at the thought of losing your life, but because you have put yourself in that situation. You are determined to survive . . . survival is the result of being angry with yourself for being a bloody fool! I have very often been in a situation in which I did not think I would survive, but by God, I would go on trying. I was going to play the bloody game right down to the bottom line, because it's fun. . . . Also, for the time being, it's all we have.

Such an acute sense of participation in life is perhaps a rare occurrence for most individuals and is often relegated to periods of potentially chronic or fatal illness. A holistic approach to health care is one which encourages individuals to seek life-styles which enable them to achieve their highest potential for well-being.

II

Toward a
New Medical Model

According to Thomas Kuhn in *The Structure of Scientific Revolutions* (1962), every dominant paradigm eventually moves to the limits of its methodologies and ceases to be creative. At that point there is an increasing body of information that it cannot incorporate and alternative paradigms come to the fore. Among the scientific revolutions he describes are the study of mechanics after Newton's *Principia* and astronomy after Copernicus.

Medicine, based upon Newtonian physics, has adhered for some time now to one mode of scientific inquiry with inherent assets and often unacknowledged limitations. The underlying paradigm on which basic research is founded has the effect of determining what are considered to be legitimate versus spurious clinical practices. The accepted clinical procedure has a subsequent impact on such pragmatic issues as licensing, public policy, and third-party reimbursement plans such as private medical insurance and Blue Cross. All too often, an innovation in treatment is set up as another area of specialization rather than being seen as an indication that clinical practice should be reevaluated. Preventive approaches such as stress management, dietary factors, and exercise point to such a reexamination. Holistic approaches to health parallel the insights of quantum physics in that both supplant the Newtonian reductionist view of the world with the quantum perspective of a dynamic universe. From this new

23

paradigm derive the philosophical and scientific roots for the practice of holistic medicine.

According to the Greek atomists of 300 B.C., inert atoms were moved by an external force often assumed to be spiritual in nature and fundamentally separate from matter. This perspective is the basis of the distinction between spirit and matter as well as between mind and body. Such a formulation was and continues to be efficacious in specific realms of physics. However, when applied to the biological and behavioral sciences, this dualism leads to some devastating consequences. Within these areas of inquiry, a dualistic model has resulted in ignoring or misunderstanding the principles of interaction between unobservable forces and tangible matter.

This classical dualism which was to culminate in Newtonian physics began its long reign over the social sciences when it was formalized in the philosophy of René Descartes in his *Traité de l'Homme*. Descartes based his theories upon a fundamental division of reality into two separate, independent realms. One was that of mind, the *res cogitans*, and the other was matter, or *res extensa*, in what has become known as Cartesian dualism. With this model, scientists could treat matter as inert and totally separate from themselves. Furthermore, the material world could be viewed as an elaborate machine comprised of assembled parts. From the second half of the seventeenth century to the end of the nineteenth, this model dominated all scientific thought.

For biology, such a concept led to the formulation that a living organism could be regarded as a machine comprised of separate and separable parts. In the eighteenth century, this concept was most succinctly stated by La Mettrie, who compared the human organism to an intricate clock:

> Does one need more . . . to prove that Man is but an Animal, or an assemblage of springs which all wind up one another in such a way that one cannot say at which point of the human circle Nature had begun? . . . Indeed, I am not mistaken; the human body is a clock, but immense and constructed with such ingenuity and skill that if the wheel whose function it is to mark the seconds comes to a halt, that of the minutes turns and continues its course (La Mettrie, *Man, the Machine*, 1748).

Paralleling the influence of the Newtonian paradigm among scientists was the attitude of the Christian Church, which, approximately five centuries ago, rescinded its stance against the dissection of the human body (Rasmussen, 1975). Prior to this, the Church had viewed the body as a vehicle of the soul through this material world into the next. Accompanying the revision was a tacit interdiction against scientific investigation of man's mind and behavior, which were to remain the sole province of the Church. This truce between Church and science resulted in the view that both inert and biological entities could be analyzed into a series of mechanistic parts with cause-and-effect relationships. A central assumption was that the whole could be entirely understood through a fine analysis of its parts and ultimately the whole could be synthesized from knowledge of those parts. Having served as the basis of scientific inquiry up to the present time, this view has had a profound impact upon medicine. "With mind-body dualism firmly established under the imprimatur of the Church, classical science readily fostered the notion of the body as a machine, of disease as the consequence of breakdown of the machine, and of the doctors' task as repair of the machine" (Engel, 1977). Actually, it was as recently as 1858, with Virchow's publication of *Cellular Pathology* (trans. 1940), that medicine moved from the realm of theological and philosophical debate into that of rationalistic science. Medical research focused increasingly on minute aspects of biological processes and systematically excluded psychological and psychosocial variables. Such an approach has led to considerable progress and was consistent with seventeenth- through nineteenth-century science and philosophy. However, it is increasingly evident that to limit all research and clinical applications to such a paradigm is no longer tenable and is anachronistic to twentieth-century science and philosophy.

Natural scientists have long realized that any theory is limited in its application and is only an approximation of reality. Unfortunately, that observation has been lost to many in the behavioral and medical sciences, who are still emulating anachronistic models. It is not that Newtonian models are incorrect and quantum theories are right, but that each is valid for a certain range of phenomena. Beyond this limited range, any singular theory becomes inaccurate and needs to be extended, revised, and integrated with other perspectives. Such a necessity is now mandated in medicine. Biological models of medicine arbitrarily exclude considerations of emotions, consciousness, and psychosocial variables in order to focus upon specific areas such as the biochemistry of infectious diseases. This is an acceptable and commendable research strategy. However, specialization (reductionism) tends to be self-perpetuating, especially when it is as successful as the biomedical approach has been. Consideration of the relationship between mind and body, psychosocial and biochemical aspects of disease, and other interacting systems has been neglected because of these arbitrary conventions and exclusions.

Emerging from quantum physics and its attendant philosophy is a new point of view wherein "the universe is no longer seen as a machine made up of a multitude of objects, but rather as a harmonious 'organic' whole whose parts are only defined through their interrelations" (Capra, 1977). The physics of subatomic particles has thrust upon science the formidable task of revising and extending previous concepts of reality. Among these revisions are many of profound import for the development of an holistic approach to medicine. Perhaps the most fundamental insight has been the recognition that subatomic particles do not exist as objects fixed in a specific space and time. At this level, Heisenberg noted that objects exhibit "tendencies to exist" (1958). More recently, Henry Stapp of the University of California at Berkeley has extended this concept and emphasized that this tendency or probability to exist is not even a probability that a "thing" exists, but rather it is a "probability of interconnections" (Stapp, 1971). An object "observed" at the quantum level is not an identifiable object but is an intermediate system dependent upon the preparation of the experiment and the subsequent means of measurement. Interactions of a quantum nature are of subtle energies that do not conform to Newtonian physics. Just as the physicist approaches the limits of Newtonian physics when dealing with subtle energy systems, biomedical researchers confront these same limits and need to revise their long-standing neglect of psychological and psychosocial energies. Just as properties of quantum objects cannot be defined independently of preparation and measurement, people cannot be separated from their context and interactions with others.

In biomedicine as well as physics, the observed and the observer are in inextricable interaction. No longer is an object an inert and passive entity but rather is in continual interaction with both environment and observer. Heisenberg's uncertainty principle states that it is not possible to measure accurately both the position and velocity of a fundamental particle since measurement of one negates the other. In a more poetic moment, Heisenberg stated, "Natural science does not simply describe and explain nature; it is a part of the interplay between nature and ourselves" (1958). Physicists have attempted to resolve this problem by requiring that the experiment and measuring instruments be separated by a large distance so that the observed object is free from influence while traversing the distance from the experiment to the area of measurement. Unfortunately, in principle, such a distance would have to be infinite. Since this is impossible in practice and still does not resolve the uncertainty of the actual moment of observation, quantum physicists acknowledge that all their concepts and theories are approximations. In the biomedical sciences, great distances cannot be considered and clinical trials always involve close interaction between the observed and the observer.

Concepts of etiology also change when one moves from a Newtonian to a quantum perspective. In the Newtonian model, disease taxonomy moves in discrete stages from symptoms to groups of symptoms, then syndromes, and finally an identifiable disease with a specific pathogenesis and a specific, rational treatment to follow (Fabrega, 1972, 1975). Such an approach has merit but often may not hold up in actual practice. In addition to this caveat, it has a major defect in its logic. Ultimately it is based upon the identification of the smallest isolable causative component, i.e., a specific bacteria or virus. However, it is not at all clear that such an initial causative agent is applicable in any of the noninfectious afflictions of civilization. In an excellent article entitled "The Need for a New Medical Model," George L. Engel has noted this flaw:

> Thus the presence of the biochemical defect of diabetes or schizophrenia at best defines a necessary but not a sufficient condition for the occurrence for the human experience of the human disease, the illness. More accurately, the biochemical defect constitutes but one factor among many, the complex interaction of which ultimately may culminate in active disease or manifest illness (Engel, 1977).

Not only is it possible for a causative agent to be present in the absence of disease, it is also equally possible that a disorder be manifest without an attendant perturbation at the biochemical level. Extensive data from Kerr L. White and his colleagues in the Department of Preventive Medicine at the University of North Carolina have focused upon varying rates of hospital utilization based on factors other than standard medical reasons. Over a period of four years, White examined the hospital admissions records of 1,000 adults per month in the United States and England and found admissions to vary with age, sex, and the seasons. Discussing the data, White points out that entry into medical care systems depends not only upon the "mechanisms of disease" but also upon the "social, psychologic, cultural, economic, informational, administrative, and organizational factors that inhibit and facilitate access to and delivery of the best contemporary health care to individuals and communities" (White, Williams & Greenberg, 1961). Their conclusion is that more emphasis needs to be placed upon "recognizing medicine as a social institution, in addition to disease as a cellular aberration."

An essential and as yet unanswered question is how psychosocial factors, in interaction with biochemical, environmental, and genetic predispositions, allow a disorder to remain dormant or become manifest. Consideration of psychosocial factors was the major impetus behind the development of psychosomatic medicine. Early pioneers such as Walter B. Cannon and Hans Selye sought to bridge the gap between the biological and psychological approaches to medicine. Progress has been slow, partially due to a tendency to fall back on reductionistic, mechanistic models that are simply inappropriate for many of the problems, such as cardiovascular disease, under consideration. From within medicine itself there are strong objections. As voiced by H. R. Holman:

> While reductionism is a powerful tool for understanding, it also creates profound misunderstanding when unwisely applied. Reductionism is particularly harmful when it neglects the impact of nonbiological circumstances upon biological processes (Holman, 1976).

Later in the article Holman states that such false assumptions can be directly linked to such pragmatic issues as unnecessary hospitalization, overuse of drugs, overuse of diagnostic tests, and excessive surgery. While our scientific philosophies may seem ephemeral, their impact is not.

As we mentioned before, issues often raised in discussions about expanding the present medical model is the fear that an organic disease would be mistakenly diagnosed as a psychosocial problem and improperly treated. While this is a valid and serious concern, it contains a false assumption. That is, if standard examination procedures for organic involvement are negative, then the symptoms are considered to be purely psychosocial in nature. The belief that biomedical screening procedures should be considered prior to psychosocial factors is not necessarily valid. There are cases of organic brain damage or tumor for which psychological testing can be more accurate than the electroencephalograph. Often a misdiagnosis can be discovered or a diagnosis clarified by psychological evaluation. It is simply false to assume that such approaches are oblivious to organic involvement. Numerous studies have demonstrated that a certain percentage of patients referred by physicians for psychotherapy have been misdiagnosed. Two psychiatrists, Stephen M. Saraway and Lorrin M. Koran from the State University of New York, have collected data indicating that "in 4 percent of consultations requested of the psychiatric liaison of a large teaching hospital, we found that the referring physician had erroneously diagnosed obvious organic diseases as psychiatric, believing incorrectly that the patient's symptoms were imaginary" (1977). Other researchers have reported similar findings such as: (1) 3.5 percent of 285 patients referred to a private psychiatric practice had unrecognized organic disease (Wingfield, 1967); (2) one out of every 100 patients referred to a psychiatric ward died or required surgery for a missed organic condition (Stokes, Nabarro & Rosenheim, 1955); (3) 2 percent of 7,500 patients admitted to a private mental hospital in Ireland had an undiagnosed organic condition responsible for their psychological symptoms. Other studies indicate that this is a rather common phenomenon. With such data, it is hardly necessary to be apologetic about the necessity of considering and evaluating psychosocial factors, if for no other reason than to make organic diagnosis more accurate. While attempting to account for these cases of missed diagnosis, Saraway and Koran emphasize the need to consider the entire context of the observer and the observed in the act of diagnosis. Some possible reasons for misdiagnosis include:

> . . . an attempt to deny the existence of a symptom, in an unconscious attempt to avoid responsibility for a situation that threatens the physician's self-esteem. . . . The wish for unrealistic perfection or omniscience or for ready answers or immediate solutions to all clinical problems. . . . We have presented these cases to demonstrate how physicians' unrecognized emotional reactions to their patients may result in the erroneous diagnosis of somatic organic disease as psychiatric (Saraway & Koran, 1977).

When the physician role-model implicitly or explictly demands the demeanor of certainty at the expense of patient care, then such a system requires alteration. Diagnosis occurs in a context in which the attitude and belief system of the doctor is as much a part of the process as the interpretation of laboratory tests. As we said before, these observations are not an indictment of the biomedical paradigm as such, but serve to point up the need for a synthesis of physical and psychosocial factors in a more comprehensive medical model.

Concepts derived from relativity theory also bear directly on medical research and practice. Space has been shown not to be three-dimensional and time not to be a separate entity. They are inseparably interconnected in a four-dimensional continuum referred to as "space-time." The separation of space and time are so absolutely central to Newtonian physics that the advent of the relativistic paradigm necessitated a fundamental change in our understanding of nature. Another insight from relativity theory is that mass is a form of energy and that energy is stored in mass. For modern physics the fundamental particles are no longer three-dimensional "basic building blocks" but bundles of energy. Relativity theory gives matter an inherently dynamic aspect since matter and energy are inseparable aspects of the same space-time reality. As biomedical science moves further away from the identifiable solids of everyday reality, these concepts complicate experimentation. At the level of reality of organs, skeletal structures, and muscles, for example, the reality of objects is a useful approximation. However, as research attempts to move to increasingly subtle levels of biochemical analysis, this approximation no longer holds true. Objects and organs consist of molecules, which are structured of atoms, which are comprised of elementary particles in a dynamic pattern of constant change. Summarizing this extraordinary convergence of quantum and relativity theory, Fritjof Capra has noted:

> Quantum theory has shown that particles are not isolated grains of matter, but are probability patterns, interconnections in an inseparable cosmic web that includes human consciousness. Relativity theory, so to speak, has made the cosmic web come alive by revealing its intrinsically dynamic character; by showing that its activity is the very essence of its being (Capra, 1977).

Numerous other concepts in quantum physics bear directly upon research concerning the nature of human consciousness and the development of holistic medicine, and these are discussed more fully in *Toward a Science of Consciousness* (Pelletier, 1978). Intrapsychic and psychosocial factors influencing states of disease or health do not exist as identifiable objects and because of this they are given second-class status in a purely biomedical orientation to health care. Yet from modern physics has come a clear mandate for the necessity of considering the variables of human consciousness in attempting to comprehend fully the nature of reality.

Western medicine has long viewed the body as a machine that could be analyzed in terms of its pasts, as in the eighteenth-century model of La Mettrie's "intricate clock." With its focus upon pathology, the present medical model attributes the ultimate origin of illness to biological factors. Until now, a number of assumptions governed the relevance of clinical interventions. Disease is conceptualized as an outside organic entity that invades the body and attacks a particular part (Veatch, 1973). Illness is seen as the result of an invasion of the host by an overwhelming quantity of this pathogenic element. The physician's role, therefore, is to select a pharmaceutical or surgical intervention aimed at the afflicted part. Another assumption is that the appropriate treatment for an illness is a biochemical agent that will counterattack the causal agent and neutralize it (Dubos, 1959). Generally such interventions are performed without consideration of the body as a whole or the patient's state of mind (Powles, 1973). Since bodies are considered to be essentially the same and personal consciousness is not considered to be a significant variable, then the same intervention is applied to different patients as long as the organic symptoms are the same.

Finally, the most striking assumption of all is that knowledge dictating treatment is complex and known only to the specialist. The patient is therefore seen as a passive recipient of the intervention, preferably without interference or resistance, since the doctor knows best (Blum, 1960; Hayes-Bautista & Harveston, 1977). A patient is seen as a disabled mechanism, and the job of the clinic or hospital is to "classify, confine, and immobilize" the patient (Carlson, 1975). Thus, the person is viewed much like an automobile, both being machines requiring repair with the major qualitative difference being degree of complexity. Unquestionably this approach has merit in crisis intervention and in infectious diseases, i.e., when there is clear evidence of trauma or organic pathology. However, when the issue is prevention of the increasing incidence of "afflictions of civilization," then more subtle psychosomatic and psychosocial variables are involved and the crisis intervention model no longer holds true.

Recently George L. Engel proposed an alternative model for medicine in terms of a "biopsychosocial model":

> To provide a basis for understanding the determinants of disease and arriving at a rational treatments and patterns of health care, a medical model must also take into account the patient,

the social context in which he lives, and the complementary
system devised by society to deal with the disruptive effects of
illness, that is, the physician role in the health care system
(Engel, 1977).

Inherent to this holistic approach are many psychosocial factors bearing directly upon an individual's state of health or illness. Even the
necessity of creating an unwieldly hybrid word such as "biopsychosocial" is testimony to the fragmentation in health care research and
delivery systems.

Generally, the presence of an abnormality is regarded as a specific diagnostic criterion for a disorder. However, a laboratory test
might be positive and yet the disorder not be evident (Engel,
1969). Diabetes is a disorder with clear diagnostic indicators but
whether a person actually manifests physical impairment due to a
deficiency of insulin depends upon numerous psychosocial and
stress influences. When a disorder is actually manifest, how it is reported and what effect it has upon an individual requires consideration of psychosocial and environmental factors. This new model
first of all takes a phenomenological view of disease and sees it as a
neutral occurrence in an individual's lifetime. Ultimately, whether
the disease is manifested or not or whether its course is positive or
negative will therefore depend virtually entirely on how that patient integrates the problem within the framework of his or her
individual life. An extreme example would be a diagnosis of cancer.
Between that first diagnosis and the time when the patient returns
for further evaluation is a critical period. Patient reactions vary
from deep depression and rampant anxiety to a determination to
seize the opportunity and initiate positive life changes regardless of
the final prognosis.

Second, a holistic model requires that an identified biochemical
imbalance be related to particular psychological and behavioral
manifestations of the disorder. Very often the patients' verbal accounts of their illnesses are ignored and physicians rely almost entirely upon laboratory assessment. A patient's experience of a disorder determines his response to that illness, according to research
by Dorrian Apple, who found that people sought medical care when
"(1) symptoms are of recent onset, and (2) discomfort disrupts normal
functions" (1960). From these findings it was also evident that dis-
rupting symptoms, although important to the patient, were not necessarily those which a physician would find relevant to diagnosis or
treatment. Related research has indicated that patients evaluate

their health quite differently from medical students. Patients tend to use feeling well as a criterion, while medical students use an absence of symptoms (Baumann, 1961). The same research concludes that health is defined differently, depending upon an individual's age, education, and socioeconomic background, and that health programs and interventions need to be targeted differently for these different groups. These variables need to be considered in order to improve the understanding between doctor and patient in reporting the nature and extent of a disorder. Communications from patients about their experience of the disorder often mix descriptions of physical sensations and psychological reactions to these threatening signs. For a comprehensive understanding of a patient's disorder, an initial interview needs to consider the psychosocial as well as physiological aspects of the presenting complaint. This can be readily accomplished by a professional skilled in interview methods. The information should be an important part of the physical examination (Angus, 1976). Such interviews often reveal patients who have had a chronic condition for their entire adult life and yet never had the pathophysiology or nature of that condition simply and clearly explained. An illness often contains an important personal message since it is an unequivocal indication that a person has exceeded his or her ability to adapt to the stress of a particular life-style. When a patient is given the opportunity, he or she can become an active and responsible "colleague of the health professional [who] must therefore be respected in the process of health care" (Miller et al., 1975). Educating patients regarding their disorder is a delicate but important task. It can serve as a means of alleviating anxiety by reducing an ominous disorder to a comprehensible problem.

A new medical model must also recognize the role of life stress. In interaction with biochemical imbalances and genetic predispositions, stress is a major determinant of the time of onset, the severity, and the course of treatment of a disorder. Research indicates that stress and environmental factors have a clear impact upon a wide range of disorders including, for example, mammary tumors (Achterberg, Simonton & Matthews-Simonton, 1976; Fox, 1976). On the other hand, positive psychosocial factors have been demonstrated to mitigate the onset of disease even in the presence of a genetic predisposition (Ader, 1973). It is evident in any clinical practice that symptoms vary greatly in their severity within the same patient given the same treatment, and any intervention needs to be considered in light of its psychosocial context. Only recently have such concepts been considered valid for scientific inquiry, and yet preliminary results indicate they might ultimately be the most important determinants of health.

A striking example of the influence of stress upon disease comes from research that links death rates to psychosocial factors. Perhaps the first concrete evidence that crowded human environments contribute to higher death rates and elevated blood pressure has been gathered by Garvin McCain and his colleagues from the University of Texas at Arlington. Results of two studies by these researchers indicate a direct correlation between increased death rates and blood pressure elevations and the intensity of crowding. Their research involved an examination of death rates over a twenty-six-year period among inmates of a state prison and patients in a maximum security psychiatric hospital in the same state. According to the prison research, which dealt primarily with inmates forty-five years of age or older, there was a doubling of the death rate in years when there was more crowding as compared with low-crowding years, as well as concomitant increases and decreases in blood pressures (McCain, Paulus & Cox, 1977). Previous animal and human research had linked crowding and numerous social problems such as crime, but this appears to be the first clear link of crowding and mortality. McCain's prison research was conducted with 20,000 to 30,000 inmates, and factors such as diet, environment, health care, personal schedule and habits were matched, with the major variable being the number of inmates in a cell, ranging from six to two. Research at the psychiatric hospital also indicated a positive correlation of death rate with number of patients. As the number of patients moved from 369 to a high of 630, the death rate varied from .27 per 100 to 2.8 per 100. Undoubtedly caution needs to be taken in generalizing from prison and psychiatric environments to places of employment, neighborhoods, or entire cities, but the findings strike a note of serious concern. According to McCain:

> In retrospect, we should not have been so surprised to find the relationship between crowding and death rates since there is a precedent for this in the animal literature. The relationship of death rates to crowding might be anticipated since crowding has [previously] been shown to increase illness complaints and elevate blood pressures. And psychological stress can impair immunological mechanisms (McCain et al., 1977).

From such research it is evident that the psychosocial context of health disorders, and even death, needs to be considered in conjunction with the traditional biomedical data and that neither can stand alone.

Yet another question which must be asked in a holistic approach to health care is, When do individuals view themselves, or when are they seen by others, as ill? Much more needs to be known about patients' thresholds for perceiving, acknowledging, and describing their disorders as well as how and when they are identified by their family or peers as ill. Many people who are quite well enter the health care system although they have no need of services. There are other people who require care and yet are never perceived by themselves or others as ill and never receive adequate health care. People often deny the unwelcome reality of a potentially serious illness by dismissing early symptoms as temporary when they might in fact indicate a serious organic problem. Hypertension is asymptomatic and may be discovered only when a person who has remained untreated develops a heart condition. Returning to the classical, biomedical model, a detectable biochemical imbalance determines certain aspects of a disorder but does not determine when or if an individual is categorized as ill and accepts the role of a patient.

When a patient does accept that he is ill, then the attitude of the clinician is of utmost importance. A humanistic orientation toward a patient has been articulated as part of the philosophy of the Institute for the Study of Humanistic Medicine in San Francisco:

> A person is more than his body. Every human being is a holistic, interdependent relationship of body, emotions, mind and spirit. The clinical process which causes the patient to consult the medical profession is best understood as this whole and dynamic relationship. The maintenance of continued health depends on harmony of this whole (Miller et al., 1975).

When such an attitude is adopted, the relationship between the person and the health care professional is altered. Since the Greek physician Galen in 357 B.C., all doctors have acknowledged that the relationship between patient and clinician exerts a powerful influence on the course and outcome of the disorder. Perhaps this relationship can directly modify the experience of the illness or even indirectly affect underlying biochemical processes through the psychophysiological mechanisms involved in stress and its alleviation (Ader, 1973; Selye, 1974; Pelletier, 1977). It is likely that the relationship between doctor and patient is largely responsible for the "placebo effect" (Benson & Epstein, 1975) whereby a substance or procedure is employed with a patient but is not a specific treatment for the patient's condition. Under such circumstances it has been noted that upward of thirty percent of patients will show improvement despite the fact that the procedure had no objective value (Nolen, 1976). Any health care system that minimizes the positive relationship between doctor and patient will also lessen the effects of this invaluable asset.

Frequently, holistic methods are dismissed by attributing any positive outcome to the placebo effect. It is far more constructive to seriously consider methods by which the placebo effect can be systematically enhanced. According to Herbert Benson and Mark D. Epstein of the Harvard University School of Medicine, "The placebo effect in most instances enhances the well-being of the patient and thus is an essential aspect of medicine. . . . More emphasis on the potency of the placebo and its positive effects is needed. . . . The placebo effect demands greater comprehension and must be allowed to survive if medicine is to provide optimal care for patients" (1975). At the heart of any clinical practice is the necessity for the doctor to convey a sense of empathy and help the patient understand his or her illness. It is the responsibility of the clinician to help the patient determine the exact nature of the problem and how to resolve it. For the most part, patients enter a clinic or hospital ignorant of exactly what is responsible for their illness. They feel incapable of helping themselves. Loss of a sense of efficacy or ability to direct their lives, due to a disability, is the most basic problem any patient presents.

Doctors themselves are often no more satisfied with the biomedical system than the average patient. One general surgeon, William A. Nolen, has written a moving account of his personal experience of undergoing coronary bypass surgery in *Surgeon Under the Knife* (1977). Throughout his hospitalization, he has access to his personal knowledge and professional advisors, yet he still feels fear and helplessness. Little, if any, support is offered him for the emotional aspects of the surgery, except by his wife. At one point in his ordeal, Nolen himself comes to the realization that his symptoms were a potent message to him and that "angina is sort of a blessing; it warns you that something is wrong with the circulation to your heart. If you heed the warning, you have a chance to hold onto both your life and your health." After the successful operation Nolen acknowledges that "surgery was not only too expensive but it didn't get to the root of the problem, prevention of the development of arteriosclerosis." From his experience he advocates a preventive approach that includes diet, exercise, life-style change, and stress management.

Emphasis upon a healing relationship between doctor and patient is in keeping with the historical development of medicine as opposed to surgery.

> Surgery developed out of the need for treatment of wounds and injuries and has different historical roots than medicine, which was always close in origin to magic and religion. Only later in Western history, surgery and medicine merged as healing arts (Engel, 1977).

Contemporary medicine has forgotten its historical roots. When the healing relationship between doctor and patient is reinforced, it is possible for a period of disability to play a positive role in the patient's life. Throughout history, literature, and politics there are numerous examples of individuals such as Helen Keller, Franklin Roosevelt, John F. Kennedy, and Norman Cousins (1977), who were able to transform personal illness into a positive experience of personal value and growth. While this observation is not new, the possibility that such an outcome may not be accidental but rather may be deliberately induced is a fundamental concept in holistic medicine. A holistic approach moves from a focus on pathology to an educational approach that recognizes an individual's ability to use experience for positive change. A doctor whose repertoire spans the psychosocial and biomedical considerations is more able to support such growth in a patient.

A fifth major aspect of a holistic orientation to health care is its view of the place of medicine. Health is not seen as a subspecialty of medicine, but rather medicine is regarded as one aspect of comprehensive health care. State licensing laws allocated the "practice of medicine" solely and strictly to licensed physicians and surgeons. Additionally, the practice of medicine is defined as consisting of three key procedures: diagnosis, prescription, and treatment (California Board of Medical Examiners, 1972–1973). Current laws state that all health care treatment must be under the direct supervision of a physician except for specific practices designated within the rights of licensed psychologists, registered physical therapists, and other related professionals. For the most part, the roles of these other professionals are limited to dealing with the patient's particular health needs as defined by a physician's diagnosis, despite the fact that these other professionals frequently determine further or overlooked needs for therapy. In actual practice these distinctions are often blurred, but they do make it difficult to redefine health care away from the treatment of disease and toward the maintenance of health. Inherent in such laws is a biomedical "catch-22" wherein holistic practitioners who are attempting to broaden the scope of health care are legally limited to working within the pathology model that focuses upon disease rather than health. It is evident that either the term *diagnosis* must be differentiated from the activity of assessing a person's health care needs, or procedures defined as *diagnostic* cannot be strictly limited to licensed physicians. Unfortunately, there are already many instances of activities that could be construed as "diagnosis, prescription, or treatment" being performed by unlicensed professionals (Chow, 1977). Such practices not only represent an element of danger to public safety but are a threat to professional attempts to revise and extend our present health care practices.

It would be disastrous to try to force holistic health care into the mold of biomedicine, whose methods are preponderantly surgical or pharmaceutical. The span of holistic medicine is far broader, including prevention, life-style modification, psychological counseling, and supporting the patient as a responsible individual. Within holistic medicine, physicians would still be the sole providers of medication and the sole performers of surgery, but would work alongside other health care providers.

Recently, Roy Menninger pointed out an urgent need for both psychiatrists and physicians to practice a genuinely holistic medicine that integrates "knowledge of the body, the mind, and the environment if they are to avoid the loss of respect . . . of the public" (Brill, 1977). Under this approach, patients are not only diagnosed for disorders, but assessed to determine the particular behaviors and practices in their life of benefit, or, alternately, detrimental to their health maintenance. Giving patients information about diet, exercise, and life-style modification helps them overcome disorders produced by daily activity, habits, and stress. This is an extremely difficult task that cannot be relegated to physicians alone. William A. Nolen has succinctly stated the human quandary:

> We would like to have perfect health, but only under certain conditions. To achieve it, we don't want to give up cigarettes, stop drinking alcohol, and drive under fifty miles an hour. We all want perfect health, but only if we can have it without making too many sacrifices. We want it—but only at our price (Nolen, 1977).

All too often this realization occurs in periods of chronic disease or in the face of death. A holistic approach would educate the patient to assume responsibility.

To conclude, this is a unique time in history when basic sciences and philosophy are converging to transform man's view of himself and of the afflictions from which we all suffer. Marie Curie once remarked, "Science deals with things not people," but that time has passed. Perhaps the very problem has been that science and its technology have attempted to deal with people as things. A particularly articulate spokesperson for the "ethical imperatives" in revising health care is June Goodfield, of Rockefeller University. She points out that people of the United States spent 22 billion dollars to purchase alcohol and 12 billion dollars to buy tobacco, but allocated only 400 million dollars to cancer research in 1975. Clearly, the indulgence in self-destructive habits far outweighs the attempts at correction. Additionally, Goodfield notes that the World Health Organization estimates the total cost of remedial intervention in the major diseases of the Third World, such as leprosy, malaria, and schistosomiasis, would cost approximately 15 million dollars per year. Such discrepancies within our culture and vis-à-vis the planetary community are impossible to ignore. On the basis of her observations, Goodfield concludes:

> There is something distasteful in the sight of a highly developed society being forced to divert great resources, both financial and intellectual, to the cure of its own self-inflicted diseases. We can characterize these as diseases of choice—those which arise from excesses in its life-style, or the pollution of its environment (Goodfield, 1977).

"Diseases of choice" is a striking concept. It emphasizes that it is incumbent upon every individual to alleviate these self-inflicted disorders not only for his or her own good but also to free our resources for the pressing difficulties of the Earth as a whole.

III

Myths, Money, and Medicine

Global ecology has unequivocally demonstrated that our natural and human resources are finite and can no longer be squandered in the abuses of planned obsolescence, aggressive competition, and the veneration of profit. Of even greater urgency than the need to change our orientation to medicine at the conceptual level are the pressing issues of the allocation of limited human and financial resources in our health care system (Kisch, 1974). To this point in time, our culture has neither sought health nor seriously considered the social and economic impact of a society oriented toward healthy life-styles rather than material saturation. Such a transformation will be possible only if the environment is made safe, psychosocial factors considered more consistently and seriously, and the social order oriented to foster health and autonomy rather than to promote dependency, exploitation, and suburban monotony. But none of these contingencies will come about unless they can be demonstrated to be "cost-effective." Ultimately, holistic health care will need to prove that it is more efficient, i.e., more benefits per dollar expended, than crisis care medicine. While there are indicators that such is the case, it is certain that, as presently constituted, "the American health care industry is becoming progressively less cost-effective" (Kristein, Arnold & Wynder, 1977). Based upon an increasing number of similar observations, it is evident that a holistic approach to preventive care is both an economic imperative and a viable possibility. However, achieving that end necessitates a profound alteration in our present health care expenditures and methods of delivery, a moving away from intervention centers such as hospitals and toward public education. There must be a profound shift in emphasis, from passive patients served by a biomedical industry to individuals assuming active roles in determining their health and well-being.

Increased funding cannot resolve the shortcomings of the present medical system. Rather, funds need to be reallocated to the task of preventing the major chronic diseases manifested as the afflictions of civilization. Writing in *Science* in February of 1977, Marvin M. Kristein and his colleagues noted:

> There are two important features about American medical care that we wish to emphasize: (1) It is primarily a disease care rather than a health care system, and (2) It lacks what economists call effective market controls. . . . Unless the economic incentives can be changed to encourage reduced utilization of medical services and increase the tension to health conservation, there appears to be little hope of containing cost or of improving the well-being of our people (Kristein et al., 1977).

Underlying such concerns is the fact that medical care has become increasingly expensive and decreasingly effective simply because it is operating from an outmoded base. Many medical care researchers agree with Ernest W. Saward, an expert on Health Maintenance Organization (HMO), who stated: "The percentage of our Gross National Product spent in the health category has, of course, been rising significantly faster than the GNP itself. . . . as no tree can grow to the sky, neither can health spending become an ever-larger percentage of GNP" (1975). In 1950, 4.6 percent of the GNP was spent on health while in 1975, the figure was 8.3 percent, which translated into approximately 102 billion dollars and made medicine the second largest industry in the nation. Of that amount, forty percent was absorbed by hospitalization costs, the most rapidly escalating cost, along with nursing home care, in the entire budget. Estimates of comparable costs for 1977 range upward to 181 billion dollars with approximately seventy percent going to hospitals, physicians, and pharmaceuticals (Knowles, 1977). Because funding is not unlimited and the cost of medical services cannot keep on escalating more rapidly than national productivity, steps will have to be taken in the coming decade to revamp the entire basis upon which medical care is delivered and reimbursed.

Few would be opposed to the present large expenditures if there had been a commensurate increase in the efficiency of medical care, or if such funds had been demonstrated to have a marked effect upon the general health in our society, but this has decidedly not been the case. It is clear from examination of health statistics that the major causes of disability and mortality in our adult population—coronary heart disease, stroke, and cancer—have shown little net decline in incidence. The slight decline in heart disease mortality since 1968 has been attributed to changes in smoking habits and other developments in education and prevention rather than to increased spending on medical care (Stamler, 1975). The average cancer incidence and survival rates have changed little since 1950 except for declines in stomach cancer attributed to nutritional factors (Cutler, Myers & Green, 1975; American Cancer Society, 1976). By contrast, there are equally clear indications that preventive measures have had an impact in such areas as automobile fatalities, the third major cause of death, which decreased twenty percent since 1973, primarily because of lower speed limits and higher gasoline prices rather than improved emergency care (Cooper & Rice, 1976). Another instance is the sharp decline in infant and maternal mortality in New York State since 1970. This is attributed to the legalization of abortion, better family planning, and improved prenatal counseling, which are all aspects of preventive care (Kristein, Arnold & Wynder, 1977).

One example of the effectiveness of preventive care is the current research into the prenatal and postnatal consequences of teenage pregnancy. Medical complications of teenage pregnancy include lower-than-average birth weights to higher-than-average complications in the delivery room. A purely biomedical approach would support the development of improved infant care or more effective medications for use during labor and delivery. However, obstetrician George H. Nolan, Director of the Adolescent Pregnancy Program at the University of Michigan's Women's Hospital, has a different perspective. According to Nolan, "The overwhelming majority of physicians have little idea of the extent to which the adolescent's psychosocial problems can adversely affect obstetrical outcome" (1977). It is to those factors that he has addressed his research. Researchers in the program noted that pregnancy was the result rather than the cause of the adolescent's psychological and physical difficulties. In a retrospective study that compared 100 adolescents who received counseling in his program to 100 mature women who were not in the program but were expected to have fewer complications, Nolan found that the adolescents did consistently well during pregnancy and that complications such as toxemia, anemia, and low birth weight were below the national average for all women. There were also impressive psychosocial benefits for the young mothers. Numerous similar examples are discussed later in this chapter; the main point here is that preventive, holistic measures can be dramatically cost-effective and promise means of controlling mounting health care expenses. Inevitably, controls will need to be exerted and then both individuals and government will face political and societal decisions regarding priorities for health care spending.

Medical science and technology cannot continue indefinitely to prolong life at any cost and the United States cannot decide to expend an ever-increasing percentage of its national resources on crisis intervention. Among the new and costly developments are kidney dialysis, transplant and micro-surgery, and artificial heart-lung pumps, all of which are undoubtedly of value, but may also be regarded as heroic efforts too late in the intervention system. Acknowledging these limits is John Knowles, who has stated, "Inevitably we must meet the question: Life for what, and what cost? Moral, ethical and philosophical concerns must enter the decision-making process in all sectors of American life" (Knowles, 1973). Each decision and subsequent allocation will affect the balance between crisis intervention medicine on one hand and medicine based on preventive care on the other. Although most professionals and laymen sense this and some are acting from that awareness, the logic of moving toward prevention is not yet fully acknowledged. One of the major obstacles appears to be that the superior cost-effectiveness of holistic, preventive medicine depends on personal and social discipline, and this is a price many are slow to pay.

Biomedical and holistic practitioners have an unfortunate tendency to assume a dichotomized stance and view each other's efforts with suspicion. Perhaps some degree of polarization is an inescapable consequence when the theoretical supremacy and economic monopoly of an established system come into question. For the benefit of all involved, it is important to agree that there are no villains and that the positive aspects of each approach need recognition (Van, 1977). Cooperation is required to foster evolution in health care, and to provide maximum benefit for every patient.

One of the barriers to change in the system is the payment policies of medical insurance. Approximately ninety percent of our population is covered by medical insurance, and thus most medical care is paid for by "third parties" including insurance companies such as Blue Cross, Blue Shield, and related state programs. These systems are pathology oriented, with virtually no incentives for prevention. When most policies pay eighty percent of medical expenses but do not cover any periodic, preventive services, then "demand for care is practically infinite" (Abelson, 1976). Stating this predicament most succinctly is David Mechanic from the Center for Advanced Study in the Behavioral Sciences at Stanford University:

> Since . . . health insurance ordinarily includes few incentives for either the consumer or the physician to economize on the use of health resources, its effect is to substantially increase consumption and the overall price of medical care. . . . the incentive of the physician under such policies is to provide a maximum level of services, regardless of their value, and the pattern of insurance facilitates his ability to generate demand without a consumer backlash (Mechanic, 1976).

Expansion of government involvement through programs similarly based—e.g., Medicare, Medicaid, and National Health Insurance— will be likely to aggravate rather than arrest the problem (Arrow, 1974; Fein, 1975). Third-party payment approaches that emphasize sick care have stimulated demand for services and have been largely responsible for the extraordinary rise in medical care costs over the last ten years.

Experience with previous government programs of medical care based upon a pathology-correction paradigm has led Marvin M. Kristein and his colleagues to conclude:

> A move to national medical insurance without substantial changes in controls of the medical care delivery system may prove economically disastrous. One can readily predict ever-rising cost and higher taxes (Kristein et al., 1977).

Perhaps there is too little recognition by consumers that the well-documented overuse of the present medical care system has a direct effect upon their taxes and personal income (Bunker & Wennberg, 1973). Only when that recognition does occur will the motivation and opportunity arise for each person to exert individual responsibility in moving toward alternative health care programs.

Throughout the literature of health care are three basic classifications of preventive or curative services termed primary, secondary, and tertiary. Briefly, primary prevention is based upon the diagnosis and treatment of disease in the asymptomatic stage and upon education to promote the avoidance of disease and disability. Secondary prevention is defined as the diagnosis and treatment of disease before serious clinical symptoms have become overtly manifest. A degree of disorder is present, and the concern is to prevent or reduce the development of a more serious disease. Lastly, tertiary care consists of the treatment of severe disorders in order to prevent them from becoming worse or even terminal. Included in this category is most of the medical care given today, care which attempts to bring about curative results, alleviate suffering, restore the maximum possible degree of function, and prolong life at any cost. Rising costs unaccompanied by commensurate effectiveness in this last category have led Ernest W. Saward to anticipate the necessity of shifting emphasis in health care:

> In view of the present consumerist nature of society and our historically ever-increasing interest in equity, it appears that the fixed allocation of resources will significantly reorder the priorities from heavy spending on complex tertiary care to spending on more accessible and available primary and secondary services (1976).

While there is an increasing agreement that such a course is necessary, there have been only a few concrete attempts at implementing it. Before citing these few highly cost-effective programs, it is useful to dissect some of the myths and consequences of a continued emphasis upon tertiary care.

Among the most prevalent myths is that increased access to the existing medical care system would promote increased health. Following closely is the assumption that it is therefore necessary to expend more funds for training medical staff, especially physicians. Unquestionably there are unmet health needs, especially among the poor, which must be met first by any transformation in the health care system. Research by Forrest E. Linder and his colleagues at the National Center for Health Statistics does "confirm clearly and in quantitative terms the generally accepted idea that there is a positive relation between poor health and low income" (1966). Also, Linder's data indicate that higher education and increased family income are significantly related to the utilization of preventive care services. However, the fact that there are strong reasons for improving access to health care should be used as an argument against a revision of the nature of that care. Furthermore, it has been demonstrated in several research projects that neither the proportion of doctors in a population, nor the technology at their disposal, nor the number of available hospital beds is a causal factor in any decrease of the overall incidence of disease (Cochrane, 1974; Carlson, 1975; Stallones, 1971; Stewart, 1971). It is more evident in comparisons between various states in the United States, as well as between the United States and foreign countries, including England, that the ratio of physicians to population has little to do with the real health of the population in question (Saward, 1975). Increased access to tertiary care as it is presently constituted may very well result in decreased health as well as increased cost.

Recently, a congressional report from a subcommittee of the House of Representatives announced a disturbing fact. They concluded from their investigations that 2.4 million unnecessary surgical procedures were performed in 1974 at a cost of 4 billion dollars. Even of greater concern is the fact that these unnecessary surgeries resulted in 11,900 deaths (House of Representatives, 1976). Excessive surgery is a major problem in numerous conditions ranging from low back pain to tonsillitis (Shealy, 1977; Van, 1977). Finer analysis of such data indicates that the specific surgeries performed correlate better with the specialties of surgeons in a given area than with any other factor (Lewis, 1969). Such information creates a clear image of the psychosocial complexity of inappropriate surgery. Recommendations from the American College of Surgeons support the solicitation of second opinions. A study of 1,350 New York City union members who sought second opinions on recommended surgery indicates that only four percent actually underwent surgery following the second opinion (McCarthy & Widner, 1974). Already the United States has one of the highest rates of elective surgery in the world and with increased access in the absence of patient and professional education in these matters, this rate may go still higher. Although the results of small-scale studies such as these are not necessarily applicable to the entire population of the United States, they do justify the widely held observation that there is too much unnecessary surgery, at a great cost in dollars and human lives. In reality, the public and professional myth of a physician shortage has much more to do with access to *effective* tertiary care than to an actual dearth of practitioners. Before the future health care system moves toward increased expenditures on tertiary care, it is necessary to clarify both the applications and limitations of this one approach to health care.

Rather than expanding tertiary care, it appears to be far more imperative to utilize it more effectively while emphasizing the less costly and perhaps more effective modes of primary and secondary prevention. Two approaches to reorienting tertiary care have been researched and preliminary indications are that these are effective methods for delivering comparable or better patient care at reduced cost. First and most often cited in this context is the Health Maintenance Organization (HMO) model, which has been in existence for the past forty years. Much research has been conducted with such organizations and innumerable articles written about them. The sum of such information is that HMOs have both clear assets and definite shortcomings. The issues are too lengthy and complex to consider here, and such detail is simply not necessary. One of the foremost advocates of HMO is Ernest W. Saward, and his publications are an efficient means of exploring further details. Essentially, the two basic characteristics of an HMO are that it serves a voluntarily enrolled population for comprehensive health services and accepts a predetermined fee per person per year to deliver those services (Gaus, Cooper & Hirschman, 1975). Such a system operates at an "actuarial risk" in that it has a vested interest in minimizing use in order to stay within the fixed fees paid by subscribers. Although such an approach has admirable features, abuses can and do occur in terms of inadequate or insufficient care. Mitigating this tendency is the fact that such organizations are dependent on voluntary enrollment and adequate membership to survive, and this renders them sensitive to patient opinions. The HMO model, far from being ideal, is presented here to provide contrast to the presently pervasive system of crisis care, which has an opposite vested interest, in excessive utilization. As pointed out in congressional testimony by William Hughes of the Mount Sinai School of Medicine in New York City:

> In fee-for-service settings . . . hospitals can receive no compensation for unfilled beds and unused operating rooms; and patients may receive little, if any, insurance reimbursement for elective surgical work performed in a doctor's office. The pressures from both directions may work toward the hospitalization of patients for minor surgical problems (U.S. Government Printing Office, 1976).

In contrast to the crisis care format, there is ample evidence that utilization is significantly reduced in a wide array of facilities under HMO plans. Among such indications are: (1) a study of 8,000 Medicaid families indicated hospital use to be twice as high in fee-for-service settings as in HMO practices (Gaus, Cooper & Hirschman, 1975); (2) reduction in the number of tonsillectomies among U.S. government employees from forty-one percent under Blue Cross to ten percent in an HMO (Public Health Service, 1975); (3) use by federal employees of an HMO was forty percent less than use by those enrolled in an Aetna plan and forty-six percent less than Blue Cross subscribers (Bureau of Retirement, 1971).

There are numerous other findings of comparable magnitude. Reviewing these results, the report of the National Advisory Commission on Health Manpower concluded that "the quality of care provided . . . is equivalent, if not superior, to that available in most communities. . . . These economies appear due almost entirely to the elimination of inappropriate health care, particularly hospitalization" (1967). Another very important factor embedded in the cost reduction is that an HMO operates at a relatively high level of efficiency and requires fewer physicians to deliver comparable care. One economist, Carl Stevens, analyzed the HMO system quite extensively and has stated that if the rest of medicine operated at a level of equal efficiency there would be an excess of physicians within the next twenty years (Stevens, 1971; Saward, 1975). Whether such projections hold true remains to be proven; but there does seem to be a good deal of evidence that the delivery of tertiary care can be vastly improved at reduced cost, and that is the prime concern. Reformulation of the practices and delivery systems of crisis care programs based upon pathology correction could free substantial funds and make them available for the development of holistic, preventive care programs. In this manner, the actual need for crisis care intervention can ultimately be reduced.

In the HMO program at Kaiser Permanente Hospital in San Jose, California, a step has been taken toward primary and secondary prevention in the form of an experimental patient education program. Under the direction of psychiatrist Robert L. Harrington, this Kaiser Hospital is conducting a research and demonstration project funded by the National Institutes of Mental Health. Previous research by Sidney Garfield in the area of Health Status Categories had identified a group of patients termed the "worried well." Such persons enter an HMO hospital because they do not feel well although subsequent examination shows that they do not have any medical problem (Garfield, 1970). Other results of his study indicated that such patients use "sick care" services at an inordinately high rate despite the fact that the medical system does not provide care which is responsive or effective in meeting their real needs. Although the "worried well" make up only twenty percent of the HMO patients, they account for approximately thirty percent of the utilization of outpatient services, particularly diagnostic laboratory procedures and prescription drugs. Moreover, the evidence indicates that half of these patients seek further care outside of the HMO facility. Utilization patterns such as these place a great burden upon medical care and yield no effective results since the present complaints are not medical in nature. Data from the profiles of "worried-well" patients indicate that they characteristically move from doctor to doctor seeking an affirmation of their belief that they are ill and that medical treatment will resolve their problems. Furthermore, these patients demonstrate a higher than average vulnerability to emotional disorders or "problems in living" (Colburn & Baker, 1974), and many eventually become psychotherapy patients. Given these observations, Harrington and his colleagues at the Kaiser Hospital began a project in 1973 to see if they could provide alternative care programs which would result in a reduction in the demands of the "worried well" upon traditional medical care services. Perhaps they could be referred to alternative services where their real needs could be addressed and resolved.

Toward that end, the Kaiser Hospital began a stress assessment and intervention project as part of their routine Multiphasic Health testing. In addition to a physical examination, the patient's psychological status and life-style are also assessed, and recommendations are made for appropriate counseling. Services offered are both inside and outside the HMO itself and include a referral to one or more of the following: (1) health education provided by courses in a local community college (West Valley College), including adult sexuality and family communications; (2) health orientation through counseling with a nurse practitioner, including a bi-monthly class on stress and illness; (3) clinical biofeedback therapy; and (4) other community resources such as diet and smoking clinics. Each referral tried, deliberately and systematically, to encourage the patient to resolve the psychosocial problems that surfaced during a standard physical examination. Thus, individual responsibility for health maintenance was central:

> This was attempted by engaging him/her in a mutual effort to establish a problem-solving plan which the patient would ultimately be responsible for implementing. By approaching the patient in this fashion, his passive dependency upon the medi-

cal care delivery system was discouraged and self-sufficiency was encouraged (Harrington et al., 1977).

Procedures for undertaking this innovative approach required that 2,500 patients be tracked, beginning with the expanded Multiphasic Health Testing and continuing through their subsequent periodic appointments in the Health Appraisal Clinic. A control group of comparable size received standard multiphasic examinations but did not receive referrals or subsequent mental health assessments. An estimated twenty percent of the experimental group would theoretically be the "worried well" and would be the primary focus of the study. Assessment of each patient in the experimental group included the multiphasic examination, a medical history including a survey of professional care, an interview with a nurse practitioner focusing upon "problems in living," the Schedule of Recent Experience (Holmes & Rahe, 1967), an assessment of Life Conditions developed by the Kaiser staff, and information from the Heimler Scale of Social Functioning, which determines a patient's degree of satisfaction versus frustration with life (Heimler, 1975). During the study, the major emphasis was upon the maintenance of an individual's health, primarily through the detection and alleviation of excessive life stress, before it developed into organic pathology. Preventive care can be a reality within a primarily tertiary care system. Patients are encouraged to view the system as a resource for health care and education rather than as an intervention facility capable of meeting any and all expectations.

Throughout the Kaiser preventive care program, health is seen as having several criteria of which only one is the absence of demonstrable acute or chronic somatic and/or emotional pathology. Among the other health variables considered to indicate positive states of well-being and an "enhanced quality of living" are: (1) a sense of personal optimism about the future; (2) a relatively balanced allocation of personal resources; (3) an improved ability to cope and adapt to changing circumstances; and (4) a step-wise reduction in excessive levels of stress. The intervention teams helped the patients view themselves as "total entities" rather than separate mental and physical selves. According to Harrington and his colleagues, "The health education program development utilized this concept of the 'totality of the person' to emphasize a necessary and changing image of the health education role and its beneficial constituents to the consumer and the medical care delivery system" (1977).

There has been a tendency on the part of practitioners of holistic medicine to disassociate with hospital and crisis intervention medicine. Primarily this is due to the fact that hospitals have epitomized biomedical technology, depersonalized patient care, and self-serving bureaucracies mired in politics and profit incentives. Although that may be the dominant image of institutionalized medicine, the Kaiser program demonstrates again that existing systems can be reoriented rather than abandoned in despair and disillusionment (Saward, Blank & Lamb, 1972). Medical institutions comprise too great a portion of health care and are too ubiquitous to be ignored. Indeed, cooperation would be of untold benefit to institution and individual alike. To date, only limited data are available to assess the effectiveness of such an altered perspective. However, that is not an argument to deter further attempts, since experiments require time for their conduct and evaluation. With this qualification in mind, the preliminary results of the Kaiser Permanente Hospital published in March of 1977 are of considerable interest. Patients expressed gratitude that psychosocial factors were being considered. Most patients were impressed that so much information was yielded in the relatively few questions of a structured interview. Many reported that this overview of their lives was "unusual and valuable information" in and of itself. Patients consistently requested unequivocal, "convenient" information concerning ways to cope with the life stresses unearthed during the program. Such a demand might be unrealistic, but it does point out that health care systems of the future should find means to impart useful information and practical suggestions that can be utilized by the patient for positive life-style changes. Toward this end, the next four chapters of this book outline several effective methods by which change can be achieved.

Apart from the subjective evaluation of the program by the patients there are also data concerning utilization of the Kaiser medical facilities. The study's major hypothesis was that: "Patient behavior in, or compliance with, the medical system is improved when psychosocial risk factors are identified and relevant interventions prescribed." Within this hypothesis was the tacit assumption that a reduction in utilization would be attributed to a reduction of medically questionable visits. Unexpectedly, there was an increase in utilization from an average of 3.78 visits to 4.42 visits. Since this increase is attributable to many factors, and since these visits made different use of the facilities from previous patterns of usage, it has not been determined whether or not the increased utilization resulted in a commensurate increase in the cost of patient care. Within that unanticipated increase are actually several of the most significant findings. Overall, the psychosocial tests such as the Schedule of Recent Experience and the Heimler Schedule of Social Functioning were highly accurate in predicting that patients who showed greater stress and life dissatisfaction used the Kaiser facilities more than those who showed greater personal contentment. Examination of the increased usage revealed that seeing a nurse practitioner or doctor for follow-up added about .7 visits, while the community courses and the bi-monthly health orientation services had a minor impact.

Interestingly, the single early intervention that produced a large decrease in utilization (2.7 visits) was clinical biofeedback. Although the researchers do not yet know why this occurred, it is consistent with similar observations in other health care settings. Biofeedback allows the clinician to acknowledge the patient's symptoms as real and, more important, to explain a self-regulatory method for alleviation. Also, it was the only intervention that gave the patient a readily available means of initiating effective stress management. Once a disorder has been diagnosed, even at a primary stage, anxiety will inevitably increase until an effective intervention has been initiated, and clinical biofeedback meets precisely this need. Biofeedback increases autonomy instead of dependence. A thirty-year study of the effects of psychological counseling with problem children ranging from five to thirteen years old, in Cambridge-Somerville, Massachusetts, found that "almost without exception, therapy appeared to have had a negative, or at least a non-positive, effect on the youngsters in later life" (McCord, 1977). In interpreting these results, Joan McCord of Drexel University hypothesizes that "It's possible that people become too dependent on counselors, and therefore they do not acquire the skills of those who do not have therapy" (1977). Clinical biofeedback differs from traditional psychotherapy in that it emphasizes the development of positive skills independent of the therapy situation. Perhaps these learned skills of stress management permit individuals to utilize dependency-oriented facilities with less frequency. In any case, there are several possible explanations for the Kaiser findings on biofeedback and an array of analytic techniques will be applied to the data.

An interim report on the Kaiser preventive care program now available is only preliminary, based upon a highly limited time period of three years, and unequivocal statements regarding its effectiveness are simply not possible. At this time, however, Robert L. Harrington and his colleagues are encouraged by their results despite the fact that:

Project interventions do not immediately decrease system utilization. This may be . . . induced by increased personal contact
generated by the project. . . . Future work will focus interventions on those patients whom we can now identify as being at
high psycho-social risk. . . . It is anticipated that individually
appropriate interventions will prove cost-effective (1977).

Already revisions have been undertaken and funding has been
renewed in this innovative program. Whatever the results, it is certain that this is a highly significant study, one which shows that it is
possible to initiate a holistic medicine program focused upon prevention within an existing tertiary care facility.

Most major chronic illnesses in the United States and other post-
industrial nations have environmental and psychosocial components
that play important parts in their etiology. Given this observation, it
is axiomatic that they are, to a large degree, preventable. Basic research and clinical practice indicate that these disorders will be most
effectively eliminated by primary and secondary intervention methods. Although acute illness and injury are most evident in health
statistics, chronic conditions are often more debilitating to individuals. Also, data from the National Center for Health Statistics indicate
that chronic disorders, "because of the continuing character, exact a
greater social cost" (Linder, 1966). Recognizing that statistics concerning health care have become increasingly unwieldy, Forrest E.
Linder has suggested the formulation of a "Gross National Health
Deficit" analogous to the Gross National Product. However, he acknowledges that it would still emphasize the negative aspects of
health as all conventional measures do already. With volumes of new
literature on the crisis in tertiary care and massive health statistics
based upon pathology rather than health, the plight of those who
seek to develop a truly preventive model of health is best summarized by Edna St. Vincent Millay:

> Upon this gifted age, in its dark hour,
> Rains from the sky a meteoric shower
> Of Facts . . . they lie unquestioned, uncombined.
> Wisdom enough to leech us of our ill
> Is daily spun, but there exists no loom
> To weave it into fabric.
>   —"Huntsman, What Quarry?"

This plight is shared by medicine and the whole of contemporary science (Pelletier, 1978). Values provide direction and order data into meaningful patterns. Questions regarding purpose and direction of individuals, societies, and planetary ecology cannot be resolved by more technology. Humankind must determine where the course of evolution is going before we will know what means to create in order to reach that end. Issues such as these are fundamental to the present crisis and medicine is caught up in a true dilemma.

A few observers have noted that the undue negative emphasis is simply because disease can be more readily measured than health (Goldsmith, 1972). Holistic approaches to health care are hampered by the fact that the very measures by which their effectiveness would be evaluated are based upon outmoded concepts. Many statisticians now acknowledge a finding by the Canadian physician H. N. Colburn of the Health and Welfare Department that "traditional methods of examining data in broad classifications tend to obscure etiological factors and the importance of behavior" (Colburn & Baker, 1974). In 1973 a large and distinguished committee chaired by Philip M. Hauser undertook to evaluate the data of the National Center for Health Statistics, which have significant impact on decisions of funding allocations. One of their numerous conclusions and recommendations noted that "mortality was a sensitive indicator of health status when the infectious diseases were a major health problem. It is still of value in certain situations. But indices of morbidity are greatly needed today for program planning and evaluation, particularly for assessing the effectiveness of programs aimed at primary prevention. Indices sensitive to changes in lifestyle and the quality of life will become increasingly significant" (Hauser et al., 1973). When statements such as these are issued by a conservative task force given the onerous task of evaluating evaluations, then a substantial revision of our entire approach to health is perilously overdue.

Taking the lead in moving toward a national emphasis upon preventive care has been the government of Canada. Under the direction of Marc Lalonde, the Canadian Minister of Health and Welfare, Canada has instituted a change which, according to Lalonde, "resembles a cultural revolution much more than an administrative reform" (Lalonde, 1975). Approximately fifteen years ago, Canada instituted a universal, prepaid, public, medical insurance program and necessity dictated that prevention rather than crisis intervention be the focus under such a system. In 1974, Lalonde and the Canadian government issued one of the most important statements ever compiled regarding preventive care at an individual and institutional level: *A*

New Perspective on the Health of Canadians. Canadians have relied upon the observations of Thomas McKeown, professor of Social Medicine at the University of Birmingham Medical School:

> ... in order of importance, the major contributions to improvement in health in England and Wales were from limitation of family size (a behavioral change), increase in food supplies and a healthier physical environment [environmental influences], and specific preventive and therapeutic measures (McKeown, 1971).

Elsewhere McKeown has noted, "Past improvement has been due mainly to modification of behavior and changes in the environment and it is to these same influences that we must look particularly for further advance" (1973). To accomplish this, Lalonde and his colleagues introduced the concept of the "Health Field," which divides health into the four elements of "human biology, environment, life-style, and health care organization" (Lalonde, 1974). An immediate result of this classification method is that it gives "a more balanced view of health issues, which are usually dominated by biological concerns" (Laframboise, 1973). In essence, this model is an ecological view of health as a "dynamic interrelationship" with an emphasis upon quality of life rather than quantity of disease (Hoyman, 1975). Following extensive analysis of the factors that contribute to a high incidence of disease, the Canadian task force cited poor eating habits, excessive use of alcohol, cigarette smoking, lack of exercise, careless driving, and the urban and work environments.

All of these factors were later affirmed by the publication *Forward Plan for Health* (1975) from the U.S. Department of Health, Education, and Welfare, which was heavily influenced by the Canadian approach. Underlying both of these comprehensive documents is the assumption that life-style and the physical and social environments are the dominant influences determining mortality and morbidity in the twentieth century. For implementing a national health care program, the Canadian report contains a list of seventy-four distinct projects ranging from "informing, influencing and assisting both individuals and organizations so that they will accept more responsibility and be more active in matters affecting mental and physical health" to such pragmatic concerns as "consultation with the Department of Justice in respect to the laws against driving while impaired by alcohol." Lalonde and his colleagues state that theirs is a working document intended to clarify and organize a "map of the health territory" in order to identify funding priorities without adding to existing levels of taxation.

Authors of this bold document are not naive about the difficulty of actually implementing such a program in totality, but recognize that "many of Canada's health problems are sufficiently pressing that action has to be taken on them even if all the scientific evidence is not in." They call for adopting a stance of "Moi Sui," which is Chinese meaning "to touch, to feel, to grope around" and is certainly a healthy acknowledgment that they do not have answers but are not afraid to seek them out. Lalonde and his group have formulated nine simple hypotheses that are as yet scientifically unproven but appear sufficiently valid to warrant positive action:

1. "It is better to be slim than fat."

2. "The excessive use of medication is to be avoided."

3. "It is better not to smoke cigarettes."

4. "Exercise and fitness are better than sedentary living and lack of fitness."

5. "Alcohol is a danger to health, particularly when driving a car."

6. "Mood-modifying drugs are a danger to health unless controlled by a physician."

7. "Tranquility is better than excess stress."

8. "The less polluted the air is, the healthier it is."

9. "The less polluted the water is, the healthier it is."

Not only do the authors of the report advocate moving ahead to implement programs on this basis, but they actually decry the eternal, scientific "yes, but" by noting that it is the very excuse that allows so many individuals to ignore such findings and to continue a self-destructive life-style hazardous to themselves and others.

To demonstrate the consequences of acting on such simple principles, it is useful to focus on the first one: weight reduction. This hardly seems a justifiable emphasis when compared to the incidence of cancer, but that is another myth of modern medicine. Another Canadian official, H. L. Laframboise, Director-General in the Health and Welfare Department, has stated this most succinctly:

It has been reliably estimated that if obese individuals were reduced to ideal weight, the average life expectancy in the United States would increase 7 years or more. The significance of this is illuminated when one calculates that if all forms of cancer can be removed, the average life expectancy of the people of the United States would increase by only two or three years (Laframboise, 1973).

Statistics such as these help to dramatize what has been emphasized throughout this chapter, that everyone wants good health but that our willingness to pay the price through personal and social discipline is thwarted by many myths and practices in our culture. At a popular level, Alvin Toffler's *Future Shock* focused attention on the price paid in poor health by individuals living a "net negative" life. These people have to absorb the impact of excessive change or have to live under a set of values that clash with basic individual beliefs. By contrast to the United States, Sweden leads the work on many significant indicators of health status, the result of their willingness to value and implement preventive care programs (Laframboise, 1973). Rather than emphasizing prevention and self-care, the United States has placed its faith in hospitals, biomedical technology, and medical expertise while ignoring destructive life-style habits until too late.

It is increasingly possible for health care professionals to use knowledge about personal health risks to advise individuals and society about how they can change attitudes, actions, and environments to ensure healthful living. Refining the process of identifying risk patterns has been the main research focus of L. Robbins and J. Hall of the Methodist Hospital of Indiana in Indianapolis. They have ranked mortality due to specific diseases within five-year age groups and have proposed the concept of "stage of life" as a means of specifying the most likely causes of death for specific age groups (1970). Their research and that of others indicates that at age twenty the leading causes of death for men and women are accidents. For males at age forty-five the causes become heart attack and lung cancer (Colburn & Baker, 1974). By age sixty-five, heart attack, stroke, lung cancer, chronic bronchitis, and emphysema are the leading causes of death for men. There are some striking differences in disease patterns and types for women but no comparably clear etiological factors as yet. Most of the disorders in the age sixty-five group are attributable mainly or in part to cigarette smoking and thus are potentially preventable. Overall, the data illustrate quite clearly that most health hazards for most age groups are both predictable and related to life-style. This will be a very important factor in the next chapter, which relies upon similar data to refine these predictions even further.

Recent innovations in screening for heart disease and certain forms of cancer may provide an alternative to the annual physical as a more effective early-detection system. In expanded secondary prevention programs hundreds of individuals can be screened by tests such as spirometry for emphysema, breath thermography, Papanicolaou (Pap) smears for cancer of the cervix, and other relatively inexpensive procedures. One device is an automated sphygmomanometer, or blood pressure device, linked to a simple computer, which was introduced in 1976 to 1,300 public facilities such as malls and factories by a Florida company. For a fee of fifty cents, individuals place their arms in a vinyl cuff and receive an accurate blood pressure reading. Except for hypertension screening and control, whose cost-effectiveness has been well established, screening procedures for early disease detection are not very widespread. A more elaborate system is "Canscreen," offered by the Preventive Medicine Institute of the Strang Clinic in New York City (*Biomedicine,* 1977). For thirty-five dollars, a one-hour evaluation of a patient's cancer risk factors is conducted, including laboratory tests with immediate results and an examination by a registered nurse with specialized training in cancer detection. Screening procedures can make the effects of self-destructive behavior clearly evident, but what happens next is the critical issue. Rather than limiting such procedures solely to tests and evaluations, they can be used as educational experiences so that a positive result will not aggravate the problem even further.

Evidence for the benefits of changing life-styles that enhance health derives from myriad sources. One unlikely source is John Plag, Director of the U. S. Navy Center for POW Studies in San Diego. Plag studied seventy-eight returned Vietnam prisoners and matched them in age, rank, education, and number of flying hours with the same number of fliers who were not captured. According to his results, the ex-prisoners were far healthier than the group of fliers who had returned to an average civilian life-style. Prisoners had significantly less glandular problems, heart disorders, deafness, genito-urinary problems, bone and joint involvements, and ill-defined conditions such as headaches. In interpreting this outcome, Plag attributes these findings to the fact that, although their conditions were extremely harsh, the ex-prisoners apparently benefited from an average of five years on an austere diet, with no alcohol, very limited smoking, and rigorous fitness programs while in confinement. Plag concludes that "the results are intriguing, particularly for heart disease and high blood pressure, where the non-prisoners have four times as much" (Plag, 1977). Among the negative consequences for the ex-prisoners were a high divorce rate of thirty percent upon their return, some parasitic infections, and widespread dental problems. Even though these data reflect an extreme instance, they do indicate that even in the midst of extreme stress certain life-style changes can have a significant effect in establishing some degree of physical health.

Research data with other unique groups of individuals also indicate that similar health habits under less harsh conditions produce similar outcomes. Studies of Mormons and Seventh Day Adventists indicate that they have significantly lower incidences of cancer and lower mortality rates than comparable populations. Actually, the rate of coronary artery disease and myocardial infarction has been half as high among male Seventh Day Adventists as among white males in general (Wynder, Lemon & Bross, 1959). Findings such as these have been attributed to life-styles that include abstention from tobacco and alcohol and maintenance of a conscientiously nutritious, often vegetarian diet, and moderate physical activity. Not only is there a lesser incidence of specific disorders and increased life expectancy, but accounting by Medicare and Medicaid in Utah indicates a significant reduction in utilization of medical facilities and a subsequent decrease in expense of health care (Cooper & Worthington, 1973). After reviewing much of these same data, Marvin M. Kristein and his colleagues have concluded that prevention can be cost-effective: "It can be said unequivocally that a significant reduction in sedentary living and overnutrition, alcoholism, hypertension, and excessive cigarette smoking would save more lives in the age range forty to sixty-four than the best current medical practice" (Kristein, Arnold & Wynder, 1977). Responsibility for primary prevention rests more with the individual and society at large than with the medical care system as it is presently constituted. Of utmost importance is that high-risk individuals become aware of the dangers of their life-style without attaching guilt or stigma. Then they can be provided with every opportunity to participate in programs of nutrition, smoking cessation, and hypertension management.

All too frequently, individuals acknowledge intellectually that certain behaviors are self-destructive and others are conducive to health, but lack the consistent reinforcement to change from one to the other. Complicating matters is the fact that under a preventive approach, most people would not be ill, and yet their traditional set would be not to seek help or change unless they were. Extensive research on motivation has indicated that individuals will seek help depending upon two conditions: "First, the degree to which the individual believes that he is susceptible to a given health problem or disease and second, the extent to which he believes that contracting such a disease or problem would have serious consequences for him" (Rosenstock, 1960). Beginning in 1972, a research team of eleven staff members of Stanford University initiated a two-year study to determine the effects of an extensive mass media campaign directed at the prevention of heart disease. At the outset of the research, they acknowledged that education and exhortation have had a long history of failure, particularly when attempting to produce permanent changes in diet and smoking habits. Nevertheless, their goal was to "develop and evaluate methods for achieving changes in smoking, exercise, and diet that would be both cost-effective and applicable to large population groups" (Farquhar et al., 1977). Their experiment was conducted in three northern California towns. One served as a control group and the other two were given extensive mass media campaigns, with one population receiving additional face-to-face counseling for a small subset of high-risk people. People from each of the communities were assessed at the beginning of the study, at one year, and at two years after the start of the program. Indices included knowledge and behavior related to cardiovascular disease and to etiological factors such as diet and smoking. Also, the researchers measured physiological indicators of risk such as blood pressure, weight, and serum cholesterol. All of the mass media and counseling efforts were designed to produce awareness of the probable causes of coronary disease and offered instructions in specific methods that would reduce the risk. The mass media campaign consisted of fifty television spots, three hours of television programming, over 100 radio spots, several hours of radio, weekly newspaper columns, advertisements, billboards, posters, and printed materials to the participants. Dietary information recommended reduced intake of saturated fat, cholesterol, salt, sugar, and alcohol. Also, the media urged a reduction in weight and an increase in physical activity. Cigarette smokers were educated on the need for, and methods of, ceasing or reducing their daily cigarette consumption.

Results of the Stanford study indicated that there was a "substantial and sustained decrease in risk" in the two treatment communities over the two years. There was an actual increase in the risk of cardiovascular disease in the control community that did not receive the media campaign. In the community in which there was face-to-face counseling the initial improvement was greater but at the end of the second year the decrease in risk was comparable for both treatment communities. Further data analysis indicated the changes in knowledge, behavior, and physiology observed in the first year were not only maintained but even improved in the second year of study. John W. Farquhar and his colleages concluded, "These results strongly suggest that mass media educational campaigns directed at entire communities may be very effective in reducing the risk of cardiovascular disease" (1977). Announcements such as this are bound to raise the spectre of George Orwell's *1984* with its dismal prophecy of media manipulation. For those individuals who are concerned about the manipulative aspects of a media campaign aimed at improving health, it is important to bear in mind that present commercials manipulate people toward pills, overeating, drinking, fast driving, and a host of other hazardous life-styles. Inherently, television viewing encourages sedentary habits. That spectre is minimized by the fact that a 1977 national poll by the Newspaper Advertising Bureau asked individuals to choose from thirty-four subjects for emphasis in an ideal newspaper. Among the highest priorities were "health, nutrition, and environment" (Nunn, 1977), suggesting that people are clearly interested in these matters but find that effective information is lacking. Every individual can still be free to engage in destructive behavior, but at least the weight of the media will be shifted toward the preservation of life. Researchers have indicated that these impressive results could be improved even further through the use of media to coordinate more interpersonal instruction in "natural communities" such as towns and factories. Also, these results have suggested the delivery of more specialized training and counseling about weight reduction and smoking avoidance. Many of their conclusions are quite similar to those noted by Robert L. Harrington in the Kaiser Hospital program in San Jose. Concluding the report, Farquhar and the other researchers noted most significantly that "Prevention of the premature cardiovascular disease epidemic of industrialized countries will require national purpose, planning, and action. It seems that part of this effort—i.e., persuading people to alter their lifestyles—can be achieved at reasonable cost" (1977). Primary prevention can be a reality at a cost comparable or less than present expenditures. Everything indicates that it could be of significant effectiveness in reducing the incidence of the afflictions of civilization.

Such programs demonstrate that effective health care must reach beyond the boundaries of biomedicine and pathology. Objectives of a holistic approach would cover a wide scope, including education concerning smoking, motivating the food-processing industry to reduce saturated fat content and increase essential amino acids, encouraging the use of alcohol level detectors to curb driving while intoxicated, and not least, ridding the environment of toxic substances. Furthermore, there is a need to establish economic incentives for prevention because the present and proposed health insurance systems provide no such inducements to maintain health. Writing an editorial in *Inquiry,* which is published by Blue Cross, A. I. White gave an impassioned critique of the inadequacy of the present health care system. White called for the major thrust of prevention to be toward: (1) improving the environment; (2) allowing easy access for all to health care; (3) more emphasis on screening, health care, and preventive maintenance; and finally (4) concentration by physicians on "curative care," which is their specific area of expertise (1974).

Lists such as these are virtually infinite, but it must be evident that prevention involves every aspect of our society. To take an extreme example, recent research indicates that a marked increase in suicides disguised as motor vehicle accidents occur after a prominent suicide is given great publicity. Professor David Phillips from the University of California in San Diego has reported, "It seems that suicide stories which are covered on the inside pages have no noticeable effect on the nationwide suicide rate, but suicide stories which are covered on the front pages do" (1977). Working from California Motor Vehicle fatality records, Phillips established that between 1966 and 1973 the number of deaths rose an average of 9.12 percent in the week following a highly publicized suicide. Actually, the proportion of the increase correlated closely with the total circulation of the newspapers carrying the front-page story. This study is cited only to emphasize the scope and complexity of prevention, and the intensity of self-destructive behavior.

Ultimately, responsibility resides with the informed individual. Again, an editorial in *Science* by John H. Knowles states this point of view most succinctly:

> I believe the idea of a "right" to health should be replaced by that of a moral obligation to preserve one's own health. The individual then has the "right" to expect help with information, accessible services of good quality, and minimal financial barri-

ers. Meanwhile the people have been led to believe that national health insurance, more doctors, and greater use of high-cost, hospital-based technologies will improve health. Unfortunately, none of them will (Knowles, 1977).

Knowles's point cannot be emphasized enough. Once it is acknowledged, the choice for each person is to remain the problem or become the solution.

If no one smoked cigarettes or consumed alcohol and everyone exercised regularly, maintained optimal weight on a low fat, low refined-carbohydrate, high fiber-content diet, reduced stress by simplifying their lives, obtained adequate rest and recreation, understood the needs of infants and children for the proper nutrition and nurturing of their intellectual and affective development, had available to them, and would use, genetic counseling and selective abortion, drank fluoridated water, followed the doctor's orders for medications and self-care once disease was detected, used available health services at appropriate times for screening examinations and health education-preventive medicine programs, the savings to the country would be mammoth in terms of billions of dollars, a vast reduction in human misery, and an attendant marked improvement in the quality of life. Our country would be strengthened immeasurably, and we could divert our energies—human and financial—to other pressing issues of national and international concern (Knowles, 1977). Clearly, we do not die as often as we kill ourselves.

IV

From Pathology to Prevention

Four measures consistently cited as central to holistic, preventive medicine are appraisals of health status, life-style change, and management of stress, diet, and exercise. Each of these components is fully explored in the next four chapters. Most clinical students find courses in preventive care to be simply boring. Usually they are either a repetition of the obvious or focus upon problems over which they as clinicians have no control, such as smoking, automobile accidents, suicide, polluted environments, malnutrition due to poverty, and related factors. These problems become even more unwieldly when approached on an institutional or political level, which are not within the scope of the discussion here. We will focus upon certain effective measures by which individuals can assess and control their own health. Each involves individual responsibility in combination with expert guidance. Among the most striking recent examples of this approach is the experience of Norman Cousins's "Anatomy of an Illness (as Perceived by the Patient)" (1976). Cousins details the course of his recovery from ankylosing spondylitis, a degenerative disease of the connective tissue of the body. The recovery involved his own active participation and therapies well outside the scope of established medicine. The experience will be examined later in greater detail, but his conclusion is a good introduction to this orientation to individual responsibility:

> The life force may be the least understood force on earth. William James said that human beings tend to live too far within self-imposed limits. It is possible that these limits will recede when we respect more fully the natural drive of the human mind and body toward perfectibility and regeneration (Cousins, 1977).

An approach which works to support this life force, for the patient rather than against the disease, is the essence of a holistic approach to health care.

In primary prevention, the first step is to make high-risk individuals aware of the risk they run. Only after this recognition is the person likely to engage in activities designed to lower that risk. Two major obstacles that have hampered preventive programs were noted by Irvine H. Page of the Cleveland Clinic: "(1) to prove beyond doubt that such modalities as exercise, low-fat diets, and a 55-mile-an-hour speed limit are cost-effective, and (2) to persuade a pleasure-loving, affluent, and undisciplined society to accept the necessary warnings" (1976). The first problem has already been considered in Chapter III, but the second is the more formidable one. "It is time that politicians and public alike realize that preventive medicine is seldom an issue that doctors can influence except through giving advice usually neither wanted or accepted" (1976). Often what a patient needs to do in order to restore or maintain health is more than evident, but, all too frequently, the recognition is not implemented. Our culture has progressively eroded the concept of individual responsibility while giving disproportionate attention to individual rights, especially regarding access to a system of conspicuous consumption. While it is important for health-care professionals to protect health by dealing with both psychosocial and physical environmental factors, it is of at least equal importance to emphasize actions that people can take for themselves. Unfortunately, many patients have come to expect or even demand an instant cure on the order of instant coffee.

For individual patients a reliable health status appraisal can often provide strong motivation to change self-destructive habits. At the present time, there are no definitive methods of obtaining an accurate assessment of the risks involved in a particular individual's life-style. Before more reliable indications can be developed, it is necessary to acknowledge both that such a need does exist and that effort needs to be expended in testing and improving existing methods. One system of personal risk assessment presented later in this chapter is not definitive (many of its deficiencies are already evident), but it is a useful model worthy of further evaluation and development. For many years, approaches to prevention were handicapped by the lack of an adequate means of clearly showing patients the detrimental results of self-destructive behaviors. How to quantify such intangibles was and remains a major issue, for individuals are not strongly inclined to act when such behavior will affect them only in the future, if at all. A complementary problem has been the lack of a means of demonstrating the potential benefits of positive behaviors. Among researchers and clinicians involved in preventive care, it is widely agreed that such positive life-style orientations are of great benefit. To note again the conclusion of Marvin M. Kristein and his colleagues: "It can be said unequivocally that a significant reduction in sedentary living and overnutrition, alcoholism, hypertension, and excessive cigarette smoking would save more lives in the age range 40 to 64 than the best current medical practice" (Kristein, Arnold & Wynder, 1977). The issue is motivation, or how to elicit an individual's participation in measures to ensure his or her health.

One organization oriented toward the establishment of preventive health care is the Society of Prospective Medicine located at the Methodist Hospital of Indiana. Two physicians there, Lewis Robbins and Jack Hall, developed the assessment known as the Health Hazards Appraisal, to be discussed later. During 1975, more than 40,000 appraisals were reported to the Methodist Hospital by physicians, medical schools, residencies, health educators, health clubs, and departments of public health. A four-stage program of patient care was initiated with periodic assessments and improvements in procedures. First, an individual is given an assessment of his ten-year chance of survival. Data used in this ten-year assessment indicate that there are different causes of death and disability which an individual will face in the next ten years based upon his age, sex, and race. Given this information, the doctors know how susceptible this patient is likely to be over the next decade to each of the twelve leading causes of death. For example, a white female between ages forty-five and forty-nine has the highest risk in the next ten years from heart attack, cancer of the breast, stroke, cancer of the intestines and rectum, and fifth, chronic rheumatic heart disease. Each five-year age group has a different risk for different disorders. In order to make these general guidelines applicable to a given individual patient, a computer assessment is required. This is derived from the administration of the Health Hazard Appraisal mentioned above, which compiles present risks and estimates future risks to a person's health. In the patient brochure, the hospital program notes, "What I (the doctor) want to get through to you is simply this: Whether you live or die is often squarely in your own hands, and because we face risks all the time does not mean we cannot do something about them" (Krehl, 1978). Included in this assessment are such aspects of life-style as weight, cigarette smoking, exercise, and an array of psychological factors. Health Hazard Appraisal systems are one of the most important instruments now being developed for preventive medicine. The second step in the program when the health risks have been identified is the choice of preventive procedures to reduce these risks. Patient and practitioner plan this together. The assumption is that "if a person can alter certain risks he or she can join a group which had predicted lower mortality" (Colburn & Baker, 1973). Third, a "health management program" is set up in which other individuals are engaged to help the patient maintain health. This may require the involvement of other members of the family, other health agencies, or a team of health practitioners.

Last and very important, there is the question of timing, since all of the risk factors cannot be changed simultaneously. Actually, when a patient first acknowledges the psychosocial causes of his particular risks, he frequently becomes quite disturbed for a brief period of time. Psychotherapists refer to this phenomenon as the "get worse-get better syndrome" and know that it has a fairly predictable timing. When this crisis period does occur, the skill of the clinician helps the patient move from recognition to recovery and fosters a positive outcome. As an individual moves through a risk-education program, there is certain to be more than one problem area and certain to be more than one means of intervention. The individual is encouraged to move along one step at a time and is not asked to undertake any measures other than those which are reasonable and practical. Emphasis is upon pacing and critical timing in arresting that individual's predisposition toward disability or more severe psychosomatic disorders. During the program, a comprehensive profile of the patient is drawn, which makes it possible to detect dysfunctional systems in an individual before they lead to more severe pathology. In the patient brochure at the Methodist Hospital the goal is stated simply: "It is my job as your doctor, to help you get safely through the coming years—treating you as a whole patient." The patient's profile helps to identify the most appropriate methods of intervention. Many of these interventions are straightforward measures, modification of excessive stress, reduction of excessive weight, and so on.

One of the people most active in the development of The Health Hazard Appraisal is John W. Travis. His publications (1978 and 1979) clarify many of its applications. Overall, the assessment attempts to address itself to medical, psychological, sociological, and behavioral characteristics that may predispose an individual toward a premature psychosomatic disorder or death. Reproduced below is a copy of the adapted HHA used by the U.S. Public Health Service Hospital in Baltimore, under the agency of the Department of Health, Education, and Welfare.

There are limitations to the applicability of the HHA, and patients need to be selected rather than using the system indiscriminately. Appraisals are most useful for individual at high risk: heavy drinking, which raises the risk of death in motor vehicle accidents; heavy smoking; no exercise; and/or obesity. While this profile may seem rare, it is unfortunately all too common. If a patient is at high risk and under age thirty-five, two printout appraisals can be done. One is for the person's present age and the other for age forty-five. This method demonstrates to the patient his risks in an age group where deaths caused by these behaviors are high. In the accompanying information letter it is noted: "Even though your risk seems insignificant now, if you continue your high-risk behavior, this is how your chances will look at age 45" (Reichard, 1975). Scoring younger people in this manner is more effective, since motor vehicle deaths far outweigh other causes in the younger groups and thereby dilute the impact of the grim statistics connected with the high-risk behaviors. However, even below thirty-five, individuals can lessen their life expectancy by many years by lack of exercise or failure to wear seat belts. The research of pathologist Robert R. Kohn of Case Western Reserve University in Cleveland reveals that the age-dependent mortality from all diseases "doubles about every eight years as one grows older" (Kent, 1976). The importance of detecting early tendencies toward disorders that increase in likelihood with age is clearly evident.

Health Hazard Appraisal

Dear Patient:

Your answers to the questions that follow will allow us to attempt to give you clues to some of the greatest risks to your survival over the next 10-year period of your life. By compiling your present risks and estimating your future risks, we may be able to help you begin a series of procedures to reduce these risks.

Please answer every question. There are a few questions that inquire about race or religion. They are asked only because they are associated with different risks in certain diseases.

INSTRUCTIONS FOR COMPLETING THESE QUESTIONS
PLEASE USE A PENCIL ONLY

* Mark a cross in the box ☒ opposite your answer.

* If you change an answer, please erase the cross completely before marking your corrected answer.

* Be sure to answer every question.

PLEASE USE A PENCIL ONLY

Name |_|_|_|_|_|_|_|_|_|_|_|_|_|_|_|_|_|_|_|_|_|_|_|_|_|_|_|_|_|_|
First   MI   Last

Patient Number |_|_|_|_|_|_|_| Location Code |_|_|_|_|

RACE: SEX:
☐ Black   ☐ White   ☐ Other   ☐ Male   ☐ Female   Age |_|_|

Weight |_|_|_|_| (lbs)   Height |_|_|_| (inches)

K. Please do not write in box

A. Have you ever been told by a physician that you had high blood pressure?

    ☐ No   1 ☐ Yes

B.P. |_|_|_| / |_|_|_| Present

B.P. |_|_|_| / |_|_|_| Highest (Optional)

Cholesterol |_|_|_|_| Optional

Triglycerides |_|_|_|_| Optional

Diabetic	☐ No	1	☐ Yes
controlled	☐ No	2	☐ Yes
Emphysema	☐ No	3	☐ Yes
Murmur	☐ No	4	☐ Yes

Have you ever had a heart attack or do you have angina?

    ☐ No   2 ☐ Yes

Converted skin test or chest X-ray positive within 12 months   ☐ No 5 ☐ Yes

Abnormal ECG* in past 3 years   ☐ No 6 ☐ Yes

Have you ever had a stroke or "shock"?

    ☐ No   3 ☐ Yes

* Vent. hypertrophy, Block, I° ST or T changes

Is your natural mother living?   4 ☐ No   5 ☐ Yes   6 ☐ Don't know

What is her present age or age at death? vM _____ Yrs

If dead, did she die of heart disease?   ☐ No 7 ☐ Yes

Is your natural father living?   8 ☐ No 9 ☐ Yes 10 ☐ Don't know

What is his present age or age at death? vF _____ Yrs

If dead, did he die of heart disease?   ☐ No 11 ☐ Yes

B. Have you ever had an ECG (EKG, electrocardiogram, heart tracing)?

☐ No   ☐ Yes   If yes, was it not normal in the past 3 years?

☐ Normal ₁☐ Not Normal

Please mark the one answer that best describes how much you exercise, including your work.

₆☐ Climbing less than five flights of stairs or walking less than 1/2 mile four times per week, or other equal exercise.
₇☐ Climbing 5 to 15 flights of stairs of walking 1/2 to 1-1/2 miles four times per week, or other equal exercise.
₈☐ Climbing 15 to 20 flights of stairs or walking 1-1/2 to 2 miles four times per week, or other equal exercise.
₉☐ Exercise greater than any of these.

C. Have you ever had rheumatic fever (inflammation of heart and/or joints)?

☐ No   ₁☐ Yes

Have you ever had a heart murmur?

☐ No   ₂☐ Yes

Do you take penicillin or medicine like it to prevent heart infection or rheumatic fever?

☐ No   ₃☐ Yes

D. Have you ever been told that you had diabetes (too much sugar in the blood)?

☐ No   ☐ Yes   If yes, mark all correct answers:

₁☐ I follow a diet for diabetes.
₂☐ I take insulin (shots) for diabetes.
₃☐ I take pills for diabetes.
₄☐ None of these.

Have your natural parents (mother or father) brothers or sisters had diabetes?

☐ No   ₅☐ Yes

E.   Have you ever had a chest X-ray?

       ☐ No   ☐ Yes   If yes, was it normal in the past 12 months?

                                ☐ Normal ₄☐ Not Normal

F.   Do you now smoke?

       ☐ No   ☐ Yes   If yes, mark all correct answers:

                            I smoke:
1 ☐ Cigarettes – 2 or more packs per day.
2 ☐ Cigarettes – 1-1/2 packs per day.
3 ☐ Cigarettes – 1 pack per day.
4 ☐ Cigarettes – 1/2 pack per day.
5 ☐ Cigarettes – less than 1/2 pack per day.
6 ☐ Cigars or pipe – 5 or more per day
     (combined total).
7 ☐ Cigars or pipe – less than 5 per day
     (combined total).

G.   Did you formerly smoke, but no longer do?

       ☐ No   ☐ Yes   If yes,

                            How long ago did you stop? vǫ____ years ago.
                            If less than 1 year   ____ months ago.

                            If you did smoke, mark all correct answers:

                            I smoked:
1 ☐ Cigarettes – 2 or more packs per day.
2 ☐ Cigarettes – 1-1/2 packs per day.
3 ☐ Cigarettes – 1 pack per day.
4 ☐ Cigarettes – 1/2 pack per day.
5 ☐ Cigarettes – less than 1/2 pack per day.
6 ☐ Cigars or pipe – 5 or more per day.
     (combined total).
7 ☐ Cigars or pipe – less than 5 per day
     (combined total).

H.　Have you ever been told you had lung trouble or breathing trouble?

☐ No　　☐ Yes　　If yes, mark all correct answers.

1 ☐ The trouble was emphysema.
2 ☐ The trouble was pneumonia.
3 ☐ I had tuberculosis (TB, consumption).
4 ☐ I am being treated for tuberculosis now.
5 ☐ None of these.

Have you had a skin test for TB (tuberculosis, consumption) in the past year?

☐ No　　☐ Yes　　If yes, mark all correct answers:

6 ☐ It was negative or normal.
7 ☐ It became positive or not normal this year.
8 ☐ It was positive this year and also before that.
9 ☐ None of these.

J.　In the past 6 months have you had bleeding from your rectum (where your bowel movements come out)?

☐ No　1 ☐ Yes

Have you had a finger examination of your rectum (where your bowel movements come out) in the past year?

☐ No　2 ☐ Yes

Have you had an examination of your rectum or colon by your doctor with a lighted instrument in the past year (sigmoidoscopy)?

☐ No　3 ☐ Yes

Have you ever had polyps or growths in your intestine or rectum (not piles or hemorrhoids)?

☐ No　4 ☐ Yes

Do you have ulcerative colitis (bloody diarrhea with pus and mucous and sores inside the rectum)?

☐ No　　☐ Yes　　If yes, mark how long you have had it:

5 ☐ More than 10 years.
6 ☐ 10 years or less.

L.   How many total miles per year do you travel in a car as a driver or passenger?

VL   ____,000   miles per year.

To help you in estimating the number of miles you drive or ride, the national averages for the following categories of driving are listed below:

Driving to and from work - 8,000 miles per year.
Driving to and from shopping and other personal business – 4,000 miles per year.
Driving to and from school and church – 1,000 miles per year.
Driving to and from pleasure, recreation and miscellaneous – 5,000 miles per year.

How many of these miles are on a freeway, expressway, toll road or other similar limited access highway?

1☐ Most (75% or more)   2☐ Some (25%–74%)   3☐ Little (0–24%)

When in a motor vehicle (car), do you wear a seat belt or shoulder harness?

☐ No   ☐ Yes   If yes, mark when you wear it:

4☐ Less than 10% of the time.
5☐ 10–24% of the time.
6☐ 25–74% of the time.
7☐ 75% or more of the time.

M.   Mark any of the medicines you are now taking:

1☐ Mood elevators (pills for depression)
2☐ Amphetamines (pep pills, diet pills like dexadrine)
3☐ Tranquilizers, sedatives, nerve or sleeping pills (Miltown, Librium, phenobarbital, nembutal, seconal, etc).
4☐ Narcotic pain pills (Demerol, codeine, morphine, etc.)
5☐ Antihistamines or allergy pills.

Mark any of these that you do:

6☐ Drive a racing car, dune buggy, or snowmobile.
7☐ Drive a motorcycle.
8☐ Fly a private plane.
9☐ Sky dive.
10☐ Skin dive.

N. Do you now drink any alcoholic beverages (beer, wine, whiskey, gin, vodka etc)?

☐ No   ☐ Yes   If yes, mark the one correct answer:
I drink:
1 ☐ 2 or less drinks per week.
2 ☐ 3 to 6 drinks per week.
3 ☐ 7 to 24 drinks per week.
4 ☐ 25 to 40 drinks per week.
5 ☐ More than 40 drinks per week.

Did you formerly drink any alcoholic beverages (beer, wine, whiskey, gin, vodka, etc.) and no longer do?

☐ No   ☐ Yes   If yes, mark the one correct answer:
I drank:
6 ☐ 2 or less drinks per week.
7 ☐ 3 to 6 drinks per week.
8 ☐ 7 to 24 drinks per week.
9 ☐ 25 to 40 drinks per week.
10 ☐ More than 40 drinks per week.

P. Do you worry or feel blue much of the time?

☐ No   1 ☐ Yes

Do you often feel alone and lonely even when there are others around you?

☐ No   2 ☐ Yes

Have you lost your appetite or have you had very much less desire to eat?

☐ No   3 ☐ Yes

Do you have trouble with waking up too early or being unable to stay asleep?

☐ No   4 ☐ Yes

Have you ever seriously considered killing yourself?

☐ No   5 ☐ Yes

Has anyone in your immediate family (parents, brothers, sisters) taken his or her own life (committed suicide)?

☐ No   6 ☐ Yes

Q. Do you carry a gun or knife other than a pocket knife? (This includes carrying a weapon in your work.)

☐ No   1 ☐ Yes

Have you ever been arrested for serious crime like robbery or attacking someone?

☐ No   2 ☐ Yes

Do you think how you live (your economic and social status) is:

3 ☐ Low   4 ☐ Medium   5 ☐ High

R. Have you ever had cancer or a malignant tumor?

☐ No   ☐ Yes   If yes, mark where the cancer or malignant tumor was located:

1 ☐ Colon-intestines (large bowel).
2 ☐ Breast.
3 ☐ Lung.
4 ☐ Rectum.
5 ☐ Stomach-esophagus.
6 ☐ Prostate.
7 ☐ Ovary.
8 ☐ Hodgkins disease or lymphosarcoma.
9 ☐ Leukemia.

MEN STOP HERE

S.   Has your mother or sister had breast cancer?

☐ No   1 ☐ Yes

Do you examine your breasts each month to detect cancer?

☐ No   2 ☐ Yes

Do you go to the doctor for a breast examination at least once each year?

☐ No   3 ☐ Yes

Do you have X-rays of your <u>breasts</u> at least once a year (<u>not</u> chest X-rays) for cancer?

☐ No   4 ☐ Yes

Has your uterus (womb) been removed?

☐ No   ☐ Yes   If yes, was it removed for cancer?
                                  5 ☐ No   6 ☐ Yes

Has your cervix (neck of womb) been removed?

☐ No   ☐ Yes   If yes, was it removed for cancer?
                                  7 ☐ No   8 ☐ Yes

Have <u>both</u> your ovaries (sex glands) been removed?

☐ No   ☐ Yes   If yes, indicate age removed: vs _____ yrs.

T. Do you have vaginal bleeding (bleeding from your birth canal)?

☐ No   ☐ Yes   If yes, mark all correct answers about when the bleeding happens:

1 ☐ Between menstrual periods.
2 ☐ During or after sexual intercourse.
3 ☐ My periods have stopped, but I still have bleeding once in a while.
4 ☐ I am taking female hormones (estrogens) and I only bleed when I am off these hormones.
5 ☐ I am taking female hormones (estrogens) but I bleed whether I am taking them or not.
6 ☐ None of these.

Have you ever had sexual intercourse?

☐ No   ☐ Yes   If yes, mark when you began:

7 ☐ Before 20 years old.
8 ☐ Between 20 and 25 years old.
9 ☐ After 25 years old.

U. Have you ever had a Pap (cancer) smear?

☐ No   ☐ Yes   If yes, mark all correct answers:

1 ☐ Some were not normal in the past 5 years.
2 ☐ Three or more were normal in the last 5 years.
3 ☐ One was normal within the last 12 months (none not normal).
4 ☐ One was normal within the last 5 years (none not normal).
5 ☐ I don't know the results.
6 ☐ None of these.

Are you Jewish? (The risk of cancer of the cervix is much less for women of Jewish descent.)

☐ No   7 ☐ Yes

Upon completion of this Health Hazard Appraisal, the booklet is computer-scored. A sample of the computer printout follows the appraisal. Comparing that individual to others of his or her own peer group yields a determination of the potential risks to that person (Geller, 1974). Basically, the program determines whether the person is above or at an average in terms of risk as compared to his or her peers. After this assessment is obtained, the individual is given a health-hazard age, which might be the same as, or in excess of, his or her chronological age. For example, an individual of age fifty may in fact have a health-hazard age of sixty in the sense of being engaged in sufficient negative life-style activity at the present time to decrease longevity by ten years. At this point the individual simply has the information that he or she is in fact living in a high-risk manner. This situation is analogous to the stage in clinical biofeedback when a patient is first passively aware of an internal biological function, such as heart rate and regularity, before actively attempting to regulate that function. The Health Hazard Appraisal also takes the next step. Contained in the computer printout is a series of recommendations for reducing these health hazards and improving life expectancy.

The form of computer printout and interpretation shown above is based on the system used by the U.S. Public Health Service Hospital of Health, Education, and Welfare (Travis & Reichard, 1978). Based upon the HHA responses, it is determined that John Q. Patient is a fifty-one-year-old white male who gets little exercise, smokes two packs of cigarettes a day, has emphysema, is sixty pounds overweight, does not wear a seat belt, has less than two drinks a week, and does not get an annual proctosigmoidoscopy. These facts are called prognostic indicators. From them the sample printout is generated. Each area of information is identified by number and an explanation for each number follows:

1. These are coded input data obtained from the questionnaire and appear at the top of the form for reference purposes.

2. Chronologic age—51: The patient's actual age.

3. Appraisal Age—60: Our patient stands the same chance of dying in the next ten years as does a man of 60. It does not say he will die nine years sooner—he may die

JOHN Q. PATIENT,123456,WM51,WT205,HT68,BP150/90,BHO/O,CH280, ❶
A5,VM87,A9,VF80,B4,E4,F1,H6,J1,K3,VL12,L2,L4,N1,P1,P2,P3,ZZ

HEALTH HAZARD APPRAISAL   2/23/73 HSR ❺   BALTIMORE, MD.

JOHN Q. PATIENT   123456 ❷   CODE RECOMMENDATIONS   BENEFIT
CHRONOLOGIC AGE 51 YRS ❸   E   EXERCISE PROGRAM   3.6 YRS
APPRAISAL AGE 60 YRS ❸   Q   QUIT SMOKING   2.6 YRS
COMPLIANCE AGE 52 YRS ❹   W   LOSE 60 POUNDS   1.4 YRS
FOR COMPARABLE AGE AND SEX,   R   YEARLY PROTOSIG   .4 YRS
PATIENT RISK IS 2.1 TIMES
AVERAGE ❼   S   WEAR SEAT BELTS 100%

                              TOTAL RISK REDUCTION ❻   8 YRS

CAUSE DEATHS/100K RISK TO PATIENT (AVERAGE RISK 1)
OF DEATH AVG. PAT.   0   1   2   3   4   5
        ❽   ❾   ❿   :......:......:......:......:......:......:
                          :
HT DIS 5874 18679   :XXXXXXXXXXXXEEEEEEEEEQQQQQWWWW
                          :XXXXXX❶❶XXXXXEEEEEEEQQ❶❷QQWWWW ❶❸
                          :XXXXXXXXXXXXEEEEEEEEEQQQWWWWW
                          :XXXXXXXXXXXXEEEEEEEEEQQQQQWWWW
                          :XXXXXXXXXXXXEEEEEEEEEQQQQQWWWW
                          :
                          :
CA LUNGS 1040 2392   :XXXXXXXXXXXXXXXXXXXXQQQQQ
                          :XXXXXXXXXXXXXXXXXXXXQQQQQ
                          :

```
CAUSE   DEATHS/100K RISK TO PATIENT (AVERAGE RISK 1)
OF DEATH AVG. PAT.        0        1        2        3        4        5
                          :........:........:........:........:........:

STROKE      666  1131     :XXXXXXXXXXXXXXXXXXXQQ
                          :        :
CIRRHOSIS   567  113      :XA      :
                          :........:
M V ACC     373  216      :XXXXSS  :
                          :        :
SUICIDE     324  324      :XXXXXXXXXXX
                          :        :
EMPHYSEMA   314  734      :XXXXXXXXXXXXXXXXXXXXXXQQQQQQ************K3*DISCLAIMER ⓮
                          :        :
CA INTEST   303  909      :XXXXXXXXXXXRRRRRRRRRRRRRRRRRR
                          :        :
PNEUMONIA   247  653      :XXXXXXXXXXXXXXXXXXXXXQQ
                          :        :
RHEUM HT    191  19       :X       :
                          :........:

OTHER ⓯    4336  4336
TOTAL ⓰   14290 29507 ⓱
THESE DATA SHOW ONLY RISKS OF DEVELOPING DISEASES. IF ANY OF THESE DISEASES
EXIST, THEIR RISK FACTORS BECOME MEANINGLESS.

***DISCLAIMER, EVIDENCE OF THIS DISEASE WAS GIVEN IN THE QUESTIONNAIRE. THUS,
THE RISK OF DEATH IS GREATER THAN THE APPRAISAL AGE INDICATES.

D SCALE ELEVATED. ⓲
```

tomorrow or he may live to be 90—but his chances of dying are that of a person nine years older than he actually is. Note: Risk is converted into "years" to make it easier for patients to understand. For example, 29,640 deaths per hundred thousand people in the next ten years has less meaning to a layman than a "60-year-old white male's risk of dying." These conversions are made from mortality tables, which show ages and the corresponding number of expected deaths per hundred thousand persons for the next ten years.

4. Compliance Age—52: If he makes all the changes shown in the "Recommendations" column at right (5), his "age" will be 52. He will have the same risk of death as a 52-year-old. In other words, he can "gain back" eight of the nine years of his excess risk.

5. Code Recommendation Benefit: Here a code letter is assigned for each recommended behavior change. These letters are used in the bar graphs below. The corresponding reductions in risk are shown, expressed in years. Again, the "years" are conversions from the number of expected deaths and are used for simplicity.

6. Total Risk Reduction—8 Years: This is the difference between the appraisal and compliance ages, and is the sum of the different behavior change recommendations.

7. For Comparable Age and Sex, Patient Risk Is 2.1 Times Average: This is another simplification of the mortality statistics and says John Q. Patient is 2.1 times as likely to die as his "average" counterpart. It is obtained by dividing the total expected deaths for patients with these characteristics (number 17 below) by the total expected deaths for the average white male aged 50–54 (number 16 below).

8. Cause of Death: This column shows in rank order the ten leading killers for 51-year-old white males.

9. Deaths/100,000—Average: These are the number of expected deaths associated with each disease. The data are taken from the National Center for Health Statistics and reflect the 1968 United States mortality experience. The first number in the column shows that 5,874 deaths

from heart disease can be expected per 100,000 white males 51-years-old in the next ten years. Similarly, 1,040 deaths from lung cancer and so forth for each of the ten disorders.

10. Deaths/100,000—Patient: This column shows the adjusted mortality figures for John Q. Patient. The first number in this column means that for 100,000 51-year-old white males with the same prognostic indicators, 18,679 are expected to die in the next ten years. This is 3.2 times as great as the number of expected deaths for the average 51-year-old white male. 3.2 is the risk multiplier for heart disease for John Q. Patient, and is shown in two components by the bar graph explained below.

11. XXXXXXXXXXX: These "X" marks indicate the irreducible portion of the risk of dying of that particular cause. The number of lines of X's and other code letters for each cause of death reflects the relative importance of that cause of death. Five lines means more than 30 percent of all deaths are from this cause; four lines mean 20–30 percent of all deaths; three lines equals 10–20 percent; two lines equals 5–10 percent; one line equals less than 5 percent.

12. EEEEQQQWWW: This is the reducible risk broken down into the behaviors which can reduce it. The letters come from the "code" column above in number 5. The combined irreducible and reducible risk make up the total "risk multiplier" for heart disease and is read as 3.2 from the scale above.

13. The width of the bar (5 rows) reflects the importance of each cause of death.

14. ******K3 Disclaimer: Evidence that John W. Patient already has emphysema was given on the questionnaire by question K-3. Hence his risk of developing emphysema becomes meaningless.

15. Other: All other causes of death are lumped here together. None account for more than 1 percent of the total deaths.

16. Total—14,290: The sum of this column equals the number of expected deaths per 100,000 for 51-year-old white males in the next ten years.

17. Total—29,507: The sum of this column equals the number of expected deaths per 100,000 in the next ten years for a cohort of patients with the same prognostic characteristics as John Q. Patient.

18. D-Scale Elevated: This is a depression scale which does not always appear on the printout. When it does appear, it means that a patient answered three out of four of the questions P1/P4 positively. It is an indication to look for masked depression if not evident clinically.

This example demonstrates that out of nine of these excessive years of risk, 3.6 years might be recoverable for that person by an exercise program, another 2.6 years might be recoverable by stopping smoking, and another 1.4 years by losing sixty pounds, and so on. Thus, the computer breaks down the years that are recoverable and points out to the person the specific area in which he should alter his life-style to decrease his health risk. Included in this risk-reduction procedure are such recommendations (item 5) as start an exercise program, quit smoking, lose sixty pounds, have a yearly physical checkup including a proctosigmoidoscopy, or simply wear a seat belt all the time while driving. Very often it is possible to decrease the excessive risk by as much as 90 percent. This assessment is still in the preliminary stages, and research is ongoing. Possible applications of the HHA are currently being evaluated experimentally in the program of preventive care initiated by the government of Canada (Colburn & Baker, 1973). While further development is required, the HHA can serve as a prototype for the standardization of other low cost, minimal time, health status assessments.

Inherent in this appraisal system is the assumption that the etiology of a disorder is a long developmental process, one that can be altered toward increased health rather than disability. The developmental stages that underlie this appraisal system are strikingly parallel to the neurophysiological stress profile as applied in clinical biofeedback (Pelletier, 1975, 1977). John W. Travis, one of the developers of HHA, describes a series of seven stages (Travis, 1978). Stage one is no-risk category, which constitutes the early part of life, when an individual is least likely to have a severe disease. At this point the HHA is not particularly applicable although it can reveal tendencies toward ill health that may result in premature disability or death in future years. Stage two is termed an "at risk" category wherein conditions such as age or environmental pollution may make an individual vulnerable to a disease. During this time prolonged exposure to negative psychosocial or biological elements in the environment can reach the critical point at which they begin to adversely affect an individual. At stage three a particular physical agent or psychosocial situation is present and is determined to be causing excessive stress in the person. The patient might smoke or engage in another activity known to be a precursor of, or to precipitate the tendency toward disease, and this places the individual in a higher state of risk. *Mind as Healer, Mind as Slayer* (Pelletier, 1978) contains a detailed examination of the neurophysiological and psychosocial factors found in this most critical stage. In stage four there are definite clinical signs of disease, but the individual is as yet unaware of it. Evidence of a disorder at this stage may be discovered during a routine physical, for instance an elevated blood pressure reading or an abnormality noted in an X ray. During stage five there are clear symptoms, such as pain, blood in the urine, or psychological signs that lead the individual to a physician or psychotherapist. At stage six there is disability, and at this point the individual has usually already sought medical care, since he is now in a stage of acute pain, disease, or disorder. If this stage is not adequately treated, then life-threatening disease in stage seven may result in death.

Practitioners usually do not concern themselves with the disease process until it reaches stage four. Most frequently, stage four begins when a routine examination picks up evidence of a disorder. In a preventive approach, however, there are at least two earlier stages to any disorder that must be considered. A Health Hazard Appraisal makes it possible to uncover disease stages two and three and to initiate preventive measures. During stage four, multiphasic testing in conjunction with a psychosocial appraisal can be of further use in introducing psychological, sociological, and situational variables into the traditional medical examination. Obviously, at stages five and six the need is for traditional medical care.

Even when an early appraisal system uncovers unequivocal signs of risk, the most fundamental problem to be resolved is how to motivate the individual to undertake health preservation measures. No amount of data will induce change by itself. It is still possible for the patient to dismiss the excess hazards because they are in the future. Even the numerical values can be too abstract and easily ignored (Mechanic, 1976). Information must be discussed with the

patient and agreement reached about appropriate life-style alterations. A potent combination is the use of the HHA, which projects
long-term risk, and the Schedule of Recent Experience, which is
widely available (Holmes & Rahe, 1967; Lecker, 1978; Pelletier,
1977) and specifies the likelihood of a disorder becoming manifest
within one year or less. When a patient is counseled regarding potential and immediate risks, with alternatives clearly posed, then the
possibility of an effective early intervention is greatly enhanced. At
present, there are several systematic means of determining a patient's emotional status, life situation, and personality (Tornstam,
1975). One is known as the Psychological Systems Review (PSR) by
Harold R. Ireton and Donald Cassata (1976) from the Department of
Family Practice at the University of Minnesota in Minneapolis.
Through the structured interview of the PSR, it is possible to obtain
a detailed psychosocial history in conjunction with a routine physical.
From their research Ireton and Cassata have concluded, "An essential attitude is the physician's willingness to view the patient's presenting symptoms and signs as possible indicators of emotional distress as well as organic disease *at the outset*" (1976). PSR offers a brief,
systematic means of gathering psychological background to help in
counseling the patient away from self-destructive habits.

According to the Health Hazard Appraisal brochure,

> . . . a copy of the appraisal should be given to the patient with
> an adequate explanation of its meaning. If possible, the spouse
> should be present when a high-risk individual is counseled,
> since investment on the spouse's part will help the patient make
> the needed changes. Compliance with the recommendations is
> difficult to achieve with many individuals, but the satisfaction
> of seeing some patients respond positively rewards the user of
> the HHA (Travis & Reichard, 1978).

An individual's entire life-style should be considered if appropriate
changes are to be encouraged. As has been noted, these life-style
changes are not slight or superficial alterations that can be easily
undertaken. All too often, leisure time for relaxation or health maintenance receives negative reinforcement from the people around
the individual. It appears as self-indulgence, narcissism, or, very simply, laziness. Many individuals in our credit-fixated society believe in
the eternal tomorrow, when they will alter or rectify life-styles that
they know are destructive, paying their debts later. Unfortunately,
"later" comes all too soon. It is incumbent upon individuals to rectify

their life-styles on an ongoing daily basis rather than wait for the elusive future. All of the computer assessment systems are excellent approaches to a complex problem but also can veil the essential issue which is that an individual outcome cannot be determined by statistics. One person can violate every tenet of health care and live illness-free, while another individual lives an exemplary life plagued by ill health. Demonstrations of statistical risk are valuable only in that they serve to turn an individual's attention toward considering certain aspects of his life-style. Specific disabilities relate statistically to particular stressors and only demonstrate the mechanics of what is occurring. By analogy, the reason for an automobile accident will not necessarily be determined by assessing the mechanical damage to the car. One of the clearest and most important messages from all meditative systems is to live in the now, to appreciate each moment in and of itself without reference to the past or anticipation of the future. People who have achieved this orientation and are living in the immediate present as fully and completely as possible generally have also developed the increased self-awareness which is at the heart of the holistic approach to preventive care.

Traditional preventive medicine consists of immunization, arresting the spread of disease through epidemiology and public health measures, multiphasic examinations, monitoring health care organizations, and related measures. The primary orientation is toward detection of signs, symptoms, and disabilities. As necessary as such an approach is, it still functions within a biomedical model, viewing health as the relative absence of pathology. Holistic approaches move beyond this neutral position to work toward increasing health and optimum health.

A striking feature of actuarial tables in the United States is the mortality of males compared to that of females. Among the causes of death with the highest male-to-female differences are respiratory malignancies, other bronchopulmonary disease, motor vehicle accidents, suicide, cirrhosis of the liver, and arteriosclerotic heart disease. According to researcher Ingrid Waldron, "These causes of death with clear behavioral components are responsible for one third of male mortality, and arteriosclerotic heart disease is responsible for an additional forty percent of excess deaths among males" (Waldron & Johnston 1976). Most of these statistics suggest that males in our culture indulge in more self-destructive behaviors than females. In an issue of the *New England Journal of Medicine,* John W. Rowe of the Harvard Medical School examined the factors contributing to the fact that life expectancy for women in the United States is eight years longer than for men. His data mirror that of Waldron in noting that forty-five percent of excess male mortality can be attributed to arteriosclerotic cardiac disease and fifteen percent to lung cancer and emphysema, which are all at least partly related to smoking (Rowe, 1977). Accident and suicides account for another fifteen percent of the sex differential in mortality. Rowe has stated, "Analysis of sex-specific mortality rates for major causes of death suggests that, in a sense, men kill themselves off." More and more evidence has linked this health gap to different "learned health care behavior," resulting from different sex roles. Charles E. and Mary Ann Lewis also noted in the same journal that "men are reluctant to seek care or adopt behaviors that would diminish these risks . . . by six years of age, males perceive themselves to be less vulnerable or susceptible than females of the same age" (Lewis & Lewis, 1977). Women generally perceive health care to have greater benefits. Concluding their article, the Lewises noted, "Men could benefit enormously if their sex-role changes carried with them some of the protective effects associated with a diminished 'macho' stance."

Significant opportunity for life-style change comes with middle age. That period can be the occasion for major life changes in a positive direction. Writing in *Geriatrics,* Lawrence Greenleigh has noted that the way people handle personal crisis in middle years can set the pattern for dealing with problems in later life. Among the problems faced in middle years are reevaluation of marriage, relationships to children, widowhood, sex, financial status, and particularly sex role changes (1976). Greenleigh has suggested a "midlife assessment" that can help people transform crises into periods of continuing personality development. Moreover, these transition periods can be made positive by recognizing the explicit life issues of middle age. Such changes are not within the realm of medicine per se but a vital part of comprehensive health care. Motivation for change can increase in midlife. Motivation appears to depend upon how frightened a patient is that a given disease will happen to him. When friends and contemporaries succumb, the dangers are brought close to home.

It would be possible to dismiss many of the concepts of preventive holistic medicine as unscientific, prophetic, and impractical were it not for the fact that they are empirically testable and, to the extent they have been tested, demonstrably effective. In traditional clinical research, a patient is determined by various measurements to be in a state of disease, a treatment is performed upon or with that patient, then the same variables are once again assessed to determine if that intervention has had the desired effect. Similar evaluations can be applied to new approaches to health care. Many of these issues are addressed in an articulate manner in the *Journal of the American Medical Association* entitled "What Is a Health Care Trial?" by Walter O. Spitzer, Alvan R. Feinstein, and David L. Sackett (1975). These physicians distinguish two sorts of trials. First, a "Health Service Trial" is one in which medical or surgical interventions are assessed. As an alternative, they propose a second trial, the "Patient Care Trial," in which an assessment of the patient's life history and performance subsequent to medical intervention are assessed.

In this latter approach, the traditional variables are considered, but also included are psychological and sociological factors and more personal data about the individual patient. Walter O. Spitzer and his colleagues illustrate this distinction between the two trials by citing two well-designed and well-executed series of research studies concerning the effects of tonsillectomy and adenoidectomy on children. In both studies the principal treatment consisted of the removal of tonsils and adenoids. For the traditional therapeutic trial (the Health Service Trial), the main variables assessed in one study were weight change, the frequency of attacks of sore throat, tonsillitis, colds, and other factors (Mawson, Adlington & Evans, 1967). Contrasted to this is the Patient Care Trial, in which the assessment included these variables plus data such as the use of medical service, days of confinement to bed, and absence from school. Essentially, this approach is concerned with how well the patient is performing, as well as the immediate effects of the surgical procedure. Emphasis is restored to the quality of a patient's life following an intervention. Examples of other data that can be included in a Patient Care Trial are ability to return to work following a heart attack, cost of hospitalization, and emotional state. The research team concluded:

> The omission of socio-personal data has made the results of many therapeutic trials difficult to interpret in clinical practice. For example, in studies of pharmaceutical agents for coronary artery disease, therapeutic accomplishment is often reported as a change in frequency of anginal attacks or in supplemental usage of nitroglycerin. A practicing physician may want to know, and is usually unable to find, any information about the occupational capacity, physical function, and general comfort of the treated patient. In the case of chemotherapy for advanced cancer, the customary emphasis is upon survival time and tumor magnitude. The patient's physical and emotional

states are seldom described, and the assessments are rarely, if ever, concerned with the way the patient's family is affected in terms of energy, costs, and morale. Expensive or hazardous new forms of surgery, radio-therapy, are often tested in therapeutic trials that are sound in their scientific logic but sometimes depersonalized by restrictions in their scientific data (Spitzer et al., 1975).

It is evident from the work of Walter O. Spitzer and others that broader attention needs to be given to the risks, the costs, and the benefits of therapy before treatment and prevention of pathology can be comparatively assessed. Also, Spitzer and his colleagues noted, "Many hypotheses about cellular, intracellular, and molecular phenomena can be scientifically tested in a sheltered laboratory environment and need not pertain to human reality. Hypotheses about the care of people, however, cannot receive a complete scientific investigation if the comparison of therapeutic efficacy does not include the total effects of the treatment on people." While modern medical technology has produced major innovations in therapy, it has also spawned massive problems as medicine becomes increasingly dehumanized. By extending the scope of scientific evidence to include psychosocial considerations, it may be possible to restore a therapeutic balance that serves the needs of both science and humankind.

Health status appraisals such as the Health Hazard Appraisal, Schedule of Recent Experience, Psychological Systems Review, and related methods introduce several specific psychosocial considerations into a holistic approach to health maintenance. However, it is of utmost importance to acknowledge that there are still more subtle and complex variables that determine the balance between health and illness, life and death. Recent research suggests that predictive instruments such as the SRE may not predict or relate to illness and health in any way other than the most general. The annals of medicine are replete with instances of individuals moving apparently inexplicably from states of pathology to optimum health (Alvarez, 1961; Achterberg & Lawliss, 1978; Perry, 1962). As dramatic as these instances are, there may be many more individuals who undergo this process and yet never appear in medical records. Critical stages of psychosis or physical disease need not be the only teachers of this lesson, unless individuals persist in being dull students. Often severe disorder seems to lead to a profound reexamination of the individual's life. Such cases are reminders of the powerful regenerative capacity of the human organism.

Most recently, in the paper noted earlier, Norman Cousins (1977) detailed his recovery from critical illness and offered great insight into the process of self-healing. After a demanding schedule in Leningrad and Moscow, he found himself in a state of "adrenal exhaustion," which he later determined to have been a precondition of his "progressive and incurable" collagen disease. After a brief hospitalization, Cousins drew conclusions such as "a hospital is no place for a person who is seriously ill," and the "hospital's most serious failure was in the area of nutrition," and, "it was unreasonable to expect positive chemical changes to take place so long as my body was being saturated with and toxified by painkilling medications" (Cousins, 1977). Rather than passively lamenting his plight, he undertook extensive personal research and initiated positive self-care. Initially, he had to redefine his relationship to his doctor. Moving from a position of dependence to a shared relationship like a "partnership," he was encouraged by the doctor "to believe I was a respected partner with him in the total undertaking." With the aid and advice of his doctor, Cousins recovered, and his recovery is a model of ideal holistic medicine. Cousins reasoned that if stress had negative effects upon the body, then perhaps positive emotions such as "love, hope, faith, laughter, confidence, and the will to live" might have "therapeutic value." Toward the end, he moved out of the hospital to his home, rented films of "Candid Camera" and other comedies to watch, and found that joyous laughter enabled him to have at least two hours of pain-free sleep. Also, he initiated a slow intravenous drip of Vitamin C that reached twenty-five grams by the end of one week. He found the combination of being out of the hospital, laughter, and Vitamin C resulting in prolonged periods of restful sleep and a sense of recovery. After months of slow recuperation, he was able to resume his work at the *Saturday Review* and his mobility improved over the ensuing year.

Reflecting upon his recovery, Cousins came to three important conclusions: (1) "the will to live is not a theoretical abstraction but a physiologic reality with therapeutic characteristics"; (2) "my doctor . . . knew that his biggest job was to encourage the patient's will to live and to mobilize all the natural resources of body and mind to combat disease"; and (3) "since I didn't accept the verdict, I wasn't trapped in the cycle of fear, depression, and panic that frequently accompanies a supposedly incurable illness." Each of these three aspects of Cousins's recuperation and optimum health are dismissed all too frequently under the rubric of placebo. They are at the heart of all healing rituals and need to be systematically researched and enhanced rather than denied. Patients can learn how potent their own self-healing capacity can be. Through approaches such as clinical biofeedback, Autogenic Training, Jacobsen's Progressive Relaxation, and meditation, these factors can be systematically learned and enhanced. "Respectable names in the history of medicine like Paracelsus, Holmes and physicians have suggested that the history of medication is far more the history of the placebo effects than of intrinsically valuable and relevant drugs" (Cousins, 1977). Cousins's movement from pathology to health illuminates such phenomena as "placebo," "will to live," "spontaneous remission," or even "miracle cure." These, says Cousins, demonstrate "the ability of the patient properly motivated or stimulated, to participate actively in extraordinary reversals of disease and disability."

Recent research by Howard L. Fields and his colleagues at the University of California School of Medicine in San Francisco has actually demonstrated a biochemical mechanism by which the consciousness of the individual produces the placebo effect. In an experiment with oral surgery pain patients, these researchers demonstrated that patients could produce analgesia to pain by activating the discharge of endorphins which are "endogenous opiate-like substances" (Levine, Gordon & Fields, 1978). Furthermore, when patients were given naloxone, a medication known to reverse the action of opiates, the people who experienced pain relief from placebo analgesia began to experience pain. Results such as these lend clear evidence that the action of will as manifested in the placebo response involves observable biochemical alterations.

Concepts such as consciousness and will have a particular meaning in this context. Frequently it is used to denote "free will," viewing the self as separate from the rest of the world. In this sense it is possible to distinguish a free decision, which originates inside oneself, from a nonfree decision imposed by external circumstances. That distinction does not hold true in most meditative traditions (Kennett, 1972; Tulku, 1977). Acknowledged teachers of meditation emphasize that "will" is a function of an isolated ego, i.e., one adhering to the illusion of separation. During the course of meditation, during hospitalization or a near confrontation with death, many individuals assume or have participatory attitudes thrust upon them and the issue of asserting free will becomes meaningless. Paradoxical terms such as passive-volition or *mushin*, meaning "no mind" in the Zen tradition, which are reminiscent of "horseless carriage" or "wireless telegraph," are a close approximation of this experience. An individual participates in and cooperates with a higher and more subtle order of knowledge leading to optimum health.

With sensitive use of health assessments it may be possible to engage in patient education years before a health crisis arises. Concepts of healing and regeneration can be introduced so that they are not alien to either health professionals or patients. Then when patients do become ill, it is possible to elicit their participation. Optimum health cannot be measured solely by physical fitness and lack of illness, but involves a subtle philosophical attitude toward life itself. When life is viewed as an ongoing process, each moment and each event becomes a potential experience of positive learning and growth. Warner Wilson of the University of Alabama reviewed studies of "avowed happiness" and concluded that "health does show a relationship to happiness, even in populations that are quite healthy on the average" (1967). Numerous other factors such as education, finances, extroversion, religion, job morale, and modest aspirations were also found to be interconnected determinants of overall life satisfaction. More recently Lisa Berkman from the University of California at Berkeley studied health behavior in 700 people over nearly a decade. From her dissertation data, Berkman concluded that "friendship, family ties, and membership in social and religious groups correlates with physical health and longevity" (1977), with friendship and family ties being the best predictors. By contrast, highly isolated people run a risk of death that is two to four times higher than their "involved" counterparts.

A fundamental philosophical revision is taking place in our paradigm of medicine. Central to this revision is the concept that all stages of disease are psychosomatic in etiology, duration, and in the healing process (Pelletier, 1977). Contemporary medicine and holistic approaches to health care exist in a complementary relationship. Western individuals are unfortunately predisposed to viewing these two systems as vying for dominance rather than seeing them as having different areas of applicability. Both are necessary and supplement one another in a fuller approach to optimum health. Chinese philosophy represents this mutual interdependence in the Yin-Yang symbolism in which all oppositions are complementary aspects of the same whole. Holistic medicine draws upon such philosophical wisdom as well as the profound implications from recent innovations in quantum physics (Capra, 1976; Pelletier, 1978). From the point of view of both Chinese philosophy and quantum physics the universe is one enormous, interrelated process, from the galaxies, to this

planet, to the mountains, trees, animals, molecules, atoms, and subatomic realm. From macrocosm to microcosm, it is evident that there
are meaningful patterns from which single aspects cannot be separated or considered in isolation (Young, 1976). Outstanding among
the attempts to communicate this perspective is a recent book entitled *How to Grow a Lotus Blossum* (1977) by J. Kennett, of the Shasta
Abbey of Sōtō Zen in Mt. Shasta, California. During the autumn of
1975, Kennett became ill with diabetes, hypertension, water reten-
tion, and cardiac irregularity. By April of 1976, she became too ill to
continue her duties as abbess of the Shasta Abbey. When she consulted a physician, she was informed that she would die of a heart
attack within three months if her condition did not improve. A week
later she was forced to confine herself to bed as well as having her
main disciple decide to leave the Abbey. As Norman Cousins did, she
boldly undertook a year of disciplined self-care and emerged in a
state of health even greater than she knew before her disorder. For
the first four months, she meditated with concerted intensity in an
Oakland Zen Temple. Not even her physician was allowed to disturb
her and she decided to cease all medications. She relied solely upon
her meditation, a few simple foods, and herbs. After leaving the
Oakland Temple, she returned to the Shasta Abbey where she continued her recovery for a full year. During that time she experienced
a major Kenshō, which is translatable as enlightenment experience,
realization, or understanding. Her book is a deeply personal chronicle of a profound religious and healing experience. One passage
describes her moment of Kenshō with vivid intensity:

> When I am in the blackness of despair my kidneys and bladder
> become sick and, if I remain in this state, may become diseased.
> . . . When I become angry or frustrated I tense up the liver and
> gall bladder and cause the rending of the hara with its resulting
> disharmony of body and mind, constant rebirth, old age, disease
> and death. . . . When the brain tries to decide what to do the
> result is catastrophe and dis-ease of every description for every
> organ in the body is affected by the fear, despair, grief, worry,
> doubt, anger, frustration and sadness that result from its mis-
> takes. . . . I was in this place and would have died there if it had
> not been for my faith in my Kenshō. *All* men can find the tiny
> hole of light, which is faith, if they will but look up . . . then the
> dark pillar turns to light and the spirit ascends . . . body and
> mind are one, heaven and earth are one, 'forsaking self the
> universe grows.' This book began as how a Zen Buddhist pre-

pares for death and has become how a Zen Buddhist prepares for life (Kennett, 1977).

In considering these profound insights, it should be kept in mind that these meditations were not undertaken to cure her illness since that is not in keeping with the Zen tenet that meditation has no goal other than itself. Nevertheless, this moving document of her one-year journey back to health has immediate implications for contemporary science and medicine.

V

Between Psyche and Soma

When Louis Pasteur and Robert Koch revealed the existence of tuberculosis bacilli to their colleagues in the 1890s they were rebuked because according to the prevailing opinion of that period tuberculosis was a product of social and environmental factors. By contrast, when contemporary researchers assert that an infectious disorder involves psychosocial and environmental dimensions, their data are suspect since the prevailing model is based primarily upon microorganisms. At the turn of the century Pasteur's "germ-theory" was directly contradicted by the physician Claude Bernard, who postulated the existence of the "milieu interieur" (1957), the organism's internal environment, which could be isolated from the external environment with all of its indeterminate and unpredictable influences. Throughout the history of medicine there has been controversy concerning the internal versus the external determinants of health and disease, and today the debate is more evident than ever, despite its fallacious foundation in Cartesian dualism. *Divided Legacy: A History of the Schism in Medical Thought* (1977) by Harris Livermore Coulter, documents these opposing points of view from 450 B.C. to A.D. 1914. Coulter identifies the two contending paradigms as the "Empirical," or the approach that considers the whole organism and its environment, and the "Rationalist," which emphasizes isolatable, physiological processes subject to the laws of logic. It is evident that these two paradigms will remain artificially separate as long as they are believed to be mutually irreconcilable. A true advancement of the understanding of disease and health requires that they be integrated.

From the previous chapter it is evident that psychosocial, environmental, and biological factors in complex interaction determine what is observed as illness or optimum health. All of these factors must be considered in the implementation of the stress management approaches which are the focus of this chapter. After a health assessment is obtained, the first obstacle to be surmounted is how to implement the necessary life-style modifications. The very attempt to alter self-destructive patterns, however, may induce further stress. Yet there are means of implementing change without incurring further disability, and these means are largely contingent upon individual adaptation to stressors. Among the most pressing issues in current research and clinical practice is not if, but how, excess stress induces disease. Unanswered questions remain regarding who becomes ill under stress, why the same stress triggers different disorders in various individuals, and why others remain totally unaffected and healthy under stress (Greenberg, 1977).

Investigations have focused upon the psychophysiological interactions which might be responsible for the observed individual variability in susceptibility to disease. A few researchers have begun to consider adaptation to stress or "ability to rally after a challenge to adapt" (Audy, 1973) to be a more predictive aspect of health than the simple absence of stress (Beckman, 1971; Luborsky et al., 1973). Much of this information was considered at length in *Mind as Healer, Mind as Slayer* (Pelletier, 1977), particularly regarding the neurophysiological responses to stress internal to the individual.

Although Pasteur's invaluable contribution has served as the basis for medical research in the decades that followed his work, it has become increasingly evident that the analysis of microorganisms provides only a partial knowledge of the etiology of disease. One physician, John Cassell of the Department of Epidemiology at the University of North Carolina, has cited numerous instances in which the known characteristics of bacteria and viruses have failed to explain —to use examples wherein they should have been most clearly applicable—the transmission of cholera from isolation to a raging epidemic; the waxing and waning of influenza; the inability to produce cholera in healthy, human volunteers by feeding them the cholera vitrio; and the varied susceptibility to tuberculosis. Even when viral infection is evident, as David Mechanic has noted, the link between the actual infection and psychosocial factors is exceedingly complex and includes such possibilities as:

> (1) that stress contributes in some fashion to the incidence of infection; (2) that the condition, itself, is a significant source of distress and weakens the person's incentive; (3) that the condition serves as an excuse to relieve distressful obligations and helps avoid social sanctions for nonperformance of responsibilities; (4) that the condition allows the person to justify to himself his failure to adequately meet social responsibilities; (5) that the distress of the condition becomes merged and confused with other existing feelings of distress so that the individual cannot differentiate clearly the source of his distress and attributes causality to the viral respiratory condition; (6) or all of these (Mechanic, 1976).

In a recent interview Lewis Thomas, author of *Lives of a Cell,* was queried about the role of microorganisms in disease: "You mean to say that we ourselves cause disease, not the bugs?" "That's right," he replied. "I believe that microbes are mostly amiable and useful. . . . We've only come to believe they are implacable enemies since Pasteur's time" (Edson, 1976). From observations such as these and others, Cassell has concluded, "Not only are answers . . . unlikely to come from further studies of microorganisms alone, but this model of causation gives very few useful leads as to what other factors need to be studied" (1964). Actually the very concept of a single "cause" of a disorder needs to be considered carefully.

In an excellent article entitled "Unified Concept of Health and Disease," George L. Engel has underscored the mistaken assumption that medicine tends to see microorganisms such as the tubercule bacillus as "the cause of" rather than "the necessary condition for" a disease such as tuberculosis (1960). Articles by both Cassell and Engel review the medical literature that documents the inadequacy of single-cause formulations or even multicausal considerations when these are limited to physical factors with other "factors within the host often ignored or minimized" (1960). By contrast, Engel proposes a psychosomatic approach to etiology in which both physical and psychosocial factors are considered: "We define etiologic factors as factors which either place a burden on or limit the capacity of systems concerned with growth, development, or adaptation; or as factors which, by virtue of their physical or chemical properties, have the capacity to damage cells or parts of the body." Such an approach is of major significance since it clearly acknowledges the reality of both organic and psychosocial elements in pathology. Critiques of psychosomatic approaches frequently note that such methods are purely psychological and often ignore physical influences. This is a valid criticism only in the extreme situation of a patient who engages in a myriad of futile introspective techniques when the problem is organic with a clearly indicated pharmaceutical or surgical resolution. One has to admit that there is little fruitful research or clinical practice at either extreme and the "Empirical" approach is as liable to become imperviously dogmatic as the "Rationalist."

In a multicausal framework, stress appears to be the single most important factor predisposing an individual toward the development of disorder. Yet the stress factor is double-edged, for when individuals perceive themselves as utilizing stress rather than being passive victims, then the same negative stressors "may under certain circumstances be neutral or perhaps even beneficial" (Cassell, 1964; Selye, 1977). James Barrell of the University of Florida and Donald Price of the National Institutes of Health found evidence indicating that stressful events may be less significant than the individual's strategy for dealing with them (1977). Under laboratory conditions, twenty-two subjects were stressed by electrical shocks given at random intervals during experimental sessions while heart rate and electromyographic (EMG) readings were recorded. From these results, Barrell and Price differentiated two types of responses. Ten subjects were "confronters" who actively prepared for the stressor and showed significantly higher EMG activity in trapezius muscles, and eleven were "avoiders," who "simply attempt to escape the situation through denial"; these demonstrated lower EMG's than the confronters and were more passive according to subjective reports. "Avoiders" demonstrated significantly higher heart rates than the confronters. (One subject showed a mixed response.) Barrell and Price suggest that the EMG response of "confronters" is related to a normal increase in somatomotor activity whenever an individual needs to search out and cope with threatening situations. By contrast, the increased heart rate of the "avoiders" may be related either to fear or general anxiety. Ultimately the elevated heart rate is more conducive to severe cardiovascular disorders. Evidence such as this, and more will be cited later, indicates that how an individual learns to manage stress is more critical to his well-being than any impossible and undesirable attempts to avoid stress.

There is no need to explicate the complex neurophysiology, biochemistry, and immunological response to stress here, since these are well covered in the numerous excellent books. Among these are Walter B. Cannon's classic (although somewhat dated) *Wisdom of the Body* (1932); Hans Selye's pioneering insights in *Stress of Life* (1956) and *Stress without Distress* (1974); and A. T. W. Simeons's *Man's Presumptuous Brain* (1961), containing his evolutionary theory of stress susceptibility. More recent data concerning psychosomatic factors in stress and stress alleviation are discussed in the author's *Mind as Healer, Mind as Slayer* (1977). After analyzing stress research with laboratory animals and clinical trials with patients, it is my opinion that the effects of stress depend primarily upon four factors: (1) how much stress reactivity is evoked; (2) the duration of that reactivity, especially when the stimulus is an often repeated one; (3) whether there exists a baseline condition of long-term, undifferentiated, unabated neurophysiological reactivity; and (4) whether the stressor activitates the pituitary or the adrenomedullary system more vigorously. Furthermore, all of the fundamental genetic, familial, environmental, physiological, biomedical, and psychosocial factors are involved in all states of disease or health. Whether health or disease, or a specific form of disease, is manifest in a particular individual is dependent upon the relative weight of each of these, but all are present and need to be considered. Also, from the sources cited above it is abundantly clear that stress is not inherently destructive and is, in fact, often highly beneficial. Both researchers and clinicians have misinterpreted findings and drawn the erroneous conclusion that the less stress the better. Nobelist Hans Selye emphasized the variability of individual adaptation in an interview in *U.S. News and World Report* when he stated:

> If a person is a stress seeker . . . and his body is falling apart, the last thing I would ever diagnose is that he be imprisoned on a beach for three months. He will do nothing but run up and down the beach and think about Wall Street. He might as well be on Wall Street and learn to accept the type of person he is and develop the disciplines that will help him live in harmony with the stress of his life (Selye, 1977a).

In other words, the absolute quantity of stress appears to be less significant than the temperamental orientation of the individual. People who push or are forced to go against their nature, rather than any absolute amount of stress confronted, appear to be most likely to develop disorders, mild ones such as chronic headache or more severe disorders such as cardiovascular disease and cancer (Selye, 1977b).

Most research concerning stress indicates that there is no single causal, predictive connection between specific sources of stress such as marital disagreement or frustration by an employer and specific disorders such as peptic ulcer or hypertension. Implicit in all the concepts of a multicausal context (Bateson, 1972) in which a disorder becomes manifest is that particular life events or circumstances take on significance depending upon the developmental history of the organism, whether animal or man. An often quoted example of this phenomenon, emphasized by Rene Dubos in *Mirage of Health* (1959), concerns cancer of the breast in mice. Although under natural conditions breast cancer occurs very rarely in this species, breeding can produce a strain of mice genetically predisposed to breast cancer. However, the actual incidence of cancer is highly variable, ranging from zero to virtually 100 percent depending upon: exposure to a virus from the lactating mother; the sex of the offspring, females being more susceptible; injecting estrogen into males, which increases susceptibility; placing the mice on a low-calorie diet, which drastically reduces incidence in both sexes; and varying levels of environmental stressors. Numerous researchers have investigated the interactions between neurophysiology and immunology that might account for these observations (Solomon, 1960; Solomon et al., 1974). This cancer phenomenon has been frequently observed, but it was not until 1977 that a similar phenomenon concerning circulatory disease of arteriosclerosis was reported. Edmund C. Lattime and Helen R. Strausser of Rutgers University reported in *Science* the results of their research indicating that laboratory rats, under conditions of a specific stress, multiple pregnancies, developed a type of immunological alteration conducive to arteriosclerosis. They noted one critical aspect of immunological activity, phytohemagglutinin M or PHA, was "depressed as much as 400 percent from that of the controls" (1977). Based on their very sophisticated procedures, which differentiated the activity of three basic cells of the immune system, they concluded, "We suggest that this model of arteriosclerosis might be included in the same category of disorders as some autoimmune or viral conditions that manifest immune complex deposition in tissues as well as significant immune suppression" (1977). Data such as these are invaluable in attempts to link stress with the specific neurophysiological and immunological mechanisms in the body. From this and subsequent research, it is clear that any single factor or subset of factors creates the necessary but not the sufficient conditions for the development of a psychosomatic disorder.

With this extremely important point in mind, it is possible to appreciate precisely what is common to the epidemiological studies relating life-stress events and the development of subsequent disorders. Numerous research projects based primarily upon the innovative research of Richard H. Rahe and Thomas H. Holmes from the Department of Psychiatry of Washington School of Medicine in Seattle (Rahe et al., 1964) have indicated that many, if not all, disorders have their onset in a multicausal context of mounting frequency of social stress. Among the findings of such projects are indications that persons suffering from bereavement (Rees & Lutkins, 1967; Parkes, 1972) or facing job loss (Jenkins, 1972) have higher than average rates of morbidity and mortality. Also, there are both retrospective and prospective studies indicating that increased incidence of illnesses such as tuberculosis, inguinal hernia, leukemia, nonfatal coronary occlusion, and others, occurs among individuals reporting many life changes during the preceding months (Rahe, 1973; Rahe et al., 1970). From all these research findings it is clear that, even though negative life events have more impact, the major factor disposing toward illness is not whether an event is commonly thought of as negative ("death of a spouse") or positive ("job promotion") but whether the individual is required to undergo too much adaptation in too brief a time period. A demonstration of this comes from research by Bett Pesznecker and her colleagues, who obtained questionnaires from 577 patients regarding incidents prior to their development of an illness. Among all the variables that were assessed, the single best predictor of subsequent health status was "magnitude of life change" (Pesznecker et al., 1975). That common factor is highly significant, for it is possible that individuals can be forewarned of such an accumulation and can learn adaptive strategies. After all, not all people with the same profile develop disorders.

An extremely important research project by Harold J. Wershow and George Reinhart of the University of Alabama challenged this entire concept in a paper entitled "Life Change and Hospitalization —A Heretical View" (1974). Their study began as a didactic exercise to teach medical students the importance of psychosocial factors in the etiology of illness. Using the Holmes and Rahe SRE Scale with eighty-eight patients admitted to a Veterans Administration Hospital, they were surprised to find little correlation between high "life change unit scores" and hospitalization. Some patients with no discernible changes in their lives became ill or were hospitalized. These researchers believe there is a link between stressful life events and illness; but they emphasize, in concert with other researchers, that the high degree of individual variability is obscured by averaging data. From their observations, Wershow and Reinhart drew an important conclusion, "We would suggest that, among other steps, deviant cases be sought out, those who handle life changes well and those who break down on what seems to be little provocation, to learn more about coping mechanisms. When the mechanisms of successful and unsuccessful coping are known, they can perhaps be taught and then we can really get on to some elements of primary prevention in medicine" (1974). While scales such as the SRE are useful in a general sense, their real applicability is as an indication of tendency and not as a warning of impending trouble. They are educational tools that enable the patient to become aware of his precarious situation in order to initiate positive adaptation. According to the observations of George L. Engel, the identification of the type and number of conflict situations "delineated individual psychological vulnerabilities and thereby defined the types of life circumstances most likely to be threatening for such persons, and hence to initiate the sequence of responses that might culminate in a final common pathway and disease onset" (Engel, 1974).

Perhaps the most striking link between stress and individual adaptation is evident in sudden death syndromes wherein a seemingly well individual dies within minutes or hours of a significant life event. Two of the most fundamental factors governing actual onset of an illness or even sudden death have been described as "fruitless struggling" and "giving up, each with different psychophysiological implications and biochemical concomitants" (Schmale, 1972). Among animals or men, loss of the ability to predict and maintain a degree of control over their environment or an inability to garner the necessary psychosocial resources for meeting particular life circumstances are highly significant in swinging the balance between health and illness, life and death. Throughout history there are reports of people dying suddenly while in the throes of great fear, rage, grief, humiliation, and even joy. In 1942 Walter B. Cannon considered this phenomenon and its psychophysiological mechanisms in his classic study of "voodoo death." This subject of sudden death has intrigued clinicians over the centuries and has been addressed recently by George L. Engel. Beginning in 1965, he collected newspaper clippings of 275 cases of sudden death, including 172 men, 89 women, and 14 unidentified by gender. Analyzing these reports, Engel created four categories: (1) most common (135 deaths) was a traumatic event in a close human relationship; (2) next (103 deaths), involved situations of danger, struggle, or attack; (3) then (21 deaths), loss of status, humiliation, failure, or defeat, all of which involved men only; and (4) last (16 deaths), those who died at moments of great triumph or personal joy. Among the most striking examples is Lyndon B. Johnson's fatal heart attack the day after the newly inaugurated Richard M. Nixon's announcement of a complete dismantling of the Great Society programs. Another is the case of a fifty-nine-year-old college president who was forced to retire by pressure from the board of trustees. As the ex-president concluded his address, he suffered a fatal heart attack. His personal friend and physician rushed to administer aid and also collapsed and died of heart failure. Equally extraordinary are the deaths under conditions of joy, such as a fifty-six-year-old minister who was so elated to speak to President Carter that he suffered a fatal heart attack.

One common denominator emerged from all the cases, that "the victims are confronted with events that are impossible to ignore, either because of their abrupt, unexpected, or dramatic quality or because of their intensity, irreversibility, or persistence" (Engel, 1977). Most of the individuals perceived themselves as no longer in control of self or situation and entered a pronounced state of giving up, helplessness, and hopelessness. In virtually all cases, the immediate cause of death was the derangement of the cardiac rhythm. In the *New England Journal of Medicine* cardiologist Bernard Lown and his colleagues of the Harvard School of Public Health detailed the case history of a thirty-nine-year-old man who experienced episodes of ventricular fibrillations in the absence of demonstrable cardiac disease (Lown et al., 1976). From this case, the literature review, and subsequent discussions, it is evident that neurophysiological processes can induce heart failure under extreme emotional circumstances, even if there is no prior history of disease. Drawing upon the so-called "flight-fight mechanism" identified by Cannon, Engel notes that this process of mobilization is accompanied by an equally strong "conservation-withdrawal mechanism" in preparation for disengagement and inactivity. Engel postulates that psychological conflict and uncertainty may invoke both responses simultaneously. Rapid shift between one and the other may have dire effects upon the maintenance of effective functioning of the heart and circulation, leading to "lethal arrhythmias."

These observations have clear implications. One is that general physicians and other clinicians can anticipate or provide psychological intervention during significant life events such as retirement, the anniversary of a close relative's death, or periods of general emotional upheaval, particularly with older patients. Engel cautions physicians that tranquilizers frequently prescribed during periods of emotional stress may actually increase the likelihood of arrythmias in some people, as has been demonstrated to be the case with laboratory rats by Joseph P. Buckley of the University of Pittsburgh (Taylor, 1970). This is of particular importance since data from a major 1970 to 1971 NIMH National Drug Survey indicated that "about 90 percent of all minor tranquilizers are prescribed by nonpsychiatrists, usually general practitioners" (*Behavior Today*, 1974). As alternatives to prescribing potentially lethal tranquilizers which do not resolve the underlying situation even when effective, methods such as basic psychotherapy, relaxation training, biofeedback, and a host of others are noninvasive, considerably safer, and usually more effective. Such methods promote the activity of the individual's own self-regulatory systems and not only correct a fundamentally pathological process, but may lead to enduring adaptation strategies and the evolution of optimum health.

From another research perspective comes a unique insight into the problem of psychosocial and environmental stress. This is found in the work of Gordon Rattray Taylor, who wrote the important book *The Biological Time Bomb* in 1968. Following the book, Taylor published a series of articles in which he explicated the phenomenon of "population crash," which is evident in animal populations. One example he cites begins with four or five Sitka deer released on a half-mile square called James Island in Chesapeake Bay in 1916. In 1956, John Christian, who was head of Animal Laboratories of the Naval Research Institute at Bethesda, Maryland, noted the population as 300. Suddenly, in the first three months of 1958, over half of the deer died. Through the next year the deaths continued until the population leveled off at about eighty, which is normal for a "population crash which reduces the original population by about two-thirds" (Taylor, 1970). Population crash had taken place when the density was only one deer per acre with an adequate food supply. Christian compared the autopsies of deer shot in 1956 and deer that died after the population crash and found eighty-one percent showed enlarged adrenal glands as well as hemorrhages of the adrenals, thyroid, brain, kidneys, and fatty degeneration of the liver. All of these are symptomatic of prolonged stress reactivity. Of particular importance are the pathological alterations of the endocrine system adrenals, which also is a major factor in human stress reactivity, discussed later in this chapter. Among Taylor's reports are innumerable instances of similar phenomena, and he has speculated as to why such a population crash has not occurred for the human species, which is not exempt from the laws of population growth. According to Taylor:

> The weight of this evidence, then, supports the idea that urban society already shows signs of the effects of overcrowding but hasn't reached the point at which infant mortality rises so sharply as to limit the population. This is due partly to modern medicine and to government intervention when a mother ceases to care for her children, and partly also to the fact that population densities still fall short of those at which crisis behavior becomes general (Taylor, 1970).

It is intriguing to hypothesize that perhaps the increased incidence of the "afflictions of civilization" with their unknown etiologies presage a form of population crash.

After this general orientation to stress as a multicausal process, it is possible to consider its role in the two most pervasive afflictions, cardiovascular disease and cancer. Coronary heart disease (CHD) is one instance in which psychosocial, environmental, and purely physical factors are undeniably involved. An opening editorial in *Psychosomatics* by Barney M. Dlin of Temple University stated, "We can safely say the role of stress factors and personality [in CHD], after years of study, has been accepted not only by the medical community, but even by the general public" (1977). Underlying both cardiovascular disease and cancer, the first and second leading causes of disability and death, is a prolonged state of sympathetic activity mediated through cortico-hypothalamic pathways (Pelletier, 1977). Perfectly normal responses of brief duration constitute a Type I Stress Response with transient occurrences such as elevated blood pressure, increased norepinephrine, epinephrine, glucose, and free fatty acids in the blood, and increased cardiac output, mediated by the sympathetic branch of the autonomic nervous system (Selye, 1956). Brief reactivity such as this is normal for both man and animals and usually occurs when the source of stress is immediate, identifiable, and resolvable. When the situation is resolved there is a period of compensatory relaxation or parasympathetic rebound, popularized as the "relaxation response" by Herbert Benson (1976). A Type I Response is characteristic of the response elicited by exercise and not only is it perfectly tolerable but is actually of considerable benefit in the maintenance of optimum health. Details of this positive reactivity and its deliberate induction are considered in Chapter VII.

However, very few stressors are immediate, identifiable, and resolvable, and the result is a Type II Stress Response in which each of the above-cited bodily changes remains abnormally elevated over time. Most stressors, in the course of a typical day such as unsatisfactory work conditions or interpersonal problems, are vague and may continue unresolved for weeks or even months. There appears to be a biological naïveté wherein the organism cannot easily differentiate between a vaguely perceived threat to its integrity and an immediately life-endangering situation. Since the anticipated actions of defense, aggression, or escape do not occur, the body remains prepared, geared up. Under these conditions the unabated stress reactivity produces a rising baseline; transient blood pressure elevations lead to hypertension and increased heart rate evolves into tachycardia, since there is no adequate period of parasympathetic rebound during which many vital functions actually fall below their normal baseline. In these circumstances the sympathetic system is "indifferent to the cause of stress and responds in a monotonous repetitive way to any type of stimulus to prepare . . . for fight, flight, or aggressive activity" (Bove, 1977). However, in animals, it appears that physical stressors such as electric shocks do not produce the long-term effects elicited by more psychosocial stressors such as a noxious environment. Autonomic responses to this latter type of stress produce an increased load on the heart for coronary blood flow. This is easily met under ideal circumstances, but multiple factors such as genetic predispositions, cardiovascular elasticity, condition of the myocardium, exercise history, dietary factors, and degree of atherosclerotic involvement usually reduce ideal conditions such that probability of heart failure is increased.

Recent epidemiologic data suggest that psychosocial stress factors may actually be of greater consequence in atherosclerosis than those which are now considered the leading culprits, such as hyperlipidemia, hypertension, and cigarette smoking (Russek & Russek, 1976; Syme, 1975). Data for a multimillion-dollar, multidisciplinary study involving tens of thousands of people over a period of fifteen years have identified common risk factors in increasing susceptibility to atherosclerotic disease. Arteriosclerosis is a general term for the condition in which the arteries thicken, harden, and lose their elasticity. Atherosclerosis is one type of arteriosclerosis involving the accumulation of plaque on arterial walls. From that study, the contributing factors noted are "a diet high in saturated fats, cholesterol, and calories; hypercholesterolemia; hypertension; and cigarette smoking" (Dlin, 1977). Identification of these factors correlated with coronary heart disease (CHD) does not necessarily give any indication of the etiology of the factors themselves. After reviewing this and related data, physician Barney M. Dlin notes ". . . all of these are potentially amenable to control. All are under the influence and control of the individual's life-style, and it is a person's psyche that determines how he chooses to adapt to these potentially dangerous factors" (1977). This evidence of the role of individual adaptation provides a basis for optimism in curbing the rising incidence of cardiovascular disease.

Although all of the above factors contribute to cardiovascular disease, it is important to determine their relative weight. Among the more sophisticated research designs are the studies of identical twins undertaken by Einar Kringlen of the University of Oslo in Norway. Research with identical twins is a method frequently employed to differentiate genetic and environmental or psychosocial influences. Kringlen and his co-workers screened 10,000 patients who had had heart attacks in Norway between 1971 and 1975. They were looking for identical twins who had living co-twins who had not had heart attacks. From this large number of patients, the researchers found seventy-eight people who met this criterion. Then they interviewed the patients and their twins in their respective homes. To date, half of the pairs of twins have been investigated, and preliminary indications are that the twins who suffered heart attacks experienced more life crises and generally lived a more pressured life-style. Medical records indicated that most of the heart patients actually had blood pressure and cholesterol levels prior to the heart failure only slightly more elevated than those of their twins (Kringlen, 1977).

Experiments such as these are suggestive but do not show how a pressured life-style elicits cardiovascular disease, and on this question, basic research in neurophysiology looks promising. Employing an electron microscope, William H. Gutstein and his colleagues in the Department of Pathology of New York Medical College have examined the arterial system of laboratory rats subjected to electrical stimulation in the lateral hypothalamus for periods of up to sixty-two days. That region of the hypothalamus is known to be a primary center in the regulation of affect and levels of general neurophysiological activation. All of the rats were normally fed, conscious, unrestrained, and "hypertension and hypercholesterolemia [increased concentrations of cholesterol in the blood] were not etiologic factors" (Gutstein et al., 1978). Their results indicated that electrical stimulation alone was sufficient to produce morphological changes of the aorta and major coronary arteries. These changes are similar to those observed in the early phases of both animal and human atherogenesis, which is uniformly acknowledged as a major contributing factor to coronary heart disease. These results are of special significance because of the absence of hypercholesterolemia or hypertension, factors now widely considered to be the key etiological agents. More sophisticated research is clearly required to weight each of these factors before applying these disparate data to a comprehensive profile of the etiology and prevention of cardiovascular disease.

Diet is frequently associated with disorders of the cardiovascular system and is considered in the next chapter. Despite the prevalent view that a high cholesterol and saturated fat diet is a direct contributor to increased serum cholesterol levels, recent evidence indicates that this formulation is inaccurate and that psychosocial stress factors may have more weight. Even in the classic Framingham study, hypertension was a better predictor of cardiovascular disorder than either cigarette smoking or serum cholesterol. Hypertension is generally defined as blood pressure greater than 160/95 mm-Hg (Kolata & Marx, 1976). More recently, researchers from the Department of Epidemiology at the University of California at Berkeley undertook an ingenious study to sort out the factors of diet, hypertension, smoking, cholesterol, weight, and stressful life changes. Among the researchers were Michael G. Marmot, S. Leonard Syme, and Warren Winkelstein, Jr., who studied Japanese-Americans in the San Francisco Bay area in view of the lower incidence of CHD in Japan as compared to the United States (Blakeslee, 1975). At the outset of the project the researchers expected diet alone to account for the marked increase in heart disease among Westernized Japanese. They tended to discount stress because Japanese society seemed to be as modernized and pressured as that of the United States. For the study, 4,000 Japanese-American men in the San Francisco area were given complete physical examinations and completed a twenty-four-page questionnaire. The questionnaire included such questions as number of years spent in Japan, whether they attended Japanese or American schools, their religious practices, ethnic backgrounds of their friends, and others. From their responses, the men were divided into "traditional" and "nontraditional" groups. Traditional group members were faithful to native Japanese cultural norms, remaining within a close group and living relatively quiet, noncompetitive lives. Nontraditional members seemed to have adopted the characteristic American cultural traits of being competitive, aggressive, and impatient. When the data were analyzed, the researchers were surprised to learn that diet did not prove to be the main factor nor did any one of the most frequently cited risk factors. Most evident was a clear relationship between "heart disease and the degree of change from Japanese customs to American lifestyles" (Blakeslee, 1975).

Findings such as these have also been supported by the research of two Johns Hopkins University physicians Caroline B. Thomas and Karen R. Duszynski, who collected prospective data on 1,337 medical students between 1946 and 1964 at the Johns Hopkins School of Medicine. Frequently cited are their results in regard to the personality and the development of cancer, but there were noteworthy findings about cardiovascular disease as well. More than 100 of the students had high levels of blood cholesterol when first tested, but only fourteen subsequently had coronary attacks. This does not necessarily deny the link between cholesterol and cardiovascular disease, but it does indicate that other factors are involved. Those factors seemed to reside in the psychological domain. Students who later developed CHD scored high in "depression, anxiety, and nervous tension . . . tended to suffer from insomnia, were often tired in the mornings, and had generally lower grades than did the other medical students" (Thomas & Duszynski, 1974). By contrast, the high-cholesterol students who did not have heart attacks were typically calm individuals who were low in such measures as anxiety, nervous tension, and depression. Given these data it is evident that biochemical factors such as elevated serum cholesterol levels are a necessary but not sufficient condition for the development of cardiovascular disease. Far more weight resides in psychosocial and behavioral variables.

Whether an individual grows up habituated to high saturated fats, cholesterol, calories, sedentary behavior, or excess stress is determined largely by familial and social circumstances. These circumstances and the adaptive responses of individuals lead to a group of character traits termed "Type A" by the San Francisco cardiologists Meyer Friedman and Ray H. Rosenman in their book, *Type A Behavior and Your Heart* (1974). These traits are amenable to primary prevention and the most effective means may be through the formation of optimum health patterns during childhood. Failing that, the task of secondary prevention is to recognize these traits in order to substitute more positive ones. It is a certainty that an individual's faulty adaptation patterns set up the preconditions for premature cardiovascular disease months and even years before a heart attack. From research by Barney M. Dlin and his colleagues, it is clear that the coronary occlusion itself represents the climax of a long chain of events including the failure of an individual's adaptation and disturbances in the body's biochemical systems. Most coronary patients suffered from one or more of the usual medical indications of that disorder such as (1) prior treatment of heart disease; (2) elevated blood pressure; (3) ongoing medication for blood pressure or heart problems; (4) chest pain, shortness of breath, or breathing difficulty under exertion; (5) ankle, foot, or leg swelling; (6) palpitations; and (7) feelings of being dizzy or faint (Roche, 1979). In addition to these, Dlin has added such behavioral factors as irritability; indecisiveness; sexual difficulties, especially impotence (Soloff, 1977); fatigue; insomnia; and especially emotional difficulties such as loss, separation, death, or serious illness involving the closest persons in their lives. Also there was a change in behavior for periods of months, weeks, or days prior to the actual heart attack in the form of a "last fling" such as travel, a business gamble, or an affair (Dlin, 1977).

Below is a list of Type A character traits adapted from Friedman and Rosenman. Any classification system is inherently overly simplified. Once a person is "identified" as a type there is a tendency to attribute to him or her all the characteristics, although they might be inaccurate. This list is to be used as a key for introspection. A person is asked to note the items that are consistent, not just occasional, patterns of behavior. There is no set score, for the method is suggestive, not definitive: A Type A questionnaire asks, "Do you . . . ?"

1. Always move, walk, and eat rapidly.

2. Find it difficult to restrain yourself from hurrying others when they are talking.

3. Get very irritated and upset when the car ahead goes too slowly, you have to wait at a restaurant, stand in line at the bank, perform repetitious tasks.

4. Almost always feel guilty when you relax and do absolutely nothing for several hours.

5. Feel yourself compelled to challenge anyone who is competitive.

6. Keep trying to schedule things tighter and tighter so you can get more done.

7. Frequently try to do two (or more) things at once, e.g., read while eating, sign papers while talking on the phone, dictate letters while driving your car.

8. Find yourself completing others' sentences, or hurrying them up with "uh huh, uh huh" or "yes yes, yes yes."

9. Feel impatient at the rate at which most events take place.

10. Find yourself taking over conversations or bringing the conversation around to those topics that interest you.

11. Frequently pound the table or your hand to make a point in a conversation.

12. Believe that your success is due to your ability to get things done faster.

13. Habitually clench your jaw or grind your teeth.

14. Fear that if you slow down others will be more successful than you.

15. Keep so busy acquiring or accomplishing that you don't have time to just be.

16. Value yourself, and others, more by accomplishments than personal traits.

17. Explosively accentuate key words in your sentences or hurry up the last few words in each sentence.

18. Find yourself constantly translating your accomplishments, and the accomplishments of others into numbers.

19. Have difficulty admitting any personal defect or emotional problem.

20. Find that your appointments are always so tightly scheduled that by the end of the day you are always behind.

21. Complete work being performed by others because they are not doing it fast enough.

Running through these characteristics is a sense of incessant, unrelenting time pressure combined with "the chronic struggle to grasp vaguely defined elements from the environment in the shortest period of time" (Friedman & Rosenman, 1974). That subjective state of being pressured to seek what the person cannot even define is characteristic of neurotic anxiety. Through the recognition of these factors, it is possible to initiate a restructuring of these self-destructive patterns and not only reduce the risk of coronary heart disease but develop a greater sense of internal peace. This restructuring must take place at a deep level, for it has been well-documented that psychological defenses only mask the outward manifestations of stress while actually creating increased physiological stress. An elegant series of research projects demonstrated that defenses actually reduced levels of an adrenal cortex secretion, 17-OHCS. These cortical steriods are essential in positive adaptation to stressful conditions of short-term duration but have the negative effect of decreasing lymphocyte levels in the blood when they are maintained for a prolonged period of time as in Type II stress reactivity (Mason, 1968, 1975; Persky, 1957).

When Norman Cousins documented his recovery from a degenerative collagen disease, very few people knew that his prior history included a serious coronary occlusion in 1954 and a period in a tuberculosis sanitarium at age ten. He noted his reaction to the cardiovascular disease diagnosis as "looking down two roads," one of which was to give up his activities, and the other to increase his exercise. His decision was the second road because it "might carry me for a few months or a few weeks or a few minutes, but it was my road. . . . I didn't think there was a cardiograph in the world that was smart enough to know what made my heart tick" (Cousins, 1978). Such a reaction is not in flagrant disregard of the diagnosis, for he did substantially change his life-style, but in a manner consistent with his active and involved character. Most of all he began to experience a "confidence and rapport with my own body" and exercised the most important faculty of all, his "will to live." As Cousins reflected on how he was able to integrate professional advice in a partnership with his doctors, he noted: "It all began when I decided that some experts don't really know enough to make a pronouncement of doom on a human being. And I said I hoped they would be careful about what they said to others; they might be believed and that could be the beginning of the end." For doctors and laymen alike, this is sage advice.

No single area of research and clinical application deserves more qualifications, precise differentiations, and caveats to both clinicians and laymen than the psychosomatic aspects of cancer. Although this extreme caution is frequently acknowledged it too frequently goes unheeded, perhaps because there is so pressing a need to clarify the implications of previous research results for clinical practice. At this point in time there are far more data implicating psychosocial and neurophysiological factors in cardiovascular disease than cancer, although specific mechanisms of stress reactivity might be common to both. There are indications of potentially productive lines of inquiry concerning the psychophysiological basis of certain forms of cancer but the research is far from definitive.

In August of 1976, the National Cancer Institute (NCI) of the National Institutes of Health issued a call for research proposals into the psychosomatic aspects of cancer. Along with that announcement they issued an excellent overview and critique of research in this area by Bernard H. Fox. Under the title "Premorbid psychological factors as related to incidence of cancer: background for prospective grant applicants" (1976), Fox's account provides a decisive and sobering analysis of the major research in this area, with citations of 373 publications. His initial observation is that there are currently two approaches to cancer causation: (1) "carcinogenesis . . . overcoming resistance of the body, e.g., chromate exposure leading to high rates of respiratory cancer," and (2) "lowered resistance to cancer that permits a potential carcinogen normally insufficient to produce cancer to do so, e.g., after a transplant." His analysis then makes several key points: (1) cancer is multicausal and includes factors such as physical and chemical agents in the environment, viruses, medications, genetic predisposition, dietary considerations, occupation, hormonal imbalances, and psychosocial elements; (2) types and sites of cancer are further complicating elements in defining control groups and in achieving comparability of data among studies; (3) numerous flaws of both methodology and data analysis exist throughout the body of research data (although this is not unique to this area of study); (4) those studies linking personality factors with underlying physiological mediators appear more substantial than those depending solely on personality inventories, which do not fare very well; and (5) stress and its manifestations in neurophysiological and immunological systems emerges as the single most potentially productive line of inquiry. Fox concludes by sketching a model of how research might be conducted on a developmental basis throughout the lifetime of individuals in order to detect the stages at which interactions between these multicausal agents actually emerge as cancer. His well-reasoned overview and exploration of these etiological factors is required reading for anyone seriously concerned with these aspects of cancer.

Since the publication of this paper, related research projects are proving to be highly significant. Numerous animal and human experimental studies have demonstrated that stress, psychological depression, and other psychosocial factors compromise an organism's capacity to prevent the induction of disease such as cancer or limit its spread. Both malfunctions have been attributed to interaction between the host's neurophysiological and immunological systems (Pradham et al., 1974). The most recent evidence indicates that the biochemistry of neurologic responsiveness is very similar to that of the immunologic system since both systems evolved from the same precursor cells to perform very similar functions: giving a specific response to a specific stimulus (Hibbs et al., 1977). There is a substantial body of data that defines the nature of the consciousness of an individual and the underlying neurophysiological processes of brain function (Eccles, 1970; Rose, 1973; Penfield, 1975; Pelletier, 1977, 1978). In the neurological system the stimuli are sensory perceptions, while those of the immunological system are chemicals such as proteins, lipids, and carbohydrates. Responses in the neurologic domain depend upon which of various neurons are stimulated, while those of the immunologic system would be various lymphocytes, which are one form of antibody cell of the immune system. It is well known that the adrenals, which are under hypothalmic control, secrete lympholytic corticosteroid (ACTH). In turn, the corticosteroids have a great deal to do with inhibiting T-cell competence. T-cells serve key functions in the immunological system in that they switch other immune responses on and off (Levin, 1979). Indeed, recent research indicates that the relation of glial cell to neuron activity in the nervous system is similar to that seen between lymphocytes and mararophages (Carter et al., 1975; Kaplan et al., 1976). In sum, there is strong scientific evidence demonstrating the adverse effects of stress upon the immunological system, an intricate matrix of psychosocial, neurophysiological, and immunological processes. With this research and clinical base, it is possible to begin a systematic inquiry into how cellular activity can be compromised or enhanced by psychosocial factors.

From the research of Andrew A. Monjan and Michael I. Collector of the Department of Epidemiology at Johns Hopkins University come some of the first experiments to explore both the depression and optimization of immunocompetence by stress. Noting that the immunosuppressive effects of short-term exposure to stressors have been well-established, their research focuses upon the long-term stress of the Type II variant described earlier. For their study they subjected laboratory mice to noise of about 100 db daily for five seconds every minute during a one- to three-hour period around midnight for a varying number of days. Control animals were exposed only to the normal activity of the laboratory room. When the animals were killed and their spleens removed, the researchers found that both the thymus-derived T-cells and the bone marrow-derived B-cells were depressed in quantity by the stressful stimulation. Reporting their results in *Science,* they stated that "stress-induced immunosuppression is mediated through the action of cortisone upon lymphocytes" (Monjan & Collector, 1977). Going one step further, the researchers speculated about the implications of their research for "potentiation of the immune response" and noted that "the enhancement phenomenon reported herein may be due to the elevation of one or more such circulating factors which stimulate lymphocyte reactivity . . . and proliferation. . . . In summary, we have shown that environmental stressors not only can depress immune responsiveness, but can also enhance it" (Monjan & Collector, 1977). Results of this experiment are in keeping with the findings of earlier research by Vernon Riley who was able to vary the incidence of mammary tumors in laboratory mice through varying the effects of stress. Mice placed under chronic stress had a tumor incidence of ninety-two percent while those in a protected environment had a seven percent incidence rate (Riley, 1975). Riley indicated that chronic stress produced an increase in certain hormones, noted also by Monjan and Collector, which appear to have inhibited the natural immune response of the body. As early as 1970, R. C. La Barba reviewed the animal experimental work in *Psychosomatic Medicine* (1970), and concluded that environmental stress produced a linear increase in tumor growth rates in laboratory animals. Also, La Barba quoted Soviet research which hypothesized that higher levels of the central nervous system such as the hypothalamus determined the hormonal balance and level of protective reactions of connective tissue as mediators of this tumor growth.

At this point, in sum, there is ample evidence that psychosocial and environmental stressors induce immunological compromise, which may in turn affect the pathogenesis of tumor growth. An excellent annotated bibliography of this research up to 1976 has been compiled by Jeanne Achterberg, O. Carl Simonton, and Stephanie Matthews-Simonton in *Stress, Psychological Factors, and Cancer* (1976). Inquiries concerning the relationship of stress and emotional factors to immunological dysfunction seem invariably to focus upon pathology rather than upon optimum states of function. The point is made most simply by Nobel Laureate Albert Szent-Györgyi in his recent book *Electronic Biology and Cancer:* "Cancer research has greatly been retarded by our asking why cancer grows, instead of asking what keeps a normal cell from growing. . . . Cancer was looked upon as a hostile intruder which had to be eliminated. It might be looked upon also as a cell in trouble, which needs help to return to normal" (1976). This book advances a theory of cancer based upon molecular interactions prior to oxygen, an α state, and with the introduction of oxygen, the β state. In essence, he maintains the problem resides in a "lack of oxygen" which has been found to "induce a malignant transformation in tissue cultures. It is easy to believe that a lack of O_2, which induces changes in other factors, will eventually take the cells back from the oxidative β state to the fermentative α state." When a cancer cell falls into the α state, a state of high fermentation, the problem is not its rate of proliferation but that it does not stop dividing when no further replication is required. Although Szent-Györgi's theory is complex and as yet unproven, the thrust of his research is intriguing; he seeks out the optimum levels of function in cells to determine the conditions which should be promoted to help cells maintain accurate replication. His approach is a positive one rather than being based primarily upon pathology, which, in itself, makes it innovative.

Psychological factors in the clinical management of cancer are the focus of another important study. After extensive research into the imagery of cancer patients during states of deep relaxation, Jeanne Achterberg and G. Frank Lawlis of the Health Sciences Center, University of Texas at Dallas, formulated a test, termed IMAGE-CA, which takes the subjective reports of patients and scores them in a manner which can be objectively reported and considered. Preliminary results indicate that the IMAGE-CA scores correlate highly with blood chemistry analyses reflecting disease status. For the study, Achterberg and Lawlis collected data from 126 cancer patients over one and one-half years and administered an extensive battery of psychodiagnostic tests along with the IMAGE-CA, as well as hematological analyses. From this research they determined that: "(1) blood chemistries tend to reflect ongoing or concurrent disease state; (2) there is a statistical relationship between psychological variables and blood chemistries; and (3) psychological factors are predictive of *subsequent* disease status" (Achterberg et al., 1977). Data from follow-up studies indicate that the psychological factors were better predictors of the outcome for the patient than hematological analysis. They are not considering causation at the present time but are attempting to develop a means by which clinicians can accurately assess the future trend of a patient's disease. Encouraged by these early results, Achterberg and Lawlis developed IMAGE-CA in order to provide clinicians with a means of understanding the role that patients play in their own treatment. Patients were asked to go through a relaxation procedure and focus upon their own subjective images of their cancer (Simonton & Simonton, 1978). Then they were asked to draw the images they had seen. The researchers conducted structured interviews and began to recognize fourteen scorable dimensions which were amenable to standardization and qualification. Those fourteen factors are:

> Vividness, activity, and strength of the cancer cell; vividness and activity of the white blood cell; relative comparison of size and numbers of cancer and white blood cells; strength of white blood cell; vividness and effectiveness of medical treatment; degree of symbolism; overall strength of imagery; regularity of imagery process; and clinical opinion, related to prognosis based on combined imagery factors (Achterberg & Lawlis, 1978).

Results of their research are detailed in the diagnostic manual *Imagery of Cancer (IMAGE-CA): An Evaluation Tool for the Process of Disease* (1978). Administration of the diagnostic test is relatively brief and involves listening to a relaxation and imagery recording, then drawing the visualizations, followed by a structured interview. Drawings of the imagery plus results of the interview are then scored along these fourteen dimensions and appear to be an accurate assessment of a patient's prognosis.

Interpretation and scoring are complex but the book is quite complete with sample drawings and transcribed cases. Achterberg and Lawlis did note that there were some common elements in the imagery which were indicative of a positive prognosis. These images included "white knights," "Vikings," "large, powerful animals especially dogs and bears," which were aggressively attacking the cancer cells. Overall, the positive imagery rarely described "mechanical devices" such as "vacuum cleaners" or "automatic sprinklers." Patients who saw "vivid, concrete white blood cells," had a more favorable prognosis than those who saw the cancer cells as more vivid. Although Achterberg and Lawlis do not discuss the function of these images per se, it is likely that they are visual representations of the patient's will to live. Perhaps these positive images are one step removed from the sugar pill placebo that Norman Cousins suggests is "only a tangible object made essential in an age that feels uncomfortable with intangibles, an age that prefers to think that every inner effect must have an outer cause . . . the placebo satisfies the contemporary craving for visible mechanisms and visible answers" (1977). Before researchers engage in a headlong plunge into minute dissection and further quantification of imagery, it is important to note that the results of the Achterberg and Lawlis research were obtained with patients treated in a holistic manner, acknowledging both medical and psychosocial aspects of their disease. Under such circumstances, various images are "placebos" in the sense that they are functionaries of the mind in its dynamic relationship with the body. They illustrate the ancient Greek term "physis," or "healing force of the body" (Coulter, 1975). "The placebo then is an emissary between the will to live and the body. But the emissary is expendable. . . . The mind can carry out its ultimate functions and powers over body without the illusion of material intervention. . . . The placebo is the doctor who resides within" (Cousins, 1977). Eliciting and sustaining that response is the essence of the healing relationship and has been the foundation of all systems of health care.

Voluntary regulation of the excessive stress reactivity of the Type II variant is the fundamental element of virtually all systems of stress alleviation. For centuries, systems of meditation and yoga have taught individuals to induce states of deep relaxation to set the stage for altered states of consciousness. More recently, similar techniques have been used in stress management through clinical biofeedback (Fuller, 1978) and Progressive Relaxation (Jacobson, 1938). This classic tradition of inducing states of deep physical relaxation before exploring states of consciousness can also be seen in Autogenic Training (Luthe, 1977), Transcendental Meditation (Wallace, 1970), zazen, Zen meditation (Kennett, 1977), and related meditation and yoga practices. The effect of all of these approaches is a sustained period of diminished sympathetic activity with an attendant increase in parasympathetic activity. Decreased sympathetic activity is an integrated hypothalamic response that was first described by Walter R. Hess and termed the "trophotrophic response" to distinguish it from the "ergotrophic response," which is equivalent to Cannon's fight-flight activity and characterized by increased sympathetic reactivity (Hess, 1957). Neurophysiological observations indicate that the trophotrophic zone is located in the anterior hypothalamus and extends into the supra- and pre-optic areas, septum, and inferior lateral thalamus. Generally, the response is mediated by the parasympathetic nervous system and results in relaxation of the skeletal muscles, decreased blood pressure and respiration rate, and pupil constriction. As early as 1957 Hess noted, "We are actually dealing with a protective mechanism against overstress belonging to the trophotrophic-endophylactic system and promoting restorative processes." More recently, Herbert Benson has popularized this concept as "the relaxation response" (Benson et al., 1974) and noted the major physiological changes as decreases in oxygen consumption and carbon dioxide elimination, decreases in heart rate, respiratory rate, arterial blood lactate, and skeletal muscle tension, accompanied by increased alpha and occasional theta activity in the electroencephalogram. For any given system or individual, these changes vary, but there is a definite tendency for them to occur collectively.

For a patient, the neurophysiological mechanisms are less important than the practice of a stress management technique. Also, it is vitally important to recognize that none of the techniques noted above can be designated as the single treatment of choice for severe psychosomatic disorders such as cardiovascular disease, cancer, and the host of the "afflictions of civilization." These methods are best applied as one of a number of holistic interventions in which the patient assumes an active participation in inducing and sustaining a trophotrophic response (Benson, 1975). There are certain characteristics that Herbert Benson and his colleagues have identified as conducive to eliciting the relaxation response:

1. *Mental Device*—There should be a constant stimulus— e.g., a sound, word, or phrase repeated silently or audibly, or fixed gazing at an object. The purpose of these procedures is to shift away from logical, externally-oriented thought.

2. *Passive Attitude*—If distracting thoughts do occur during the repetition or gazing, they should be disregarded and the attention should be redirected to the technique. One should not worry about how well one is performing the technique.

3. *Decreased Muscle Tonus*—The subject should be in a comfortable posture so that minimal muscular work is required.

4. *Quiet Environment*—An environment with decreased environmental stimuli should be chosen. Most techniques instruct the practitioner to close his eyes. A place of worship is often suitable, as is a quiet room (Benson, Beary & Carol, 1974).

All of the above aspects are greatly enhanced when instruction in a given method is under the supervision of a trained instructor or licensed clinician. Relaxation methods are oriented toward a restoration of "homeostatic self-regulatory mechanisms" (Luthe, 1977) within the psychosomatic system but complications can arise when the techniques are undertaken improperly or without adequate supervision. Contraindications are discussed later in this chapter. Each of the relaxation procedures cited earlier does follow the basic outline of the relaxation response. In *Mind as Healer, Mind as Slayer* (Pelletier, 1977), basic instructions on achieving a Zen meditation posture was detailed in Chapter 6 and an outline of the stages and postures of Autogenic Training were explicated in Chapter 7. Since the data to support each system and instructions on practicing the basic exercises are available in my previous work as well as in full-length works on each discipline (Luthe, 1965; Kennett, 1977), the details are not repeated here. Both Zen meditation and Autogenic Training are excellent methods to use as a primary technique in the clinical management of specific psychosomatic disorders and can also be a potent adjuncts to a wide range of techniques of traditional care.

Autogenic Training is based on a well-researched method of meditation. Of all the systems noted, it is the most comprehensive and can serve as a model for all others that address themselves to clinical treatment of psychosomatic disorders. Autogenic Training developed experimentally out of the medical hypnosis work of Johannes H. Schultz, who published *Das Autogene Training* in 1932. Schultz defined Autogenic Training as exercises which are developed (Greek, *genos*) from within the self (Greek, *autos*). After working with Schultz, the Montreal physician Wolfgang Luthe translated the German publications and extended the theory and practice of Autogenics through his publications (see bibliography). Despite the extensive research data and case histories, the actual application of Autogenics has been hampered by the lack of a training manual, although courses leading to certification have been offered. In 1977 Luthe finally published such a training manual, *Introduction to the Methods of Autogenic Therapy,* which provides clear instructions for a clinician using autogenics in practice. According to the manual, "The techniques developed and used in Autogenic Therapy have been designed to support and facilitate the natural self-healing mechanisms that already exist. Thus, the emphasis is not in trying to control the natural system, but rather on helping natural systems use their inherent potentials of self-regulatory adjustment more fully." That description fits the methods of holistic medicine, which are anticipated in the development of Autogenic Training. Luthe offers instruction in applying Autogenic Training to various psychosomatic conditions, alone or as an adjunct to medical treatment. Among these conditions are cardiac arrhythmias; hypertension; respiratory disorders, such as asthma and tuberculosis; irritable colon; peptic ulcer; ulcerative colitis; obesity; genitourinary, including sexual dysfunction; musculoskeletal disorders, including rheumatoid arthritis and low back syndrome; endocrine and metabolic dysfunction, such as diabetes mellitus and functional thyroid; neurological disorders, such as headaches, neuralgia, epilepsy, cerebral palsy, and Parkinsonism; and many others; plus special clinical applications such as improved postoperative recovery.

Autogenic Training and all self-regulatory methods are noninvasive and relatively safe, although as with any therapeutic intervention, potentially serious complications can arise. Autogenics is particularly responsible in this respect, and all others would do well to emulate this model. The *Manual* contains the contraindications which render autogenic treatment improper or undesirable. Contraindications noted here are applicable to all self-regulatory therapies including clinical biofeedback and should be kept in mind by all practitioners. Among these are doubtful or impending myocardial infarction (MI) during or directly after MI; transient blood pressure elevations which need to be monitored; diabetic conditions; hypoglycemia; glaucoma; involutional psychotic reaction; paranoia; and dissociative episodes. There are specific reasons for each of these contraindications based upon research data. Also included in the *Manual* is a health questionnaire, ROCOM, which was developed by the Patient Care Systems branch of the Hoffman-LaRoche Company of Vaudreuil, Quebec. It includes a patient-administered Health History Questionnaire and a Physical Examination Form that renders medical history in an extremely compact form. Clearly there are purely educational and nonmedical applications of these methods but when they are rendered with patients, then all of the above considerations are essential. Although the emphasis here is upon the applications of Autogenic Therapy with psychosomatic disorders, the basic relaxation postures of this method are prerequisites for a second stage of training, which enters into visualization and meditation. Meditation practices in Autogenics are intended to induce an "intensification of psychic experience by increasing an individual's ability to visually experience endopsychic phenomena" (Gorton, 1959). The precise directions are not included here since they are detailed in *Autogenic Therapy*, Volume I, by J. H. Schultz and Wolfgang Luthe

(1969), and summarized in Chapter 7 of *Mind as Healer, Mind as Slayer* (Pelletier, 1977). There are six stages of meditative exercises beginning with a positioning of the eyes involving a "voluntary rotation of the eyeballs upward and inward looking at the center of the forehead," and culminating in vivid visualizations of significant people and events in the person's life, particularly regarding emotional relationships. Autogenic Training thus takes an individual beyond the healing of specific psychosomatic disorders toward a state of optimum health.

Another self-regulatory approach to psychosomatic disorders is Progressive Relaxation, developed by Edmund Jacobson, beginning in 1908, at Harvard University. His initial experiments led him to conclude that tension involved excess effort which manifested itself in the shortening of muscle fibers when fewer individuals subjectively reported anxiety. To rectify this condition, Jacobson developed a program of systematically tensing and releasing various muscle groups. When a patient could learn to attend to and discriminate the resulting sensations of tension and relaxation, he could enhance the latter and achieve a state of deep relaxation. Jacobson's studies and a description of his procedures were first published in *You Must Relax* (1934) followed by a more professionally oriented version entitled *Progressive Relaxation* (1938).

As of 1962, modifications of the basic approach were introduced, with the result being a relaxation procedure involving fifteen muscle groups. Each group was dealt with for from one to nine hour-long daily sessions before proceeding to the next group for a total of fifty-six sessions of systematic training (Jacobson, 1964). Significant modifications of this procedure were undertaken by Joseph Wolpe (1958) who used the same sequence but created a program that could be completed in six twenty-minute sessions with two fifteen-minute daily home practice sessions between clinical sessions. Wolpe's major innovation was to introduce a graduated series of imagined exposures to anxiety-provoking situations while the person remained relaxed. This method of "systematic desensitization" has proven to be of significant clinical efficacy with phobias. In actual practice, the procedures are usually of much briefer duration. Recently, Douglas A. Bernstein and Thomas D. Borkovec of the University of Illinois at Urbana-Champaign have written an excellent summary of this method for clinical use in *Progressive Relaxation Training: A Manual for the Helping Professions* (1973). Included in the manual is a 33-$1/3$ r.p.m. record describing the basic procedure in order to clarify its pacing, which is very important. The order in which the muscle groups are worked with is as follows:

1. Dominant hand and forearm.
2. Dominant biceps.
3. Nondominant hand and forearm.
4. Nondominant biceps.
5. Forehead.
6. Upper cheeks and nose.
7. Lower cheeks and jaws.
8. Neck and throat.
9. Chest, shoulders, and upper back.
10. Abdominal or stomach region.
11. Dominant thigh.
12. Dominant calf.
13. Dominant foot.
14. Nondominant thigh.
15. Nondominant calf.
16. Nondominant foot (Bernstein & Borkovec, 1973).

In the sessions, a sequence of events is followed with respect to each muscle group. That sequence is: (1) the patient's attention should be focused on the muscle group; (2) at a predetermined signal from the therapist, the muscle group is tensed; (3) tension is maintained for a period of five to seven seconds (this duration is shorter in the case of the feet); (4) at a predetermined cue, the muscle group is released; and, (5) the patient's attention is maintained upon the muscle group as it relaxes. Generally this approach works well for general anxiety, muscular tension, in a wide range of neuromuscular disorders such as spasms, and in physical rehabilitation. Progressive Relaxation is a much more limited and specialized approach than Autogenic Training but is of considerable efficacy when applied appropriately.

Both Autogenic Training and Progressive Relaxation are also useful when applied in conjunction with clinical biofeedback. Clinical biofeedback has been used increasingly to clarify psychosomatic conditions to the patient in an intelligible and effective manner. A comprehensive overview of the field was recently published in *American Psychologist* by George D. Fuller (1978). From that article and others it is clear that clinical biofeedback is an efficacious method for the treatment of neuromuscular reeducation (Basmajian, Baeza & Fabrigar, 1965), reduction of tension, cerebral palsy (Finley et al., 1976), and dental disorders such as bruxism (Rugh, Perlis & Disraeli, 1976). Although EMG (electromyographic) biofeedback is probably the most widely used in clinical practice, other methods used are the electroencephalogram (EEG), the electrodermal response (EDR), electrocardiogram feedback (ECG), peripheral temperature training (TT), as well as penile erection feedback using a plethysmograph, which indicates blood flow. Each of these instruments have been used with a wide range of disorders. Each year all published papers in the field are anthologized in an annual reader entitled *Biofeedback and Self-Control* (Barber et al., 1970) from Aldine Publishers in Chicago.

Future innovative applications of biofeedback include a clinical procedure for the normalization of thalamocortical EEG patterns in psychosomotor epilepsy (Sterman, 1977), direct blood pressure feedback (Steptoe, Smulyan & Griffin, 1976), and computer-based feedback of multiple channels of information simultaneously. Clinical biofeedback is a powerful tool yielding an unprecedented, highly accurate method of monitoring the physiological states from which psychosomatic disorders develop. Unfortunately, there is a tendency for individual practitioners to reify the instruments and become fixated on electronic gadgets, rather than recognizing the instruments as mirrors of the patient's internal state. The instruments are best used as one element of a holistic therapy that considers placebo effects, medical factors, psychosocial parameters, and the active participation of the individual.

At professional conferences, or in the literature of Autogenic Training, Progressive Relaxation, clinical biofeedback, and related approaches, it is striking how compartmentalized each of these approaches tends to be. There is little if any cross-referencing among these systems despite the fact that each has specific applications and limitations. Frequently, a shortcoming of one system is a strong attribute of another. Whereas clinical biofeedback offers accuracy in the clinic or hospital, it is cumbersome or prohibitively expensive for home practice where Autogenic Training or Progressive Relaxation are clearly preferable. Unfortunately, there can be a tendency to apply a given method when it is not clearly indicated. A conservative approach to self-regulatory methods advocates a specific intervention when clearly indicated to the best of the clinician's judgment. When all the options are kept in mind, then it is possible to achieve a comprehensive approach to the development of optimum health.

This chapter on Psyche and Soma began with microorganisms and ends on stress, for stress is the key factor responsible for altering an individual's susceptibility to disease. More than any other single contributing agent, excessive stress reactivity is the major influence in the "afflictions of civilization" (Dubos, 1965). Fortunately, the deleterious effects of stress can be mitigated through the systematic induction of periods of parasympathetic rebound which enables the entire psychosomatic system to undergo periods of profound restoration. Writing in *Doctor Zhivago*, Boris Pasternak acknowledged, "Your health is bound to be affected, if, day after day, you say the opposite of what you feel, if you grovel before what you dislike and rejoice at what brings you nothing but misfortune. Our nervous system isn't just a fiction; it's part of our physical body, and our soul exists in space and is inside us, like the teeth in our mouth. It can't be forever violated with impunity." Underlying all the systems of deep relaxation and meditation is the common element of quiet, or providing an individual with the opportunity to listen to the body and become sensitive again to inner directives. Any approach to meditation is an effective means of curbing the onset of psychosomatic disorders, but it cannot substitute for the arcane dictum to know ourselves as fully as possible.

VI

Nutrition and Health

Complex biochemical processes take place constantly in all the cells of our bodies. In order for these to continue, a variety of nutrients must always be present in adequate amounts. Beyond this single point of agreement, the field of nutrition and health fragments into a morass of strident opinions based upon little or no empirical data, and dietary prescriptions which are frequently totally contradictory. No other area of health maintenance is more subject to confusion and misinformation by both laymen and professionals than the role of diet. Clearly there is a great interest in this area of health care. According to *U.S. News and World Report* (November 28, 1977), "A Gallup Poll last year found that 88 percent of adults want to know more about nutrition. A Harris survey taken earlier this year found that only 14 percent of those questioned thought Americans ate a proper diet." Nutrition is consistently cited as a major determinant of health:

> The requirements of health can be stated simply. Those fortunate enough to be born free of significant congenital disease or disability will remain well if three basic needs are met: they must be adequately fed; they must be protected from a wide range of hazards in the environment; and they must not depart radically from the pattern of personal behavior under which

127

man evolved, for example, by smoking, overeating or sedentary living (McKeown, 1976).

Four of the seven basic factors conducive to health and longevity in the UCLA studies by Lester Breslow and his colleagues cited in Chapter I are related to diet. Individuals argue their positions on diet vehemently, self-righteously and evangelistically, as if they were political opinions. After reading one book on diet many people believe they have all the answers. After reading several other books or articles they feel less certainty since it becomes evident that the actual data agreed upon by researchers in the field of nutrition are scarce. After a more thorough perusal of the contradictory literature, an individual seems to be faced with two alternatives: being resigned to perpetual toxicity or relegated to a total fast. Relatively little scientific research has been conducted in the field of human nutrition and the important cross-correlations among existing studies have not been fully examined. Much of the existing data are based upon biochemical research conducted on tissue cultures or upon animal populations, and the applicability of these studies to the high-order complexity of human nutrition has been established only to a very limited degree (Williams, 1973; Fernstrom & Wurtman, 1974). After reviewing the field, neurosurgeon C. Norman Shealy concluded, "About all we do know for certain is that foods contain fats, carbohydrates, proteins, vitamins, and minerals, and that some sort of balance of all these elements is essential for good health" (1977). Nevertheless, nutrition is of key importance as a determinant of health and the current controversies underscore the necessity for further research.

The emphasis in this chapter is upon those common dietary factors that can be demonstrated to be conducive to an optimum state of health and not upon diet as therapy for obesity, alcoholism, psychological disturbances, or other pathologies. One of the only books which assume a holistic stance toward diet and weight loss in the context of a person's life-style is *The Holistic Way to Health and Happiness* by the physician Harold H. Bloomfield and Robert Kory (1972). Most nutrition articles and books assume a medical stance of prescribing particular diets for the prevention or alleviation of specific conditions. This is an area of considerable interest, for instance orthomolecular medicine, which uses megavitamin dosages as a treatment for severe psychosis. However, the focus in this chapter is upon defining the dietary factors which need to be considered by an individual seeking to establish an optimum state of health rather than to alleviate a specific disorder. Nutrition practices constitute that aspect of life-style which is most easily controlled by the individual. As such it may be the single most important determinant of health.

Among the medical care analysts proposing a life-style orientation to health care is Thomas McKeown, author of two highly influential books, *Medicine in Modern Society* and the most recent *The Role of Medicine: Dream, Mirage, or Nemesis.* According to McKeown: "In light of the importance of food for good health, governments might use supplements and subsidies to put essential foods within the reach of everyone, and provide inducements for people to select beneficial in place of harmful foods" (1978). In the past, nutrition has either been focused upon as a single-factor panacea or dismissed as inconsequential by traditional medicine. Given its biological necessity, on the one hand diet can be seized upon as the *sine qua non* by those actively pursuing health while on the other hand it can be seen as a passive and automatic means of achieving health: an individual simply needs to eat the proper foods and good health will ensue. Unfortunately, many nutritionists subscribe to such simplistic notions and fail to recognize first, that there is little agreement as to what constitutes optimum nutrition and second, that nutrition exists in a complex matrix of social conditions, stress, age, sex, and exercise with the end determinant being the biological uniqueness of each individual's metabolism. A major shortcoming of virtually all dietary prescriptions is the erroneous assumption that there is one diet suitable for a wide range of individuals. A leading proponent of the more appropriate concept of "biochemical individuality" (1956) is the eminent University of Texas biochemist and nutritionist Roger J. Williams, who is the discoverer of pantothenic acid and folic acid, important constituents of the vitamin B-complex. He has noted that there can be as much as forty-fold differences between the biochemical needs of any two individuals. If this range of variability applied to physical features, people would have noses ranging from a half-inch to two feet in length. Any dietary prescription needs to take into account that general principles must be adapted for each individual. Although this is a formidable task, the computer assessment methods discussed later in this chapter have made it easier. Much of the confusion and contradictory information in the field of nutrition appears to reside in the global application of ill-defined general principles. Once emphasis is placed upon assessing and supplementing a particular individual's needs, then many complex issues can be addressed.

This chapter will approach the subject of nutrition in four steps: (1) defining the biochemical constituents underlying any discussion of

diet; (2) enumerating the commonly agreed upon negative and positive influences of specific food substances; (3) an example of one
computer assessment technique which adapts these general principles to any given individual; and finally (4) a discussion of the covert
philosophical and value issues which generally determine which dietary practices will actually be adopted and which will be discarded.

To begin, there are fundamental definitions which need to be
understood. Most nutritionists differentiate between diet, which is
"the daily intake of food and drink," and nutrition, which includes
"all of the processes involved in using foodstuffs for the body's
growth, maintenance, and repair" (Cheraskin, Ringsdorf & Brecher,
1976). In addition to oxygen, water, and energy-yielding foods such
as carbohydrates, there are forty chemicals essential for human life.
Writing in his most recent book, *The Wonderful World Within You:
Your Inner Nutritional Environment* (1977), Roger J. Williams terms
these the "growth and maintenance chemicals." Neither the body
nor any cell in it can function unless every one is present and in
place. Williams emphasizes that the quantitative aspect of nutrition
is vital because of the fact that one such chemical may make up one
percent of a food while another, equally indispensable, may be present in an amount as infinitesimal as one-millionth of one percent.
For convenience these growth and maintenance chemicals are often
classified into five groups:

1. Amino Acids—isoleucine, leucine, lysine, methionine,
    phenylalanine, threonine, tryptophan, and valine.

2. Major Minerals—calcium, chloride, potassium,
    magnesium, sodium, and phosphate.

3. Trace Elements—cobalt, chromium, copper, fluorine,
    iron, iodine, manganese, molybdenum, selenium, zinc.

4. Vitamins—A, biotin, B_6, B_{12}, C, D, E, folic acid, K,
    niacinamide, pantothenic acid, riboflavin, thiamin.

5. Other—choline, linoleic acid (Williams, 1977).

These forty chemicals are known to be required for human nutrition
as well as to be involved in the metabolic processes of every kind of
living organism. Due to the strong similarities in the metabolic requirements of different life forms, people are generally protected
from the most flagrant dietary imbalances. Such a diet is not exotic
but does require a heightened consciousness of nutritional needs. As

this chapter proceeds, the principles for formulating a sound diet according to individual requirements are enumerated. Ultimately, guidelines for any individual diet should be arrived at by the person becoming first alert to his or her own practices, then as well-informed as possible concerning diet and nutrition, and, finally, engaging in consultation with a specialist in nutrition.

Frequently the first concern of individuals assessing their nutrition is with the role of vitamins. Vitamins constitute only one of the five classifications of growth and maintenance chemicals yet they receive a disproprotionate amount of attention, perhaps because the data regarding vitamins are quite straightforward and easy to understand. Notwithstanding, the concept of a vital amine is a sophisticated one. Nobel Laureate Albert Szent-Györgi, who received the prize for his discovery of ascorbic acid (vitamin C) and also has conducted extensive research on cellular respiration and muscle contraction, points out:

> The whole idea of a vitamin is paradox and difficult to digest. Everybody knows that things we eat can make us sick, but it seems utterly senseless to say that something which we have not eaten could make us sick. And this is exactly what a vitamin is: *a substance which makes us sick by not eating it. . . . It is wrong to look upon a vitamin as a substance which just combats specific symptoms. Like a lubricant, the vitamin makes the normal working of your body possible* (1977).

There is a great deal of empirical data regarding vitamins and considerable agreement concerning their essential functions in human nutrition. It is necessary to clarify the terms used in discussions of vitamins and vitamin supplements, which are set by the Food and Drug Administration (FDA) of the U.S. Department of Health, Education, and Welfare. Referring to the chart below, the column marked "U.S. RDA" stands for the United States Recommended Daily Allowance and is the amount of a given vitamin that the FDA considers necessary for maintaining good health. Actually, this "U.S. RDA" standard is subject to continual study and debate. For one thing, many nutritionists and other scientists consider the RDAs to be too low and recommend higher amounts and consumption of most vitamins. Many nutritionists point out that, contrary to popular understanding, the RDA for a vitamin is not the allowance that leads to the best of health for most people. Furthermore, the RDAs are "not recommendations for the ideal diet," according to the Chairman of the Committee on Recommended Dietary Allowances of the U.S. Food and Nutrition Board. The RDA standard is, instead, the estimated minimum amount that would prevent serious illness or death from an overt vitamin deficiency for most people. This is an extremely important point that has recently received a great deal of attention from the U.S. Senate Subcommittee on Health chaired by Senator Edward Kennedy. While testifying before that Committee, Nobel Laureate Linus Pauling stated:

> I believe that the expression "Recommended Dietary Allowance" used by the Food and Nutrition Board and by the FDA is misleading, in that the RDA's are not the amounts that should be recommended as providing the best of health, but are only the amounts, probably much smaller, that prevent death or serious vitamin deficiency disease. I suggest that the name Recommended Dietary Allowance should be replaced by the name Minimum Dietary Allowance (MDA), which represents in a better way the actual significance of the amounts (Pauling, 1978).

Later in the same testimony, Pauling further suggested that the FDA introduce a new range of quantities, which might be termed the Recommended Daily Intake (RDI), corresponding to the known amounts of "individual variability" in vitamin requirements. As an example, Pauling cited vitamin C whose RDI would range from 250 milligrams to 4,000 milligrams per day for an adult. If adopted, the RDI would be applicable to all vitamins, its values would be higher than those of the RDA because they would indicate the range of optimum daily intake. Pauling's concept of "RDI individual variability" is consistent with Williams's observations of "biochemical individuality" and both refer to a key concept in nutrition—that individual differences must be considered. Only then can nutritionists untangle the controversies arising from erroneous attempts to apply global prescriptions where they are inappropriate. Individual adaptation and response is also a key concept in stress and exercise and in the entire field of holistic medicine.

Referring to the chart below, "I.U." stands for International Unit, which is a standard for measuring the potency of a substance. "Mg" stands for milligram and "mcg" for microgram, a thousandth and a millionth of a gram respectively (31 grams equal one ounce). Information contained in this table is a highly condensed compilation of the functions, sources, and interactive factors of fifteen essential vitamins. Primary sources for this chart are the *Dictionary of Nutrition* by Richard Ashley and Heidi Duggal, *Remington's Pharmaceutical Sciences* edited by John E. Hoover, and *Nutrition Almanac* compiled by Nutrition Search Incorporated. Other substances that may be vitamins are currently under study, but not included here, since this chart is meant to be a basic guide rather than an exhaustive source. For a more complete compilation of the properties and applications of known and hypothetical vitamins, other sources include *The Heinz Handbook of Nutrition: A Comprehensive Treatise on Nutrition in Health and Disease* (1959) edited by B. T. Burton, *Physicians' Handbook of Nutritional Science* (1977) by Roger J. Williams, *The Complete Book of Vitamins* (1977), a more popular treatment compiled by J. I. Rodale, and an excellent bibliography of articles for research purposes in *Nutrition Against Disease* (1973) by Roger J. Williams. For most personal diet planning the chart provides reliable basic information.

Following closely upon any discussion of vitamins is the perpetual issue of dietary supplements. Again there is widespread and vehement disagreement. Given the dearth of longitudinal, double-blind, human subjects research in this area, the issue cannot be resolved by reference to empirical data. Although nutritional supplements may not be necessary if a well-balanced and diversified diet is consumed, it is often difficult to obtain foods sufficiently rich in the required growth and maintenance chemicals to meet even the questionable minimums prescribed by the U.S. RDA. Actually, the concept of average dietary requirements is relatively meaningless. Aside from the obvious fact that many individuals eat diets poorer than average, an increased requirement for one or more nutrients may be caused by individual biochemistry, psychological stress, surgery, all kinds of diseases, physical inactivity, pollution, aging, medicines by the hundreds, and many other factors too numerous to mention. It is difficult to plan a diet to assure this important nutrient excess. No one can or will eat optimally 100 percent of the time; so even if food lost no value either when grown, prepared, transported, or served (and it invariably does), supplements would often be necessary (Cheraskin, Ringsdorf & Brecher, 1976, p. 181). Further, many additives involved in food processing and cosmetics also detract from the food value, aside from being toxic in and of themselves (Longgood, 1960; Hall, 1974). Hundreds of preservatives, stabilizers, coloring, flavoring, and other chemical additives are now routinely processed into foods. Although these additives are usually tested for any immediate

Vitamin	Name	Need In Human Nutrition	U.S. RDA	Deficiency Disease	
A	Retinol	Essential for growth and maintenance of body tissue, strong bones and teeth, and good eyesight. (Helps to form and maintain healthy function of eyes, skin, hair, teeth, gums, various glands and mucous membranes. Also involved in fat metabolism.*)	5,000 I.U., for adults and children four or more years of age, except pregnant and lactating women, for whom the RDA is 8,000 I.U.	Xeropthalmia; Night blindness.	
B Complex	Thiamine (B_1)	Essential for utilization of carbohydrates in energy production. Promotes healthy central nervous system and mental attitude, and improvement of food assimilation and digestion.	1.5 mg.	Beriberi.	
B Complex	Riboflavin (B_2)	Essential for good vision and healthy skin, nails, and hair. Functions with other substances to break down and utilize carbohydrates, fats, and proteins.	1.7 mg.	Ariboflavinosis —lesions of the mouth, lips, skin, and genitalia.	
B Complex	Niacin (Niacinamide or Nicotinic Acid)	Essential for healthy brain functions, nervous system, and skin. Important in tissue respiration. Essential for synthesis of sex hormones.	20 mg.	Pellagra.	
B Complex	Cobalamin (B_{12})	Essential for maintenance of healthy nervous system, and for utilization of carbohydrates, fats, and proteins.	6 mcg.	Pernicious anemia; brain damage.	

(*Information provided by the Vitamin Information Bureau, Inc., Chicago, Illinois.)

Subclinical Symptoms	Natural/Food Sources	Antagonists	Toxicity Level	Miscellaneous
Eyes—Inability to adjust to darkness; dry and inflamed eyeball; sties. Face and/or skin blemishes—rough, dry, prematurely aged skin. General —Loss of smell; loss of appetite; frequent fatigue; diarrhea.	Fish liver oil; carrots; green and yellow vegetables; liver; whole milk and dairy products; eggyolk, yellow fruits.	Excessive consumption of alcoholic beverages; mineral oil; cortisone (and other drugs); polyunsaturated fatty acids with carotene (unless anti-oxidants are present).	More than 50,000 I.U. daily could produce some toxic effects.	The human body—except for diabetics and persons with impaired thyroid functions —has the ability to convert a certain portion of carotene obtained from foods into Vitamin A.
Muscles—Cramps; general weakness; tenderness in calf. General—Loss of appetite; fatigue; loss of weight; burning sensation in soles of feet.	Brewer's yeast; wheat germ; bran; liver.	Cooking heat, air, water; caffeine; food processing techniques; sulfa drugs; sleeping pills; estrogen; alcohol.	No known toxic effects.	
Eyes—burning sensation; bloodshot.	Milk; liver; enriched cereals; brewer's yeast; leafy green vegetables; fish; eggs.	Water; cooking; sunlight; food processing techniques; sulfa drugs; sleeping pills; estrogen; alcohol.	No known toxic effects.	
Nervous System— Hostility; suspicion; insomnia; loss of memory; irritability; anxiety. General— Abdominal pain; burning sensation in tongue; dry and scaly patches of skin.	Liver; brewer's yeast; kidney; wheat germ; whole grains; fish eggs; lean meat; nuts.	Water; food processing techniques; sulfa drugs; sleeping pills; estrogen; alcohol.	Nontoxic, except some side effects may result from more than 100 mg. daily.	
Nervousness; heart palpitations; inflamed tongue.	Liver; kidney; milk and dairy products; some types of meat.	Water; sunlight; acids; alkalis; food processing techniques; sulfa drugs; sleeping pills; estrogen; alcohol.	No known toxic effects.	Cobalamin, or Vitamin B_{12}, is the only vitamin that contains a mineral, cobalt.

Vitamin	Name	Need In Human Nutrition	U.S. RDA	Deficiency Disease	
---------	------	-------------------------	----------	--------------------	
B Complex	Para-Amino-benzoic Acid (PABA)	Helps to form folic acid and in utilization of proteins.	Not established.	Depression; headache; eczema.	
B Complex	Folacin, or Folic Acid	Essential for division of body cells, for production of nucleic acids (RNA and DNA) and for utilization of sugar and amino acids.	0.4 mg. (400 mcg.)	Anemia.	
B Complex	Inositol	Combines with choline to form lecithin, which in turn metabolizes fats and cholesterol. Important for healthy hair.	Not established.	Eczema.	
B Complex	Choline	Combines with inositol to form lecithin, which in turn metabolizes fat and cholesterol. Essential for healthy liver and kidneys.	Not established.	Kidney damage.	
B Complex	Pantothenic Acid; Panthenol; Calcium Pantothenate.	Essential for conversion of fat and sugar to energy, for use of PABA and choline, and vital to proper function of adrenal glands.	10 mg.	Hypoglycemia; other blood disorders; duodenal ulcers; skin disorders.	
B Complex	Pyridoxine (B$_6$)	Essential for metabolism of amino acids. Aids in blood building, utilization of fats, and normal functioning of brain, nervous system, and muscles.	2 mg.	Anemia.	

Subclinical Symptoms	Natural/Food Sources	Antagonists	Toxicity Level	Miscellaneous
Fatigue; irritability; constipation; nervousness; graying hair.	Liver; kidney; whole grains.	Water; food processing techniques; sulfa drugs; sleeping pills; estrogen; alcohol.	No known toxic effects.	
Gastrointestinal disorders.	Liver; Tortula yeast; green vegetables.	Water; food processing techniques; sulfa drugs; sleeping pills; estrogen; alcohol; sunlight.	No known toxic effects.	
Loss of hair; constipation.	Liver; brewer's yeast, whole grains; wheat germ; unrefined molasses; corn; citrus fruits.	Water; food processing techniques, sulfa drugs; sleeping pills; estrogen; alcohol.	No known toxic effects.	
Deteriorating kidneys, abnormally high blood pressure.	Brewer's yeast; liver; kidney; wheat germ; egg yolk.	Water; food processing techniques; sulfa drugs; sleeping pills; estrogen; alcohol.	No known toxic effects.	Can be synthesized in the human liver.
Restlessness; vomiting; abdominal pains; muscle cramps; burning sensation in feet.	Whole grains; wheat germ; bran; kidney; liver; heart; green vegetables; brewer's yeast.	Heat; cooking; canning; caffeine; food processing techniques; sulfa drugs; sleeping pills; estrogen; alcohol.	No known toxic effects.	
Loss of hair; water retention during pregnancy; nervous system disorder; cracks around mouth and eyes; increase in urination.	Brewer's yeast; wheat bran; rice bran; wheat germ; liver; kidney; heart; blackstrap molasses; milk; eggs; cabbage; beef.	Canning; long storage; roasting or stewing (meat); water; food processing techniques; sulfa drugs; sleeping pills; estrogen; alcohol.	No known toxic effects.	

Vitamin	Name	Need In Human Nutrition	U.S. RDA	Deficiency Disease	
B Complex	Biotin (Also called Coenzyme R or Vitamin H)	Essential for utilization of proteins, carbohydrates, and fats, and for healthy hair and skin. Aids in the maintenance of the thyroid and adrenal glands, reproductive tract, and the nervous system.	0.3 mg. (300 mcg.)	Dermatitis; depression; anemia; anorexia.	
C	Ascorbic Acid	Principal function is to maintain collagen, which is necessary for the connective tissue that holds body cells together. It is involved in wound healing, the formation of red blood cells, and is believed to be involved in disease resistance.	60 mg.	Scurvy.	
D	Calciferol	Essential for utilization of calcium and phosphorus. Necessary for strong teeth and bones.	400 I.U.	Rickets; osteomalacia; senile osteoporosis.	

Subclinical Symptoms	Natural/Food Sources	Antagonists	Toxicity Level	Miscellaneous
Mental depression; dry, peeling skin; muscular pains; poor appetite; lack of energy.	Brewer's yeast; egg yolk; liver; milk; kidney.	Water; food processing techniques; sulfa drugs; sleeping pills; estrogen; alcohol.	No known toxic effects.	Can be produced in the human body by the intestinal microflora.
Slow wound healing; loss of appetite; bleeding gums; muscular weakness; shortness of breath.	Fresh fruits and vegetables.	Heat; light; oxygen; water. Much Vitamin C is destroyed when vegetables are overwashed or cooked, and when fruit is overwashed.	No known toxic effect. Although not proven, excessive use of Vitamin C has been associated with kidney stones in some persons, and has a diuretic and/or laxative effect on some people.	Claims as to the beneficial effect of Vitamin C have been made by a number of scientists, among them Nobel Prize winner Dr. Linus Pauling. Among the beneficial effects are increased resistance to disease, particularly the common cold, less tooth decay and possible use as a general antiviral agent.
Weakening bones, including teeth; weakening muscles.	Fish liver oils; milk and dairy products; sunlight.	Mineral Oil.	25,000 I.U. daily over a long period of time could produce a toxic effect in adults.	Ultraviolet rays of the sun activate the cholesterol present in the skin, converting it to Vitamin D.

Vitamin	Name	Need In Human Nutrition	U.S. RDA	Deficiency Disease	
E	Tocopherol	Protects from oxidation Vitamin A, selenium, two sulphur amino acids, polyunsaturated fatty acids, and some Vitamin C.*	30 I.U.	Kidney and liver damage; anemia.*	
K	Menadione	Essential for formation of prothrombin, a bloodclotting chemical. Important to proper liver function and longevity.	Not established.	Celiac disease; sprue; colitis; hemorrhage.	
P	Bioflavonoids	Essential for proper use of Vitamin C.	Not established.	Combined with Vitamin C, rheumatism and rheumatic fever.	

*Nutritionists, doctors, and federal government scientists disagree as to the exact metabolic function of Vitamin E and, therefore, its defiency diseases as well. The need listed here, however, is generally agreed to by those involved with nutrition research.

Subclinical Symptoms	Natural/Food Sources	Antagonists	Toxicity Level	Miscellaneous
Muscle degeneration; enlarged prostate; red blood cell damage.	Vegetable oils; whole raw seeds and nuts; soybeans.	Food processing techniques; heat; freezing temperatures; oxygen; iron; mineral oil.	Nontoxic, except for persons with high blood pressure or chronic rheumatic heart disease.	If taking vitamin and mineral supplements, Vitamin E should be taken at least two hours before or after a person takes an iron supplement.
Diarrhea; bleeding nose.	Yogurt; eggyolk; safflower oil; fish liver oils; kelp; alfalfa; leafy green vegetables.	Aspirin; X-rays and radiation; frozen foods; industrial air pollution.	Natural Vitamin K is considered nontoxic, but more than 500 mcg. per day of synthetic Vitamin K is not.	The abundance of Vitamin K in most diets generally precludes the need to supplement food with this vitamin. Vitamin K deficiency is rare, except for newborn babies.
High tendency to bleed easily.	White pigments of citrus fruits; rutin.	Same as Vitamin C.	No known toxicity.	

toxic effects, no longitudinal research has been conducted to determine what long-term deficiencies might be associated with ingesting
these foreign substances over many years. Most nutritionists emphasize that the closer food is to its original source and the less it has been
processed, the better it will meet an individual's nutritional requirements. With reference to the acknowledged influences of genetic
predisposition toward unique metabolic processes for each person,
the authoritative *Heinz Handbook of Nutrition* states, "The typical
individual is more likely to be one who has average needs with
respect to many essential nutrients, but who also exhibits some nutritional requirements for a few essential nutrients which are far from
average" (Burton, 1976). While each individual has unique nutritional requirements influenced by genetic predispositions, some
guidelines are generally agreed upon concerning the amount of supplement required by most individuals. These nutritional supplements are listed in the table below. Data for this table were compiled
by Michael Volen and David E. Bresler from the Department of
Anesthesiology in the School of Medicine at the University of California at Los Angeles. Their conclusions are published in "A Guide to
Good Nutrition," one of a series of patient education pamphlets
prepared by the Center for Integral Medicine. CIM is a nonprofit
California corporation founded in 1974 by a group of doctors, including myself, who are concerned with the development and maintenance of health. These guidelines for daily supplements suggested by
Volen and Bresler are in keeping with the dosages suggested by
Roger J. Williams in *Nutrition Against Disease* (1973) and those in
the "Optimal Diet" chapter of *Psychodietetics* (1976) by Emanuel
Cheraskin and his colleages at the University of Alabama in Birmingham. Many vitamin and mineral preparations, containing somewhat
different combinations, are commercially available. Although the
sources and functions of vitamins have generally received more attention, minerals serve equally vital functions, e.g., building and
repairing the skeletal system and the teeth. Recommended food
sources of the minerals listed on page 144 include nuts, meats (especially liver), molasses, peas, cereal, brewer's yeast, dried prunes,
wheat germ, eggs, whole wheat bread, and sea salt. Common drinking water is one of the most important sources of minerals but artificially "softened" water can be dangerous because of its excess of salt
and its abundance of potentially harmful cadmium which competes
with and displaces zinc, a useful mineral (Shealy, 1977). There is no
single "best" combination but an individual can choose sensibly by
comparing not only formulations, using the table (p. 144) as a guide,

but also prices, which can vary widely and do not necessarily reflect superior quality.

All of the above quantities represent conservative estimates. Any vitamin and mineral supplement should always be taken before or during a meal in order to ensure that all the essential nutrients are present at the same time in the digestive tract. It is important to bear in mind that supplements are an addition to and not a substitute for a sound diet.

Some individuals may wish to modify or supplement these guidelines. Among the many debated applications of vitamin and mineral supplements far beyond the dosages cited above are: (1) vitamin C for preventing the common cold as propounded in Linus Pauling's controversial book *Vitamin C and the Common Cold* (1974). This was supported later by sophisticated research reported in the *Journal of the American Medical Association* by Judy Z. Miller and her colleagues at the Indiana School of Medicine, in which forty-four monozygotic twins were tested and the treatment group experienced cold episodes that were "significantly shorter and less severe" than the control group (Miller et al., 1977); (2) vitamin C and its possible life-extending effects for cancer patients (Pauling, 1977; Cameron & Pauling, 1976) as well as its possible prophylactic effects on cancer (Szent-Györgi, 1978); (3) magnesium given to prevent deficiencies leading to adverse effects on the heart such as premature ventricular contractions and ventricular fibrillation (Anderson, 1976; Flink, 1976); (4) vitamin E given in an attempt to retard the aging process as in research conducted by gerontologist Denham Harman of the University of Nebraska School of Medicine (Harman, 1972), or the research of Alton Ochsner, the surgeon who also noted that vitamins C and E prevent premature and dangerous blood clotting (Ochsner, 1970); and (5) diet used as therapy for neurotic as well as psychotic behavior, hyperkinesis in children (Wright, 1977), as well as adult disorders such as dyskinesia (Kolata, 1976), hypoglycemia, and other treatments being researched under the rubric of orthomolecular psychiatry. The orthomolecular or megavitamin approach to a wide range of disorders is a relatively new and controversial area which has been reviewed by Richard A. Passwater in *Supernutrition for Healthy Hearts* (1977). This list of intriguing nutrition research could be extended considerably. As controversial as such studies are, they constitute an area of definite promise that has already demonstrated significant breakthroughs. Another necessary source of information for both laymen and professionals is a publication of the United States Department of Agriculture entitled *Compo-*

VITAMINS: SUGGESTED DAILY SUPPLEMENTS

Vitamin A	7,500–10,000 units
Vitamin D	300–400 units
Vitamin E	100–400 units
Vitamin C	250–1000 mg
Vitamin B_1	2–25 mg
Vitamin B_6	3–25 mg
Vitamin B_{12}	9–50 mcg
Niacinamide	20–100 mg
Pantothenic acid	15–50 mg
Biotin	0.1–0.3 mg
Folic acid	0.2–0.5 mg
*Choline	100–250 mg
*Insitol	100–250 mg
*P-aminobenzoic acid	20–30 mg
*Rutin	25–200 mg

MINERALS: SUGGESTED DAILY SUPPLEMENTS

Calcium	250–400 mg
Magnesium	150–250 mg
Iron	10–15 mg
Zinc	0.1–0.5 mg
Copper	0.5–2 mg
Iodine	0.10–0.15 mg
*Manganese	2–5 mg

*Need in nutrition not established   (Volen & Bresler, 1979)

sition of Foods: Raw, Processed, Prepared (1963). From the definitive tables in this book, an individual can determine the calories, fiber content, vitamins, minerals, saturated fats, unsaturated fats, protein content, and even the energy value of virtually any food substance in any one of the three states of preparation. Using this information and the dietary guidelines which follow, it is possible to formulate an optimum diet. In nutrition, as much as in any other field, it is important to have truly informed consumers.

Given the basic vocabulary of nutrition, it is possible to proceed to the second step and explore the generally agreed upon positive and negative aspects of a given diet. At the moment, this is an issue of highest national priority. In 1969 the U.S. Senate created a Select Committee on Nutrition, chaired by Senator George McGovern, with a number of key members on the committee including Senators Kennedy, Humphrey, Dole, and Percy. Initially the Committee focused on the Food Stamp Program and other governmental food programs. While these matters are themselves highly controversial, the Committee took a greater risk when it addressed the more fundamental issue of the dietary choices of the United States public. Following many hearings and months of testimony by leading nutritionists and organizations such as the American Medical Association, the Committee resolved to take a position regarding what changes the people of the United States need to make in their nutritional patterns. Such a step had not been undertaken before by Congress and the results have had major impact. When the conclusions of this inquiry were made public, Senator McGovern characterized the work of the Committee as follows in his introductory remarks:

> . . . this is the first comprehensive statement by any branch of the Federal Government on risk factors in the American diet. The simple fact is that our diets have changed radically within the last 50 years with great and often very harmful effects on our health. These dietary changes represent as great a threat to public health as smoking. Too much fat, too much sugar or salt, can be and are linked directly to heart disease, cancer, obesity, and stroke, among other killer diseases. In all, six of the ten leading causes of death in the United States have been linked to our diet. Those of us within Government have an obligation to acknowledge this. The public wants some guidance, wants to know the truth, and hopefully today we can lay the cornerstone for the building of better health for all Americans, through better nutrition. . . . My hope is that this report will perform a

function similar to that of the Surgeon General's Report on
Smoking. . . . The same progress can and must be made in
matters of nutritional health . . . (McGovern, 1977).

Conclusions such as these are hardly new but it is striking that they
should have been issued by a committee of the U.S. Senate.

Results of the report were termed a "landmark" by consumer
advocates and predictably labeled an "atrocity" by the two-billion-
dollar-a-year food industry (Welborn, 1977). Actually, the McGovern
report probably would not have created such a reaction and would
have remained at the level of impotent rhetoric characteristic of so
many government reports had the Committee not proceeded to
translate their position into these specific recommendations:

UNITED STATES DIETARY GOALS

1. To avoid overweight, consume only as much energy
   (calories) as is expended; if overweight, decrease energy
   intake and increase energy expenditure.

2. Increase the consumption of complex carbohydrates and
   "naturally occurring" sugars from about 28 percent of
   energy intake to about 48 percent of energy intake.

3. Reduce the consumption of refined and processed
   sugars by about 45 percent to account for about 10
   percent of total energy intake.

4. Reduce overall fat consumption from approximately 40
   percent to about 30 percent of energy intake.

5. Reduce saturated fat consumption to account for about
   10 percent of total energy intake; and balance that with
   polyunsaturated and monounsaturated fats, which
   should account for about 10 percent of energy intake
   each.

6. Reduce cholesterol consumption to about 300 mg a day.

7. Limit the intake of sodium by reducing the intake of
   salt to about 5 grams a day (Bumstead, Carter & Field,
   1978)

Going one step further, the Committee's report became even
more specific by enumerating pragmatic measures for implementing

each of these goals and recommending the following changes in food selection and preparation:

1. Increase consumption of fruits and vegetables and whole grains.

2. Decrease consumption of refined and other processed sugars and foods high in such sugars.

3. Decrease consumption of foods high in total fat, and partially replace saturated fats, whether obtained from animal or vegetable sources, with polyunsaturated fats.

4. Decrease consumption of animal fat, and choose meats, poultry, and fish which will reduce saturated fat intake.

5. Except for young children, substitute low-fat and nonfat milk for whole milk, and low-fat dairy products for high-fat dairy products.

6. Decrease consumption of butter fat, eggs, and other high cholesterol sources. Some consideration should be given to easing the cholesterol goal for premenopausal women, young children, and the elderly in order to obtain the nutritional benefits of eggs in the diet.

7. Decrease consumption of salt and foods high in salt content (Bumstead, Carter & Field, 1978).

In practice, each of these measures would result in major changes in the diet of most individuals.

These goals are quite similar to the standards independently developed by the Norwegian Ministry of Agriculture in 1968 and subsequently incorporated into their Diet and Exercise Program (Royal Norwegian Ministry of Agriculture, 1975–1976). According to *U.S. News and World Report,* the Committee report prompted protests from the cattle industry, egg producers, sugar interests, and other food processors. Confusion has resulted for many consumers because of the split opinions of the medical and nutrition professions. From the AMA came the reaction that "insufficient evidence exists at this time to support the need for or the benefit from major changes in the national diet as proposed" (Welborn, 1977). This opinion is in direct opposition to the endorsements of groups such as the American Heart Association, American Dietetic Association, and the Society of Nutrition Education, organizations devoting considerable research and attention to the relationship between diet and health. Although the protests may have some validity, those from food producers are dubious since the profit incentive has long since usurped concern over nutritional quality. To many people it seems incredible that serious dietary deficiencies should exist at the present time but a survey of ten states sponsored by the U.S. Department of Health, Education, and Welfare during the years from 1968 to 1970, covering every region of the country, indicated some alarming deficiencies in the nutritional status of many sociocultural groups (Garn & Clark, 1975). Ernest Saward and Andrew Sorenson, while recognizing that this problem is amenable to correction through multiple means, caution, "The final consideration is the role of the individual citizens. Even with a stronger role for government, better informed health-care providers, and a more nutritionally conscious food industry, if the consumers themselves do not desire to improve their nutritional status, the best that can be expected are slight changes" (1978). Complete details of the McGovern Committee report were submitted for review to over fifty authorities and their responses are anthologized in an 869-page volume, *Supplemental Views,* available from the McGovern Committee (1977).

 Among the many controversial aspects of diet and health is the relationship between the intake of saturated fats and the subsequent development of cardiovascular disease. Factors four through six of the recommended United States Dietary Goals relate to this consideration. Suspicions that our current dietary practices in this area represent a major problem have received additional support from a thirteen-year study of the Maori, a seafaring Polynesian people who inhabit certain widely scattered islands of the South Pacific. Three different groups of Maori were selected to represent different stages of exposure to European culture, including diet. Research teams led by Ian Prior of New Zealand studied the westernized New Zealand Maori, the Maori of Rarotonga who live 2,000 miles northeast of New Zealand and are in an intermediate stage, and the Maori of Pukapuka who dwell over 3,000 miles away and live very primitively (Prior, 1977). Islanders of Pukapuka live on an 1,800-calorie per day subsistence diet of fish, coconuts, taro, flour, and rice with small quantities of fresh meat. Although some of the women were fat, none were obese and no males fat or obese. Furthermore, despite the high saturated-fat content of the staple food of coconut, the population showed relatively low serum cholesterol levels and low incidences of heart disease, gout, diabetes, and hypertension. When the Rarotongans were studied, their more Western 2,100-calorie diet consisted of canned meat and fish, taro, rice, vegetables, coconut sauce, butter, fresh meat and fish, sugar, and salt. Researchers found that twenty-five percent of the women were grossly obese, twenty-one percent of the men and thirty-six percent of the women had hypertension, and diabetes and heart disease were more prevalent than on Pukapuka. Even more striking were the findings among the New Zealand Maori who consumed an entirely Western 2,500-calorie diet with twice as much fat, sugar, and salt than their island counterparts. New Zealand Maori had a higher incidence of all the above disorders than either of the other two populations and were also afflicted by tuberculosis, which appeared to be due to the crowded and unsanitary urban living conditions.

Research data such as these underscore the problems of our national diet described earlier. "Bad nutritional status (of the too-much-fat-intake-resulting-in-obesity type) can predispose the individual to heart attacks, strokes, cancer of the gastrointestinal tract, diabetes, liver and gall-bladder disease, degenerative arthritis of the hips, knees, and ankles, and injuries. . . . Although the mechanism has not been established, it would appear that high fat intake (usually with resultant obesity) predisposes the American to both cancer and cardiovascular disease" (Knowles, 1977). Since these disorders comprise the two leading causes of premature disability and death in the United States and since both are stress-related, there is a clear mandate for individuals to lower their saturated fat and cholesterol consumption.

However, diet cannot be considered in isolation from other factors. The risk engendered by cholesterol intake is also highly dependent upon the stress factors cited in the previous chapters and upon the extremely important factor of exercise. Yet these are often completely overlooked in considerations of dietary principles in health. There is a tendency of researchers to focus upon one variable and to ignore or disparage consideration of others. Fortunately, this trend is changing. Emmanuel Cheraskin and William M. Ringsdorf acknowledge the interaction between stress and diet in *Psycho-Dietetics* (1976) by including the Holmes and Rahe Schedule of Recent Experience as a factor altering dietary requirements and affecting cholesterol metabolism. After a generation of research focusing upon the "diet-heart" problem, a recent excellent overview in the *New England Journal of Medicine* by George V. Mann pointed out, "no one has been able to prove that dietary treatments either prevent or modify the behavior of coronary heart disease," and later asserted quite blatantly, ". . . the diet-heart hypothesis is wrong" (1977).

Mann's assertion is clearly supported by the research of physician Mark D. Altschule whose careful review of the eight major studies contributing to the diet-heart hypothesis drew the same conclusion (1976). Dietary factors alone are not sufficient in and of themselves to prevent cardiovascular disease.

The most recent research demonstrates that cholesterol does not exist in the circulatory system on its own but as an attachment to more than half a dozen different substances called lipoproteins. Some of these compounds actually protect against cardiovascular disease rather than promote it. One important type of lipoprotein, low-density lipoproteins or LDL, carries cholesterol from the liver to various tissues where it serves the positive function of synthesizing cell membranes and certain hormones. From data obtained in the Framingham heart studies, it appears that individuals with high LDL levels in their blood are more likely to suffer heart attacks. However, another type of lipoprotein, high-density lipoprotein or HDL, has been demonstrated to be inversely related to the incidence of coronary heart disease (Miller et al., 1977). It is hypothesized that HDLs remove cholesterol from artery walls, preventing it from being deposited there, and thus actually protect individuals from cardiovascular disease. After examining the four major lines of evidence that refute the simplified "diet-heart" link, George V. Mann concluded that there is considerably more evidence linking exercise as a critical variable than dietary factors alone, and pointed out the evidence suggesting that fit and active people are spared the complications of atherosclerosis. In support of this conclusion he cited studies of the Maasai tribe indicating that exercise makes even atherosclerotic vessels enlarge so that the capacity of coronary vessels increases despite an increase in atherosclerosis (Mann et al., 1972); studies by Richard S. Paffenbarger indicating a sparing effect of occupational exertion on coronary heart disease (Paffenberger et al., 1977); and, the well-known "seven-country study" (Keys, 1970) indicating quite clearly the benefits of exercise in reducing coronary heart disease. Most interestingly, these studies appear to indicate that regular exercise increases HDL levels in the blood and significantly alters the utilization of serum cholesterol. In sum, while a marked reduction in cholesterol intake may be conducive to cardiovascular health, exercise may be the more critical factor. To date, no systematic trials of the effectiveness of exercise per se in preventing cardiovascular disease have been conducted. Today's runners might not know if fitness protects them against cardiovascular disease, but they do know that exercise makes them feel better. In the meantime many are following the quip of scientific savant and runner Irvine H. Page (1977), who said he still follows a low-fat, low-cholesterol diet because he has no intention of being the smartest man in the cemetery.

Inextricably tied to any discussion of limiting saturated-fat intake is the all-important issue of protein ingestion, which was not specifically addressed in the McGovern Committee Report. Proteins are fundamental to all life forms in that they are the basis of the nervous system, muscles, organs, skin, and in every vital metabolic function. Since 400 B.C. athletes have consumed diets rich in animal protein, although the origins of this practice are obscure since earlier athletes subsisted primarily on bread, cheese, fruits, fish, and wine. "Sports medicine" physician Allan J. Ryan theorizes that in the consuming of meat "there was some association with the idea that consuming the flesh of a powerful animal would give a human greater strength" (1978). That fantasy of physical prowess may continue as an unconscious influence upon those individuals who wish to emulate athletes. However, even in athletics, the desirability of a predominantly protein diet has been virtually discarded. Protein is not used as an energy source in the body except during starvation or when the diet is grossly deficient in fats and carbohydrates. From Ryan's observations published recently in *Science,* the ability of an athlete to sustain high-level performance over time is directly related to the stores of glycogen in the liver and muscles at the beginning of competition. For this reason, the practice of "carbohydrate loading" has replaced the precompetition meal of animal protein, although animal protein still occupies an important place in the athlete's diet. In carbohydrate loading, "the high-protein, high-fat diet is taken for three or more days and then followed by a high-carbohydrate diet that is low in fat and protein . . . levels of muscle glycogen are higher than those found with the high-carbohydrate diet alone" (Ryan, 1978). Thus, from athletic competition derives further evidence that a diversified diet appears to be more conducive to optimum health than based largely on animal protein.

Saturated fats are present in quantity in the diets of most Americans because of their preference for consuming animal protein, particularly red meat, eggs, and dairy products. Part of the outcry from the food-processing industry is the warning that if the McGovern Committee recommendations were carried out, the average diet would result in a lower consumption of protein. But of course protein can be found in other than animal sources. Recently an article in the *Journal of the American Medical Association* by William H. Crosby addressed the question, "Can a Vegetarian Be Well Nourished?" (1975). Based upon the data cited in the article, such is clearly possible, but great attention is required in planning a sound diet. The article noted that "the greatest risk comes from undue reliance on a single plant-food source," and recommended variety in the diet in order to ensure adequate protein. Protein is comprised of up to twenty-two or more amino acids. Of these twenty-two, the body can synthesize all but eight. These are known as the eight essential amino acids and all must be present at the same time for protein formation. Both the quantity and quality of one's protein intake are central factors in all dietary practices. All living matter is comprised of protoplasm which in turn is composed of nitrogenous compounds. Protein is the only foodstuff containing nitrogen and is therefore essential to any diet (Crosby, 1975). Foods of animal origin contain these eight amino acids in nearly optimum amounts and in available form. These "high-quality proteins" include meat, poultry, fish, eggs, and dairy products. By contrast, the quality of proteins in plant sources is generally lower than that of animal proteins, although some plant sources, notably soybeans, seeds, and most nuts, are high-quality protein. Cereal grain proteins are termed "lower-quality protein" because they lack adequate quantities of the essential amino acid lysine. Other nutrients likely to be of marginal content in purely vegetarian diets are calcium, iron, riboflavin, vitamin B_{12}, and, for children not exposed to adequate sunlight, vitamin D (Crosby, 1975). Despite these limitations, it is unquestionably possible to reduce reliance upon animal protein sources, thereby avoiding the attendant elevated cholesterol levels, without incurring nutritional deficiencies.

There are three main variations in vegetarian diets: *total vegetarianism,* which excludes all but plant foods, *lacto-vegetarianism,* which relies upon plant foods plus dairy products, and *lacto-ovo-vegetarianism,* which utilizes plant foods plus eggs and dairy products. Which of these an individual chooses to follow is usually a matter of religious, philosophical, or even economic persuasion. These considerations are not addressed here. The question is simply whether or not it is possible to obtain all necessary nutrients while practicing partial or total abstinence from animal protein sources. As a diet becomes more diversified, the probability of its meeting nutrient requirements increases. When limited amounts of dairy products such as milk or eggs are included, the risk of nutritional inadequacies is greatly reduced. However, even a strict vegetarian diet can meet all requirements if appropriate information is obtained and attention is given to food preparation. Studies of people on pure vegetarian diets from many populations of the world have demonstrated that these individuals maintain excellent health. One study reported by M. G. Hardinge and F. J. Stare concerned the nutritional intake and health status of 200 subjects in the three dietary groups noted above (1954). Based upon physical examinations and laboratory analyses, the results indicated no evidence of deficiencies and the intake of nutrients by each group equaled or exceeded the Recommended Dietary Allowances of the National Research Council. One exception was a lower level of vitamin B_{12} in the total vegetarian diet, which could have led to evidence of anemia had the studies been continued over time. This potential hazard can be overcome through the use of fortified soybean milk or a vitamin B_{12} supplement.

Since an adequate supply of the "growth and maintenance chemicals" is required in all diets, it is particularly important for strict vegetarians to acquaint themselves with the amino acid content of diverse foods. An excellent source of information on this subject is the book from the U.S. Department of Agriculture entitled *Amino Acid Content of Foods* (Orr & Watt, 1968), which analyzes virtually all foodstuffs with respect to the relative content of eighteen amino acids. The practice of balancing the amino acid content of vegetarian diets was popularized by Frances Moore Lappé's *Diet for a Small Planet.* She explains the principle of "protein complementarity," i.e., "the combination, in the proper proportions, of non-meat foods, that produces high-grade protein nutrition equivalent to—or better than —meat proteins" (1973). When cereals, which are low in lysine and high in methionine, are eaten in conjunction with a legume such as dried beans, which contains ample lysine but is short on methionine, an amino acid balance is achieved and high-quality protein is supplied. Drawing upon extensive data, Lappé's book demonstrates that diets of properly selected plant foods can be nutritionally adequate. According to Lappé, the worldwide practice of combining cereals and legumes in the food of both humans and farm animals provides viable evidence of the supplementarity of one plant protein food with another. If this complementary mixing is done judiciously, combinations of "lower-quality" protein foods can definitely provide meals of the same nutritional value as those based on "high-quality" animal protein sources. Whatever the dietary source, approximately 70 to 100 grams of protein per day is recommended for an average diet (Shealy, 1977). Thus, it is quite possible, whatever one's philosophy or life-style, to plan a nutritionally complete diet.

Returning to the McGovern Committee Report, several items of both the goals and the implementation strategies address the issues of carbohydrate and sugar consumption. Carbohydrates are a large class of substances derived from primary alcohols with the most important carbohydrates being starches, sugars, celluloses, and gums (Agnew et al., 1965). Carbohydrate foods are available in forms ranging from totally unprocessed or raw forms, as in an apple, to highly processed and refined as in a teaspoon of sugar. In the body, these substances are all reduced to simple sugars before being absorbed into the blood. From the circulatory system, they are utilized by the cells for energy or stored in the liver and muscles as glycogen for future utilization. If the body depletes this store of glycogen, then fat reserves are used for energy. Carbohydrates are essential for adequate nutrition but it is increasingly evident that most individuals consume an excessive proportion of their carbohydrates in refined forms. Even a moderate consumption of fats is essential to proper nutrition since they are the richest source of energy in the diet, yielding twice as many energy units as either carbohydrates or proteins. Nutritionists are concerned about the overconsumption of these foodstuffs, particularly highly refined carbohydrates, and the negative consequences of this behavior. According to John H. Knowles, "The removal of dietary fiber and a high intake of refined carbohydrates typical of diets in developed countries such as the United States result in a slowed transit time of food through the intestines. This is thought to facilitate the development of cancer, along with such diseases as diverticulitis, appendicitis, and even hemorrhoids . . ." (1976). Highly refined or processed carbohydrate foodstuffs contribute virtually nothing more than simple sugars and have been labeled "empty calories" (Cheraskin, Ringsdorf & Brecher, 1976). Not only do these "empty calories" not provide nutrients, they also displace other, essential foodstuffs.

Among the common sources of these excessively refined carbohydrates are precooked breakfast cereals, white-flour products such as both sweetened and unsweetened baked goods, white rice, and all highly sweetened foods such as desserts, soft drinks, and candy. Most devastating to human nutrition is white table sugar, which is estimated to contribute from twenty to fifty percent of all the calories consumed in an average diet. Until 125 years ago, sugar was virtually unused in foods. Today its consumption occupies a minimum average of twenty percent when it should make up five percent or less of one's total intake of calories. Frequently there are "hidden sugars" in foods such as mustard, canned vegetables, and innumerable other sources. Unquestionably, refined sugar is detrimental to human nutrition. Among the demonstrable effects of consuming excessive quantities of white sugar are: (1) increased incidence of atherosclerosis (Agradi et al., 1974); (2) elevated levels of cholesterol, triglycerides, and phospholids in plasma (Naismith, Stock & Yudkin, 1974); (3) suppression of immune system activity by decreasing the phagocytic capacity of neutrophils in humans (Sanchez et al., 1973); and numerous other negative effects. These have been popularly compiled in *Sugar Blues,* by William Dufty (1975). Another major source of refined carbohydrates and sugars is alcoholic beverages. Physicians frequently observe that people who abuse alcohol show signs of malnutrition, but there are also suggestions that improper diet can itself induce an alcohol craving. Investigators have induced a craving for alcohol in rats by feeding them a diet high in refined carbohydrates, low in vitamins, minerals, and proteins (Geller, 1971). Much has been written about alcoholism's effects on the body, ranging from the carcinogenic properties of alcohol to its role in causing birth defects. For this discussion, however, it is sufficient to point out that alcoholism and diet constitute a reciprocal problem and that alcohol per se is another major source of empty calories. Recently, a group of researchers from the School of Medicine at the University of Toronto reported in *Science* that chronic alcoholics who abstained from alcohol consumption for an average of five months demonstrated "functional improvement" and "partially reversible cerebral atrophy" (Carlen et al., 1978), or an ability to recover from minimal brain damage.

Rectifying the overconsumption of refined carbohydrates could lead to an increased intake of roughage and bulk in the diet through consumption of such foods as whole grains, fruits, coarse vegetables, and the excellent source, bran. Foods such as these contain indigestible fibers and other materials which aid in digestion and elimination. They lend bulk to the intestinal contents and promote the normal excretion of liver bile and the movement of waste products through the intestinal tract. An excellent overview of the research demonstrating that an increase in the roughage content of an individual's diet can be useful in preventing coronary and diverticular disease, colon cancer, and gallstones can be found in *Medical World News* (1974). From that report the researchers concluded:

> Seeking reasons for the increases in these diseases, a number of investigators have related them to a radical change in the intake of dietary fiber by the population dating from about 1850. In the past 100 years there has been a reduced con-

sumption of fiber by the general population caused by a decrease in wheat flour consumption, a more highly refined mill-
ing of flour which today has reduced the fiber content of
white bread to virtually nil, a reduction in potato consumption, and a replacement of wholemeal cereals—such as the
oatmeal porridge—with ready-made breakfast cereals that are
not only depleted of fiber but moreover are coated with sugar
(*Medical World News,* 1974, p. 37).

While many individuals are able to reduce refined sugar intake, there
is a tendency to seek out sugar substitutes and artificial sweeteners
such as saccharin. Yet there is clear evidence from both animal and
human research by two groups of Canadian researchers that saccharin causes bladder cancer (Howe, Burch & Miller, 1977). One researcher, Bernard L. Cohen of the University of Pittsburgh, has even
compared the risk of a person getting cancer from ingesting saccharin with the risk of excess body weight from ingesting sugar calories.
From his calculations, Cohen reported in *Science* that "if ingesting
a diet drink inhibits ingestion of more than one kilocalorie, its benefits exceed its risks" (1978). While some individuals may find solace
in this and others await the discovery of safer artificial sweeteners
such as the new flavonoid derivatives of citrus fruit peels, the important question is why so many individuals crave excessively sweetened
foods. One of the best sugar substitutes is honey, which is preferable
to sugar although it should also be used in moderation. Honey has a
high content of levulose, which breaks down relatively slowly during
metabolism and does not overload the pancreas as do the other
sugars. Raw honey also contains traces of essential nutrients. Rather
than seeking artificial sweeteners, it is far more beneficial that individuals learn to appreciate the diversity of tastes characteristic of
unrefined foods.

Finally, an aspect of diet not addressed in the McGovern Report
is the excessive consumption of caffeine by most individuals. Research conducted at the University of Michigan by psychiatrist John
F. Greden and his colleagues determined, from administering a wide
range of tests to 100 volunteers, that a serious "caffeinism" does exist.
Individuals who consumed 750 milligrams of caffeine daily, heavy
consumers, were compared to light consumers and were found to be
"much more frequently: female; inactive in religion; less educated;
smokers; alcoholics; and depressed" (Greden et al., 1977). Caffeine at
the 750-milligram level from sources such as coffee, cola, tea, over-
the-counter medications, cocoa, and others is the equivalent of eight

to ten cups of coffee per day. The most intriguing finding in the study was that "78 percent of the heaviest caffeine consumers were depressed on the Beck [depression] Scale but had never been treated with antidepressants. One third of those depressed high-caffeine consumers observed, however, that coffee or tea made them feel *less* depressed." From these findings it is evident that individuals might use caffeine as self-medication for depression, with the unfortunate side effects of an overdose being irritability, dizziness, frequent urination, and free-floating anxiety. Greden and his colleagues suggest that these symptoms constitute an important clinical phenomenon calling for diagnosis and treatment since "clinically significant caffeinism may exist among a large number of individuals with psychiatric problems." Related research has indicated serious consequences for the infants of mothers who use caffeine, nicotine, and alcohol during pregnancy. According to the prospective study of psychologist Ann P. Streissguth and her colleagues, each of these factors was found to decrease overall activity and muscle tone in the offspring of 1,529 pregnant women. When statistical adjustments were made for the effects of caffeine and alcohol, the caffeine use level was found to be more significant. However, Streissguth points out, "We still have much more information to analyze before the true impact on the baby's health can be determined. At this time, no permanent impact on the child's health can be inferred" (Streissguth et al., 1977). This is a welcome note of caution, since it means that at this time caffeine need not be zealously purged from an individual's diet. However, it is also important to recognize that caffeine is a potent stimulant and needs to be used accordingly. As with virtually all aspects of diet, well-informed moderation is preferable to any extreme practice.

Third among the major considerations in planning an optimum diet is the necessity of adapting these general principles to the requirements of a given individual. This issue, perhaps the most formidable task for a science of nutrition, has yet to be adequately resolved. One promising area of research involves computer assessment techniques similar to those cited in the stress reactivity research of the previous chapter. Perhaps the greatest paradox of the movement toward holistic medicine is that high-technology devices such as computers and the biomedical instrumentation of biofeedback are among the most potent tools of transformation. Sophisticated computer assessments makes it possible to consider a complex array of variables to help determine how they relate to a particular individual. According to a recent overview of the field of computer assessment, Harold M. Schoelmar and Lionel M. Bernstein noted in *Science* that "the rapid growth of biomedical information has created an available body of knowledge (facts, concepts, and their interrelationships) far greater than any individual can assimilate. . . . Computers, with their massive information handling capabilities, are looked to as potential expanders of the physician's information and knowledge resources" (1978). This approach to health care has been simplified for the lay person by two physicians, Donald M. Vickery and James F. Fries, in an excellent book, *Take Care of Yourself: A Consumer's Guide to Medical Care* (1977), containing computerlike charts for the diagnosis and treatment of the most common medical problems from common sprain to arthritis.

One of the most common and well-founded criticisms of dietary information is similar to the objections made to the Holmes and Rahe SRE Scale, regarding stress assessment. Research psychiatrists such as Mardi Horowitz of the University of California School of Medicine in San Francisco point out that assessment methods such as the SRE Scale do not adequately account for an "individual's unique response to life events" (1977) and that any consideration of individual applications needs to be based upon the consideration of multiple factors. This is particularly true of nutrition, and computer assessment methods promise to meet this criterion. A fundamental change underlying the scientific base of holistic medicine as discussed in Chapter II is a redefinition of the relationship between man and machine. What used to be an adversary relationship has evolved into a synergistic collaboration through the recognition and respect of the unique capabilities of each. Computer assessment and clinical biofeedback represent the interface of individuals and instrumentation in a humanistic technology.

In nutrition, the unique contribution of computer assessment techniques is the ability to take the first step in alteration of diet, and that is to assess the individual's initial state. Both the nutritional counselor and the individual patient need to know where they are beginning before they can determine where they wish to go. Numerous computer profile programs are available which use the basic method of an individual listing his or her quantitative intake of various foodstuffs, from which the computer generates a profile of the essential nutrients available in that diet. Unfortunately, most of these methods consider diet in a vacuum, neglecting to account even minimally for contributing factors of life-style, stress, and exercise. The most comprehensive of these attempts is the "Nutrition, Health and Activity Profile" of Pacific Research Systems in Los Angeles. (See Appendix A.) This approach is based upon the method described above but is broader: "This computerized profile will determine your dietary intake of proteins, carbohydrates, fats, vitamins, minerals, fibers, calories, etc., compare them to established requirements, and discuss their meaning and interpretation for your particular case. In fact, each major area of lifestyle critical to health and longevity will be contrasted with essential requirements for a healthier and longer life. Suggestions will be made for supplemental reading, where necessary, to further clarify important points. For those concerned with losing weight, a safe and sane approach will be discussed for losing extra pounds sensibly and keeping them off permanently. These recommendations can be carefully reviewed by your doctor and modified, as necessary, to suit your lifestyle" (Pacific Research Systems, 1979). That last sentence is a most important acknowledgment too often overlooked in clinical nutrition. Even computer programs cannot yet account for factors of individual sensitivity in keeping with Williams's concept of biochemical individuality and Horowitz's concept of individual adaptation to stress. According to Robert J. Marshall, President of Pacific Research Systems, both laymen and nutritional counselors can "access" the Profile program (which is the computer term meaning "have use of the stored data") for approximately ten dollars. Also, doctors of medicine, psychology, or related areas can obtain a special packet of information by requesting one on their letterhead stationery. Bear in mind that this profile is not cited as definitive in any sense. It is used here as an illustration of a first step toward the development of an individually based, objective, low-cost, computer-assisted method of assessing dietary factors in interaction with multiple other factors contributing to optimum health.

From this basic information, a twelve-page computer printout displays the essential nutrients ingested, compares those levels to standards adjusted to the individual's characteristics, and offers clear suggestions for implementing the indicated changes to "avoid disease and to attain your best possible health" (Pacific Research Systems, 1979). A sample printout is given in Appendix A of this book. Overall, the printout is an invaluable source of information for the individual planning an appropriate diet and, equally important, it contains extensive references to books and articles for individuals to educate themselves further. Included in the printout are sections which consider environment, any recent medical findings, and the highly significant variable of exercise. Appropriate cautions are given, for instance, to consult a physician before dietary changes are initiated in the presence of a disorder such as ulcers. The program is "designed to be educational, to point out risk factors, to teach good health habits and nutrition and is not meant to detect medical disorders or diseases" (Pacific Research Systems, 1979). In this regard, the *Nutrition, Health and Activity Profile* is compatible with the *Health Hazard Appraisal* and the *Schedule of Recent Experience* and can be used in conjunction with these latter to obtain a comprehensive overview of an individual's health status.

Of course, there are shortcomings of any system of dietary analysis in that "the recommendations" may include suggestions which a particular patient may need to adjust, such as the sources of protein in a given diet. Certain fine distinctions are not made. For example, the *Nutrition Profile* and the *Health Hazard Appraisal* are both inordinately sensitive to alcohol consumption and tend to lump together wine and hard alcohol. Recent evidence indicates that an average daily consumption of four ounces of wine, especially red wine, is beneficial for "lassitude" and "sleeplessness." Another study indicates that wine, as well as grape juice, appears to be a potent "antiviral agent" which can inactivate such viruses as "polio, herpes simplex, and various enteric viruses (which cause gastrointestinal disorders)" (Kowalchuk & Speirs, 1977). Related to these findings are data presented by Tavia Gordon and his colleagues of the National Heart and Blood Institute, who initiated a study to determine the effect of moderate alcohol consumption on serum cholesterol, triglyceride, and lipoprotein levels in the blood. From their research reported in *Lancet,* they found that moderate alcohol consumption was associated with high levels of high-density lipoproteins (HDL), which have been linked with a resistance to heart disease, and a low level of the low-density lipoproteins (LDL) thought to induce cardiovascular disease (1977). Of course, no one is suggesting that alcohol is a preventative for any disorder, for alcohol carries its own medical and psychosocial risks and such research is highly speculative. Complicated issues such as these simply underscore the need to individualize any dietary assessment and subsequent change needs to be formulated cooperatively by the individual patient and an experienced dietary counselor who is aware of recent research findings.

Related to these computer assessment programs is the evolution of low-cost, comprehensive hematological analysis. From a blood sample it is possible to detect minute levels of at least fourteen blood variables known to be early precursors of potentially severe disorders. At the present time this research is in its preliminary stages with research designed to establish standardization levels taking place under the direction of George Williams of the Institute of Health Research in San Francisco (Williams, 1970, 1977). Developments such as these have the disadvantage of being invasive, i.e., requiring blood specimens, but future research may result in a mutually enriching protocol of dietary and hematological assessment. It is possible to use these scientific data in conjunction with life-style variables to derive a reasonable program of nutrition-based therapeutics. Nutritional factors do not and cannot replace traditional medical and psychological interventions but do constitute an invaluable addition.

The fourth and last variable in an effective dietary program for optimum health is how and how well it is implemented. None of the information in the chapters of this book is of any use simply as theoretical fodder, for the real impact resides in implementation, not in intellectualization. Responsibility for implementation of any system of holistic medicine resides with each individual working in conjunction with health-care professionals. This need not be pursued with dour determination. Some very clear guidelines are offered by Roger J. Williams, who notes:

> When selecting from the large number of wholesome foods, we should consider these factors: (1) *foods chosen should be liked;* (2) *their cost should not be prohibitive;* and (3) *they should be readily and agreeably accepted by our bodies.* If this principle were generally followed, human nutrition would be immeasurably improved (1977).

Given these basic guidelines, the ultimate determinants are those of life-style.

In 1978, two cardiologists, Sven Danner and Arend Dunning of the University of Amsterdam School of Medicine, decided to investigate the rise in incidence of ischemic heart disease, which has become the number one cause of death in Holland. They selected a group of 100 Dutch people who were in their nineties and obtained from them physicals and family histories, since this group evidenced a lower incidence of coronary disease than contemporary middle-aged Dutch adults. From their research, they determined that the elders generally were of lower socioeconomic class, tended to be unskilled laborers, only two percent smoked, and only ten percent were overweight. Of particular interest to the researchers were the detailed nutritional analyses of forty of the elderly people, which demonstrated "they tended to eat less than the Dutch population as a whole but had approximately the same relative contribution of protein, fat, and carbohydrate as their countrymen. Although their cholesterol consumption was low, their relative cholesterol intake—compared with findings of recent Dutch population studies—was high" (1978). As in previous studies, the high-density lipoprotein (HDL) level was in a rather high ratio to total cholesterol. In interpreting these results, the researchers emphasized that, while the genetic factor of parental longevity was clearly important, nutritional and life-style factors appeared to be the major determinants of the Dutch elders' health. One researcher in the study, Curtis G. Hames, remarked that these people had been "spared the hazards of affluent living" and this contributed significantly to their healthy old age.

Longevity and health is an intriguing subject which is considered in depth in the last chapter. At this point the emphasis is upon the fact that individuals consuming comparable diets will experience quite different states of health depending upon the context of their life-style. Many researchers have pointed out in surveying health determinants that an individual's immediate community or family is a key determinant of health practices, especially nutrition (Litman, 1974). Within that context, individuals must take responsibility.

Heightened awareness of nutrition can lead to individual change which in turn has profound implications for society as a whole. Aggregates of individuals practicing optimum health in the ancient tradition of *mens sana in corpore sano* will determine the nature of the health-care system of the twenty-first century.

VII

A Sound Mind
in a Sound Body

Physically the human body is essentially the same as it was over a half a million years ago in the evolution from Peking Man in Java and China and Australopithecus in South Africa. Individuals living in the post-industrial period of only the last 100 years, however, have placed this body in the midst of a radically reshaped internal and external environment. Over thousands of years the body was oriented to and sustained by habitual, varied, and extensive physical activity. Suddenly, with dramatic swiftness this functional pattern has been disrupted into one of high stress and low physical activity. Whether this jarring juxtaposition is viewed from the perspective of the evolution of the nervous system and its adaptation to stress (Simeons, 1960) or in terms of extreme dietary maladaptation (Williams, 1962) the most striking area of concern is that of exercise. Technological innovations have assumed an increasing amount of the heavy labor formerly performed by physical exertion. While these developments have been positive for the most part, a tendency has arisen for individuals to assume a too sedentary life-style. Stimulation of the body's tissues and internal organs received through regular physical labor has markedly diminished. "The human body is built for action, not for rest. This was a historic necessity: the struggle for survival demanded good physical condition" (Astrand, 1979). Today the struggle for survival involves the necessity of systematically reintro-

163

ducing physical exercise as a preventive measure for alleviating the afflictions of civilization, and as a step toward reaching optimum health.

Exercise is a complex subject, perhaps even more confusing than nutrition. Of necessity, this chapter will be relatively brief since the objective assessments of exercise benefits are highly limited; there are no effective assessment methods based upon questionnaires. More than any other variable in holistic medicine, exercise is to be implemented, not contemplated. Virtually everyone is aware that regular exercise is a major contributing factor to good health. Despite this pervasive acknowledgment, there is a dearth of research. As with nutrition, exercise is an area that has been abdicated by traditional medicine and, in this case, relegated to the quasi-superstitious rituals of professional athletic training. The research that is available, however, shows exercise to be a singularly important determinant of health. In 1977, Ralph Paffenbarger of the University of California at Berkeley presented to the American Heart Association a study of 17,000 male alumni of Howard University (Paffenbarger et al., 1977). Paffenbarger studied the exercise habits of these men, whose ages ranged between thirty-five and seventy-four, for over a decade and concluded, "The protective effect of being active seemed to hold regardless of whether the men had other serious risk factors such as cigarette smoking, high blood pressure, parental heart attacks, or a lack of college athletic experience" (Lang, 1978). From the outset it is important to recognize that exercise in the context of optimum health is not only a matter of attaining a certain level of physical development but also the elicitation of a certain state of consciousness within the participant. Optimum health is a total psychosomatic state of being.

More than any other variable in preventive medicine, exercise is contingent upon the active participation of the individual. It is simply impossible for an individual to "be jogged." Nutrition is more passive and people know they must eat but exercise is inherently active and is all too often viewed as a passable option. Time spent in exercise or play is considered frivolous or even a waste since it does not necessarily promote achievement, wealth, or employment advancement. At the other extreme, exercise can become compulsive or done for irrelevant reasons. Human bodies are sometimes trained to potentially injurious performance levels, as in professional athletics, or treated as objects to be narcissistically adorned in currently fashionable athletic clothing. It is far too easy for consumers to become engulfed by the exercise equipment industry's promotion of computerized bicycle exercisers and other exorbitantly expensive paraphernalia, offering the promise of health as the newest commodity in a consumption-fixated culture. Exercise has been and can be undertaken at virtually no cost, the sole requirement being the motivation of the individual. "Every man is a builder of a temple, called his body. . . . We are all sculptors and painters, and our material is our flesh and blood and bone" (Henry David Thoreau). Exercise more than any other aspect of holistic medicine requires responsibility and active involvement as well as reorientation of an individual's life-style.

According to sports physician Allan J. Ryan, "The physical qualities that normally must be improved beyond resting or basal activity levels to permit effective performance in a sport include strength, speed, endurance, cardio-respiratory function, agility, flexibility, co-ordination, balance, and reaction time" (1978). In addition to this array of physical factors involving neuromuscular integration there is the state of consciousness of the individual participant (Leonard, 1975). That all-important element will be discussed in detail later in this chapter. All of the above qualities of physical exercise are dependent to a greater or lesser extent on the development of strength, which is achieved by the progressive overloading of selected muscles ranging from the biceps to the heart and lungs. Muscles can be overloaded by progressively increasing resistance, the number of repetitions, the frequency of repetitions, or by increasing the time during which a muscle contraction can be maintained in an extended position. Virtually all exercise, from walking to Olga Korbut's 1972 Olympic gymnastics, is dependent upon the progressive strengthening of specific muscles, emphasizing the trophic response of the central nervous system as discussed in Chapter V. However, an equally important aspect of exercise is the trophotrophic, or relaxation, response that induces deep physiological relaxation analogous to that induced during periods of meditation (Doherty, 1964). On a purely physiological level this trophotrophic phase can be considered as one emphasizing flexibility. By contrast to the trophic activity of muscle strengthening, flexibility is improved by regular stretching exercises performed with slow rhythmic movements, as in hatha yoga with its emphasis upon both strengthening and lengthening muscles. Flexibility alone can be attained by stretching muscles and ligaments but maximum improvements are best obtained "in those who have developed strength symmetrically in agonist, antagonist, and stabilizing muscles" (Ryan, 1978). Exercise is a matter of both strength and relaxation, both endurance and balance.

Exercise is central to Marc Lalonde's implementations of the Canadian "Operation Lifestyle," in keeping with the goals of a *New Perspective on the Health of Canadians* (1977). In many ways it is far more difficult to discuss exercise than stress or nutrition since there are no paper and pencil assessments which can give individuals a sense of where they are beginning. With this limitation in mind, it is possible to specify general guidelines which can be adapted to each individual in a sequence of stages analogous to those established for nutrition. Generally, exercise physiologists recommend the following four considerations:

1. A preliminary screening of medical history and exercise goals within determined limits (i.e. "target pulse");

2. Physical fitness assessments in an exercise physiology laboratory or under other supervised conditions;

3. Planning and implementing an exercise program based upon the findings of these assessments and individual goals and exercise preferences;

4. Periodic reevaluation after the exercise program has been initiated.

Each of these stages requires careful consideration in order to establish a safe and reasonable exercise program. For many individuals, phases one and two may seem inordinately conservative or wholly unnecessary. That would be true if most individuals entering upon an exercise program were reasonably fit at the outset, but that is not a safe assumption. Most people know far more about the selection of an automobile or a refrigerator than an appropriate exercise. Particular caution needs to be emphasized for those patients with a familial or active history of cardiovascular disease. Over the past five years, there has been a marked increase in public participation in sports all over the world. Among the most evident examples in the United States is the upsurge of participation in various forms of running, from brisk walking to amateur marathon races of the traditional Olympic and Boston Marathons of 26 miles up to as high as 100 miles. While this increase has generally had positive results, the potential hazards are also evident in the increase in running-related injuries to knees, legs, ankles, and feet. A physical examination can help prevent these and many other negative side effects. Such a physical is not the same as "multiphasic health testing" or any other form of periodic health surveillance for adults. There is considerable doubt about the efficacy of these and even more doubt concerning their cost-effectiveness (Currier, 1977; Saward & Sorenson, 1978). Physical exams conducted for purposes of sports or exercise participation are "directed at uncovering any factors that might make effective performance in the selected sport impossible or dangerous. The examining physician should be familiar with all pertinent aspects of the sport in question in order to be able to make a correct judgment in the matter" (Ryan, 1978). The limited goal is to detect any medical disorders which might be aggravated rather than improved by a specific sport or exercise. The individual's personal choice of a recreational sport or exercise program is an important beginning and worth encouraging, but that choice should be made with adequate information at hand.

Closely related to the exercise-specific physical is a more specialized evaluation which can be conducted in an exercise physiology laboratory. Among the variety of assessments in such a laboratory, by far the most important one is "work capacity," which involves running on a treadmill or riding a bicycle ergometer. Work capacity, a key concept in exercise, includes two key measurements, "aerobic process" and "resting pulse." Other, less essential assessments include a body composition evaluation, for which the person is weighed under water. From the ratio of body weight to underwater weight, the amount of fat versus lean body weight can be determined and lung volume can be calculated. Another assessment, based on blood chemistry tests, evaluates serum cholesterol and triglyceride concentrations. Lastly, some laboratories offer a variety of muscle strength tests which allow the measurement of muscle forces in motion.

The two most important assessments are the aerobic and resting pulse determinations. Of foremost concern in any exercise program is the heart and these tests are designed to measure both the capacity and potential of that organ. The heart is a muscle capable of improving its condition in response to appropriate exercise at any age. "Appropriate exercise" is that which moderately elevates and sustains an elevated heart rate over a prolonged period of time. During a treadmill or ergometer session, maximum oxygen consumption (VO_2max) and the electrocardiogram (ECG) and blood pressure are constantly monitored. Treadmill evaluation is considered to be the best available measure of physical fitness and also identifies any ECG abnormalities which might affect participation in an exercise program. Results from treadmill and ergometer evaluations reflect those bodily processes which require oxygen and are termed "aerobic processes" (Cooper, 1976). During the initial phase of heavy work or exercise, the muscles utilize an "anaerobic," or "without oxygen," process. Energy yield occurs in the absence of oxygen by metabolism of the energy molecules termed adenosine triphosphate (ATP) and creatine phosphate plus small amounts of glycogen. However, the ability to exercise in this manner is very limited due to the rapid accumulation of toxic by-products including lactic acid. Anaerobic motor activity dominates the first phases of exertion but the longer-duration exercise calls forth aerobic processes. When an individual performs a maximum effort for approximately five minutes the circulatory system is taxed in its capacity to transport oxygen for the aerobic processes. By monitoring this performance with an ergometer and measuring the amount of oxygen consumed, a trained specialist can derive the load placed upon the heart and circulatory system. This figure represents maximal oxygen uptake or maximum aerobic power and the greater the figure, the greater the heart's ability to perform. Generally, maximum oxygen uptake and, indirectly, cardiac functions decline for both males and females from the values obtaining during their twenties. However, research by Per-Olaf Astrand indicates that "training can increase maximum oxygen uptake by 10 to 20 percent or more. . . . studies have proved that we, with regular training, can counteract (if not completely prevent!) the decline in maximum motor power which usually accompanies increasing age beyond 20" (1979). Given this potential for rejuvenation of the cardiovascular system, the assessments obtainable from exercise physiology laboratories can be of great benefit. Contained in Appendix B is a survey of some of the major exercise assessment laboratories in the United States.

Another less complex way of measuring the heart's sustained rate over time employs the pulse, which can serve as an invaluable gauge in planning a taxing but safe exercise program. There are two places to measure the pulse: at the wrist on the radial artery and under the angle of the jaw at the carotid artery. Using the first two fingers on either of these positions, an individual counts the number of pulses that are felt in ten seconds and then multiplies by six in order to get the average pulse rate per minute. To ensure an accurate reading of the basal level, all stimulants such as coffee or cigarettes should be avoided for several hours prior to the measurement. A pulse reading taken after a period of quiet relaxation is termed the "resting pulse," and it will usually decrease approximately six months after beginning a regular exercise program. Normal resting pulse levels range from

75 to 80 beats per minute for an adult woman and from 72 to 76 for an adult male. In most cases, a woman's resting pulse over 80 or a male's resting pulse over 76 indicates need for improved cardiovascular fitness.

Using pulse measurements as a guide, Canadian physician Kenneth H. Cooper has stated two basic principles of exercise,

> After four years of searching for it, I can lay down two basic principles. If your program is limited to 12–20 minutes a day of activity, the exercise must be vigorous enough to produce a sustained heart rate of 150 beats per minute or more. If the exercise is not vigorous enough to produce a sustained heart rate of 150 beats per minute, but is still demanding oxygen, the exercise must be continued longer than 20 minutes, the total period of time depending on the oxygen consumed (1975).

Another variant of using pulse rate to gauge exercise has been suggested by Lawrence Morehouse, who developed the fitness training programs for the Skylab astronauts. Later, in the popular book *Total Fitness in 30 Minutes a Week* (1975), Morehouse and Leonard Gross suggested the following guidelines for determining the exercise pulse rate that an individual can use as his or her "target pulse" to sustain during exercise by checking it for 10-second intervals. According to their guidelines: (1) If you are in poor condition, take 150, subtract your age, and divide by six to get your 10-second target pulse; (2) if you are in fair condition, take 170, subtract your age, and divide by 6; and (3) if you are in excellent condition, take 190, subtract your age, and divide by 6. By learning to read the pulse and then referring to these guidelines, an individual can test his or her exercise pulse at regular intervals and increase it to a safe level with no side effects such as angina, dizziness, or chest pains. In actual practice, the target heart rates for individuals in excellent condition, based upon a 72 BPM resting rate for men and 80 BPM for women, are approximately those noted in the table below. Exercise physiologists generally concur that the best exercise is one that elevates oxygen consumption and engages the heart in a heightened pulse level sustained over a period of time.

This hypothesis is the basis of the *Aerobics* series of books by Kenneth H. Cooper, which offer an excellent system of gauging, implementing, and monitoring a regular exercise program. Cooper's major contribution was to convert the often expensive ergometer analysis into concise and readily available "field testing" assessments

TARGET HEART RATES

AGE	RECOMMENDED	HEART DISEASE HISTORY (Not to exceed)
20	160	150
22	158	148
24	157	147
25	155	145
28	154	144
30	152	143
32	151	142
34	150	140
36	149	140
38	147	138
40	146	137
45	143	134
50	140	131
55	137	128
60	128	120
65+	120	113

If your resting pulse is more than 12 beats per minute slower (than 72 for men and 80 for women), determine your recommended training rate from this formula:

Your Recommended Rate = .62 × (Recommended Rate in table) + Your Resting Rate.

The value you compute from this formula should be somewhat less than the value in the table.

which prescribe the precise level of physical exercise that an individual can undertake for his or her age, sex, and "fitness category." According to Cooper, "Despite their simplicity and ease of administration these field tests are almost as accurate and reliable as laboratory measurements made on the treadmill" (1975). Aerobics is an excellent, scientifically based system for the development of a regular exercise program in virtually any sport. Since Cooper's is such a comprehensive approach, it is not possible to encapsulate it adequately here. Recommended are his four books, the original *Aerobics* (1975), followed by *The New Aerobics* (1976), then a program for women written by Cooper and his wife Mildred Cooper in *Aerobics for Women* (1977), and the most recent, *The Aerobics Way* (1978), which is oriented more toward the general public. Most significant in the latest update of aerobics are a detailed "Fitness Level and Coronary Risk Profile," developed by Cooper and quite similar to previously noted computer assessment profiles; specific recommendations on appropriate equipment such as jogging shoes; consideration of dietary factors; and examples of personal record-keeping forms for gauging safe progress.

Cooper distinguishes between a "conditioned beginner" and an "unconditioned beginner." A conditioned beginner is someone who has been exercising regularly at least three times per week for a minimum of six weeks and has been given the necessary medical clearance for his or her age. For the unconditioned beginner Cooper outlines a series of "starter" programs to undertake as a preliminary to an exercise program. The following sequence of entering an aerobics program is based upon the assessment of a conditioned beginner. There are two field tests in the initial assessment. They are the 12-minute test and the 1.5 mile test. In the 12-minute test, a person runs and walks as far as he or she comfortably can in twelve minutes. Then the distance is measured. The oxygen consumption over actual distance covered is closely correlated (correlation coefficient = .90) with the oxygen consumption recorded on a treadmill. As an example, if a man covers 1.25 to 1.49 miles in 12 minutes, his oxygen consumption level is 33.8 to 42.5 Ml/Kg/Min which is equivalent to the consumption recorded under laboratory treadmill conditions. Separate charts for men and women in five age categories—under 30, 30–39, 40–49, and over 50—are then consulted. The person looks under his or her age range for the distance covered and finds an assessment of physical condition based on performance. There are five "Fitness Categories" ranging from very poor, poor, fair, good, to excellent. At the end of this process, a man or woman has a fitness category starting point, based upon age, sex, and performance in the 12-minute test, from which to initiate an entire exercise program.

Cooper also devised a 1.5-mile test in order to evaluate the physical fitness of large groups of men, such as 15,000 members of the United States Air Force. Cooper's 1.5-mile test is based upon the time in which a man is required to run 1.5 miles, which is then related to his age and fitness category to determine the initial exercise program conditions. After this assessment, a person chooses an exercise he would like to engage in based upon his medical examination and consultation with an individual trained in implementing exercise programs. When starting the program, a person is given a week-by-week safe performance level for any given activity based upon his or her fitness category. Over the course of sixteen weeks a person gradually increases his performance level. To simplify the process even further, Cooper developed a point system whereby a person is advised to accumulate a 30-point-per-week program in a series of graduated steps. For an example, a person 30–39 years old engaging in a running exercise program who scored "good" or "excellent" in fitness can start by running 1.5 miles in 19:30 minutes, five times per week, to earn a total of 15 points per week. By the end of sixteen weeks, the performance level would increase to 1.5 miles in 12:25 minutes, two times per week, for a total of 34 points per week. Although the foregoing condensed summary may make aerobics seem complicated or even mechanistic, it does represent the best widely accessible approach to establishing a safe exercise program.

From the perspective of engaging aerobic processes and maximizing oxygen consumption, Kenneth H. Cooper has definite preferences for certain exercises. According to Cooper, "The best exercises are running, swimming, cycling, walking, stationary running, handball, basketball, and squash and in just about that order. Isometrics, weight lifting, and calisthenics, though good as far as they go, do not even make the list, despite the fact that most exercise books are *based* on one of these three, especially calisthenics. Participant sports, like golf, tennis, volleyball, and others fall somewhere in between, not as good as the first group, but definitely better than the second" (Cooper, 1976). Isometric or isotonic (equal tension) exercises such as weight lifting do not produce adequate movement or demand appreciable amounts of oxygen at a sustained level. Sports such as tennis and golf produce a widely varying pulse rate not usually sustained over time. Cooper strongly advocates a running program which, "without any equivocation, is the best. It's quick and it's sure—and it's inexpensive. . . . Swimming is a close second . . . cycling is a good match for running and swimming" (Cooper, 1976). It is very important to note that Cooper's intent is to provide an optimum exercise program for an average adult, not to train a competitive athlete.

In the realm of competitive athletics, there are extensive research efforts to derive the precisely suitable type of training for a specific sport. Among training approaches is an aerobic method emphasizing long, continuous sessions at moderate speeds, a second is continuous sessions in which slow pacing alternates with bursts of rapid pacing as in speedplay (Watt, Plotnicki & Buskirk, 1972), and a third is relatively short sessions of activity broken at regular intervals by rest periods and then repeated many times, as in the popular interval training. However, this is a complex area with highly specialized applications. For most individuals the goal is to find accessible and enjoyable activities which can become a regular exercise program.

Cooper applies his point system to each of the exercises he recommends in the following way:

1. Five points' worth of exercise done daily produces a good training effect.

2. Five points should be considered the daily average for a six-day week.

3. Any variation in the daily routine is permissible as long as the week averages out to 30 points. Five days at 6 points per day is best. Four days at 7½ points per day is a good "happy medium." Three days at 10 points per day is still of value but you're close to the borderline.

4. Any variation from the 30-point week will produce more or less training effect, depending on whether the variation is more or less than 30 points' worth. In other words, 30 points per week will maintain the training effect. More than 30 will increase it. Less than 30, and you start losing it (Cooper, 1976).

Although there is some disagreement regarding Cooper's exercise preferences, his conclusions are in keeping with the present limited data concerning the necessary work required to maintain the cardiovascular system in proper condition. Cooper's is not an overly complex solution given the unwieldly nature of the problem. His method is the primary basis for the *Fit Kit* (1979), devised by the Canadian Department of National Health and Welfare. Contained in the Kit is a 33 ¹/₃ RPM record which guides an individual through a home fitness test and helps to measure progress as the person follows a recommended physical activity program. Also included in the packet is a Progress Chart; a Fit-Tips exercise wall chart illustrating various stretching exercises; a Walk-Run Distance Calculator; an Rx for Phys-

ical Activity pamphlet; and a booklet by Per-Olaf Astrand entitled
"Health and Fitness." This entire packet of information is available
by sending a check for $5.95 made out to the Receiver General at
the Mail Order Section, Printing and Publishing, Department of
Supply and Services, Ottawa, Ontario, K1A 0S9, Canada. Overall, the
Fit Kit represents an excellent example of gauging overall exercise
principles and applying them to individual differences in preference
and life-style. *Fit Kit* is consistent with the Health Hazard Appraisal
Profile and together they represent a sensitive and pragmatic program for the improvement of individual health.

Exercise research has many gaps similar to those cited in the discussion of diet. There are no definitive, objective data as to how or
if exercise has a positive effect, particularly on the cardiovascular
system. To date, the most comprehensive research compendium
assessing the effects of exercise is the imposing *Textbook of Work
Physiology* (1970) by the two Scandinavian physicians Per-Olaf Astrand and Kaare Rodahl. Despite a systematic attempt to research
the issues, Astrand has concluded, "Research in this area is very
complicated and it may take over a hundred years or more of intensive studies to demonstrate with certainty that there is or is not a
connection between cardiovascular diseases and habitual inactivity.
The question is then critical whether we should wait so long for final
proof one way or the other. In my opinion there is so much indirect
evidence that regular physical activity, or training, has a beneficial
effect on the function of the heart that the opportunity must be
seized now actively to affect health in a positive way through a
systematic improvement in physical fitness by training" (1979). Despite the many unknowns, it is possible to enumerate several basic
principles underlying any exercise program. First, consistent with all
holistic health practices, there is the necessity of active, individual
participation. In concluding his first book, *Aerobics,* Kenneth H.
Cooper emphasized, "Ultimately, however, it comes down to an
individual decision, from the top executive to the average worker.
Just how do you plan to treat your body? How do you expect it to
service you, if you won't give it the minimum amount of attention
in terms of beneficial exercise?" (Cooper, 1976). Once this is recognized, the other basic principles begin to apply. Any individual
should progress slowly in a given exercise. Many individuals may
dangerously exceed their capacity if they become discouraged at less
than professional competence during early stages. There are always
signs if appropriate levels of exercise have been exceeded. A person
might experience dizziness, faintness, nausea, constriction or pain in

the chest, severe shortness of breath, or loss of muscle control. In such instances all exercise should stop immediately. Another useful sign is heart-rate recovery. This can be gauged by taking the pulse five minutes after exercise at which time it should have returned to a rate of 120 or below. If it has not, then the exercise is too strenuous. Heart-rate recovery can again be assessed ten minutes after exercise when the pulse should be below 100. A person's breathing recovery rate should be approximately ten minutes. If an individual is still short of breath after that time, the exercise level is excessive. Also, if a person feels fatigued after exercise, this is an indication that the exercise is too strenuous. Appropriate levels should be stimulating and invigorating. Even after a program is successfully initiated, according to research by physician Warren P. Lombard of Clark University dating as early as 1892, the "power curve" of muscular strength does not increase in a linear fashion after beginning a regular, strenuous exercise program. For a period of time, the unaccustomed workload causes fatigue to overcome the effects of exercise. As exercise continues for approximately one week, the "power curve" returns to the original level and "eventually the initial efforts are surpassed" (Lombard, 1892). Actually this "get worse–get better" syndrome is noted in intellectual as well as physical activity and is also a characteristic noted with patients in psychotherapy and in clinical biofeedback. When this phase is anticipated, it is possible to avoid the discouragement which might have the effect of making an individual discontinue a potentially beneficial exercise program.

Closely related to the necessity of progressing slowly is the need for a warm-up period of five to ten minutes. This is especially indicated for people over forty. Essentially, this involves stretching exercises with slow, rhythmic movements, such as those of calisthenics or yoga. As sports physician Allan J. Ryan points out, "There is less chance of injuring a muscle if it is thoroughly warmed up before stretching and is not called on for maximum contraction shortly after it has been fully stretched" (1978). In addition to the prophylactic benefit, the stretching exercises per se serve to increase flexibility and coordination and to strengthen muscles which may not be used in the aerobic phase of the exercise. Warm-up exercises range from simple stretches to elaborate systems such as that devised by Gustaf Laurel (1963), the National Coach of Sweden, a series of twenty-one stretching exercises preliminary to jogging.

Another essential aspect of any exercise program is regularity. As Kenneth H. Cooper has stated so unequivocally, "If you can't exercise regularly, you're better off not exercising at all" (1975). Regular exercise means at least four or five times per week. Exercising on weekends only or on a sporadic basis is potentially dangerous, especially for those over forty, because the cardiovascular system may not be strengthened sufficiently to withstand a vigorous workout. Research concerning cardiovascular physiology also indicates that "cardiac patients should avoid isometric exercises and also heavy work involving small muscle groups (like pushups, chinups). Such activities load the heart abnormally since the heart rate and arterial blood pressure become higher than in dynamic work with large muscles" (Astrand, 1979). The only exception to this principle of regularity is that exercise should be temporarily diminished or suspended if a person is ill, excessively fatigued, or in the presence of any of the previously noted contraindications. Otherwise, regularity of the exercise program is absolutely essential if any of the benefits are to be maintained. Both laboratory and training research have demonstrated that "improvements achieved by training can be maintained only by repetition, which must be an average frequency . . . of approximately three times weekly, preferably not consecutive days. Failure to maintain this frequency . . . results in a decay of the improvement to the original baseline for that quality" (Ryan, 1978). Finally there should be a cooling-down period after rigorous exercise. This it is as important as warming up. During exercise such as jogging, the blood initially tends to engorge the large leg muscles. As the exercise continues, the leg muscles contract and squeeze the blood back to the heart and the rest of the body. If the exercise is stopped suddenly and completely, the blood remains pooled in the legs and extremities but there is no contraction of the leg muscles to return the blood to the heart and brain. As a result, a person can experience dizziness, fainting, nausea, or even more serious consequences. All of this can be prevented by having a three- to five-minute cooling-down period between vigorous exercise and rest. Joggers, for example, should slow to a walk, and others should slow whatever exercise they are doing to a relaxed, easy pace before stopping. This prescription for safe exercise is strikingly parallel to the procedures of Autogenic Training, Jacobson's Progressive Relaxation, and the forms of yoga and meditation, all of which point out that the proper completion of the session is as important as its beginning. Aside from the physiological value, this final phase also serves an important psychological function by becoming a ritual of closure and completeness.

As has been stated earlier, an individual does not need to achieve a professional or even a competitive level of fitness to attain an optimum level of health. In fact, the intensive training characteristic of competitive sports may often be counterproductive or detrimental to sound health. As Astrand has noted, "As far as health is concerned, it is not the absolute amount and volume of training that is important but *the work in relation to the individual's capacity.* The severe, prolonged training of the top athlete adds no health benefits to those of a submaximal training program twice a week!" (1979). When the goal is physical fitness, it would be unfortunate to subject ourselves to the same overbearing sense of achievement, competitiveness, and mastery so characteristic of Western culture as a whole. The goal is rather to attain an active life-style which has these five basic exercise characteristics, according to physician Harold M. Bloomfield: "Enough stretching, twisting, reaching, and bending to maintain flexibility and elasticity; at least two hours of standing every day; a few minutes of moderate exercise that pushes your pulse rate up to 120 and thereby forces your circulatory system to maintain a reserve efficiency; exertion of moderate physical effort once or twice daily, thus maintaining your strength and energy; and enough daily physical activity to burn at least 300 calories" (1978).

As minimal as they are, the purely neurophysiological benefits of following such a program are quite extensive. From the research of Kenneth H. Cooper, Per-Olaf Astrand, Kaare Rodahl, and others, it is possible to formulate a list of the agreed-upon benefits of a regular exercise program.

1. Replacement of intramuscular fat (marbling by lean muscle), leading to more efficient utilization of calories. Most of our calories are burned by lean body mass (muscle); fat burns nothing (Harris & Hallbarer, 1973).

2. Strengthening of heart and lungs and muscles throughout the body, thus improving general circulation. This may have the added benefit of reducing blood pressure and usually slows the heart rate (Grimsby et al., 1966; Karvonen, 1959).

3. Improved absorption and utilization of food.

4. Increased energy and stamina (Baekeland, 1970).

5. More restful sleep (Passmore & Durnin, 1955).

6. Improved appearance; more positive self-image and outlook on life (Morgan et al., 1970).

7. People who exercise regularly consume far fewer drugs, coffee, tea, alcohol, tobacco, sugar, and refined carbohydrates than nonexercisers. They find these things to be antagonistic to a healthy life-style (Ismail & Trachtman, 1973).

This list could easily be longer. There is recent evidence that jogging might be therapeutic for anxiety and depression. Considering the pervasive incidence of depression and its marginal management by pharmaceuticals, this is an area of great potential. One clinician and researcher, Robert S. Brown of the University of Virginia School of Medicine in Charlottesville, has examined the psychological effects of physical training in over 2,000 normal or depressed subjects over the past five years. Most of the subjects were college students; some were his patients and all were evaluated using the Zung Self-Rating Depression Scale. His research indicated that depressed patients showed significant improvement in anxiety and depression after eight to ten weeks of noncompetitive jogging done three times per week. An even greater improvement occurred when the patients ran five times per week. Brown has theorized that the benefits derived from jogging are truly psychosomatic. From a psychological perspective, he believes depression is "in many cases an environmentally influenced condition secondary to a lifestyle of physical immobility. . . . confinement and physical inactivity have been used as punishment for thousands of years; it may be that some people have happened upon inactivity as a form of self-punishment" (Brown, 1978). Brown also theorizes that the antianxiety-antidepressant effect is biochemical as well as psychological. His observations are based upon the research of Julius Axelrod, the Nobel Laureate who identified the neurotransmitter norepinephrine, which suggests that a deficiency of norepinephrine can induce depression. Antidepressant medications do affect this neurotransmitter, and Brown believes that jogging might naturally enhance its production. The observed antidepressant action of jogging probably involved multiple factors such as "proprioceptive feedback from the musculoskeletal system to the brain, biogenic amine facilitation, enhanced cerebral blood flow, salt loss from sweating, and hyperthermia" (Brown, 1978). Research has also focused on variations in the depressed patient's level of the metabolite 3-methoxy 4-hydroxy phenylglycol, a sensitive indicator of central nervous system activity. Pursuing this research with Brown is Frederick K. Goodwin at the National Institute of Mental Health in Bethesda, Maryland.

In a related study, preliminary research by psychiatrist John H. Geist of the University of Wisconsin Medical School indicates that eight moderately depressed patients who ran for ten weeks showed as much improvement in depressive symptoms as sixteen other comparable patients in psychotherapy. Most noteworthy in Geist's approach is that patients were encouraged not to dwell on or discuss their depression while jogging. This is consistent with the clinical practice of stress-management therapies such as biofeedback in which the emphasis is upon developing positive health rather than analyzing existing pathology. Of course, Geist cautions that these results are highly preliminary and that care needs to be taken to avert the possibility that failure at jogging might actually aggravate the depression to a dangerous degree.

Over a period of four years Jungian psychiatrist Thaddeus Kostrubala has employed "running psychotherapy" with fifty-five patients for conditions including schizophrenia, depression, and anorexia nervosa. By his own account, Kostrubala was a fat, sedentary, San Diego psychiatrist who at age forty-two decided to get in shape by starting a running program. Two years later, he completed the demanding Honolulu Marathon. Based upon his personal experience with jogging Kostrubala wrote an excellent book entitled *The Joy of Running* (1976), which emphasized the use of "target pulse" and aerobic levels of jogging. For the therapy sessions, Kostrubala has his patients run three one-hour sessions per week with himself or one of his four running co-therapists. Then he follows each session with a group or individual psychotherapy session (Higdon, 1977, 1978a, 1978b). While this form of psychotherapy might never become very popular among sedentary therapists, Kostrubala reports a high degree of positive outcome. Even more striking in his approach is the holistic attitude of the practitioner who does not stand aloofly apart from the patient and prescribe a treatment which he himself is not practicing.

"You're highly exposed in this kind of therapy," Kostrubala points out. "My patients know as much about me as I do about them. We make a pact of mutual confidence at the outset of treatment" (Brown, 1978). It is clearly evident in the moving content of *The Joy of Running* that Kostrubala has grown and benefited greatly from experiencing and participating in his own therapy. His autobiographical account is a sensitive portrayal of himself and others moving toward optimum health in middle age. As he observes a man passing him in the Honolulu Marathon he notes, "He is fifty-seven years old and this is his first marathon. As he leaves me and disappears ahead,

I am very, very proud of him. God, what a man. Dripping sweat, being polite, driving himself, helping one. I cry for him, small, wet tears. Happy tears. Grateful." Whether or not such states can be objectively assessed is of no consequence. In moments such as these, individuals exhibit the highest state of health and consciousness toward which our species is eternally striving.

Viewing exercise from the purely neurophysiological perspective, it is evident that exercise is an example of deliberately induced stress which beneficially stimulates the central nervous system. Psychologically, exercise involves a voluntary, enlightened stress response of the Type-I variant discussed in Chapter V. That response is characterized by stress reactivity which is identifiable, resolvable, and of relatively brief duration. If such a response were monitored, it would provide an invaluable means of assessing individual stress reactivity as well as progress in exercise programs. It should also be noted that, even though the emphasis here is upon the individual, it is possible to use assessment methods which would be applicable in group settings including athletic, clinical, and corporate contexts. At the present time biochemical blood analyses are used with athletes in training to monitor levels of "urea nitrogen, lactic acid, and hemoglobin, and rapidly changing factors such as blood pH" (Ryan, 1978). Using computerized microanalysis of these and related variables, it would be possible to determine at a neurophysiological and biochemical level if the Type-I response is being elicited and if it is comparable to the biological adaptation response characteristic of both man and animals. If such a response were occurring it would be characterized by a transiently elevated neurophysiological response followed by a compensatory period of parasympathetic rebound, as discussed at length in *Mind as Healer, Mind as Slayer* (Pelletier, 1977). From a biochemical perspective, this form of stress should be accompanied by an increase in adrenal cortical activity consistent with the data presented in Chapter V of this book. Further indicators would be elevated levels of urinary 17-ketosteroid and uropepsin both before and during the exercise. Furthermore, the psychosomatic factors could be detected since it is likely that both the neurophysiological and biochemical profiles would elevate more during actual competition than during practice sessions. Psychological testing could be conducted prior to and following such a study, examining variables such as depression, anxiety, repression and denial to determine further psychosomatic interactions.

One early study of biochemical reactivity due to the stress of crew racing indicated that these parameters do vary as indicated, but the research has not been replicated and confirmed (Hill et al., 1956). One interesting finding of this early study was the correspondence between the biochemical findings and the psychological makeup of at least two persons. One of the crewmen was very different from the rest of the crew in his psychological tests where he gave only eight responses to the Rorschach, showed little freedom or spontaneity or imagination on the Thematic Apperception Test (TAT), indicating blocking and anxiety. Biochemical data parallel these traits and indicate that his 17-ketosteroids were the lowest of the group, his uropepsin was below normal, and during the race day, 17-OHCS level was the lowest. Another crewman gave forty-five responses to the Rorschach, but included only one color response, which is usually associated with reluctance to expressing personal feelings outwardly. He achieved the second highest increase in 17-OHCS on the time trial and race days, his uropepsin was the highest noted, and the 17-ketosteroid level was also the highest. His biochemical profile appeared to reflect his psychological makeup of being "calm on the outside while barking on the inside" (Hill et al., 1956). Further data from such studies would assist both researchers and laymen in assessing the psychosomatic effects of regular exercise.

Both the psychosomatic and the purely physiological benefits of exercise have applications in business settings. In 1973, David R. Koerner recognized that physical fitness programs could reap cardiovascular system gains, especially among individuals who have recovered from myocardial infarction. His concern was if those benefits be demonstrated in industry-based physical fitness programs. To inquire into this issue, Koerner examined the exercise program developed for executives of the Xerox Corporation. He compared employees enrolled in the program to unenrolled employees by having them undergo treadmill testing. Of the two groups, the exercise program executives were able to perform for longer time periods, had lower maximal and resting heart rate, took more time to achieve maximal heart rate, and took less time to return to a normal resting heart rate. All are indicators of a superior state of physical fitness. Overall, Koerner concluded, "The exercise regimens utilized here produced the desirable cardiovascular benefits which warrant the continuation and promotion of the fitness program" (1973). Research such as this could be enhanced by the addition of neurophysiological and biochemical data of the type suggested above. Most research regarding exercise has naturally focused upon the cardiovascular system and has gathered impressive results. It would also be possible to consider the effects upon the immunological and neuroendocrine system, with possible applications to the prevention of a wide range of psychosomatic disorders. In the words of the Fit-Kit of the Canadian Department of Health and Welfare, "Physical activity is nature's tranquilizer" (1979).

Before turning to the all-important factor of the internal experience of exercise, it is useful to consider the interaction between exercise and diet. Nutrition and diet do not exist in a vacuum but rather in the context of complex metabolic processes constantly occurring within the body. Apart from research by Astrand, there are very few data available concerning this important subject. From their limited research Astrand and his colleagues have noted, "A person with a sedentary occupation and little body movement during leisure needs 1,500–2,500 kcal a day depending on body size. . . . the appetite is often set for an energy supply *greater* than we need. . . . if a person takes in 50 kcal/day more than he needs, his annual surplus would be 18,000 kcal, corresponding to nearly 7 pounds of fat. This could lead to a seventy-pound weight increase in ten years" (1979). With most modern eating habits, an intake of approximately 2,000 kcal per day is necessary to supply the body's requirements for the essential nutrients. Many individuals not only choose a diet in excess of the above limits but also consume excess amounts of fats, refined carbohydrates, and sugar, as noted in the previous chapter. Since the contemporary diet tends to have a preponderance of foods low in vital substances, the risk of subtle malnutrition and psychosomatic disorders increases. To aggravate the problem further, the dietary habits that individuals establish between the ages of twenty-five and thirty tend to create a pattern difficult to modify in later life. Similar observations have been made by Kenneth H. Cooper who cited three pertinent studies. One study compared the diets of 150 pairs of Irish brothers of whom one had emigrated to the United States while the other remained in Ireland, where they ate larger amounts of food and higher fat diets. Despite this, their more active life-style resulted in the Ireland brother weighing less and having a much lower incidence of cardiovascular disease. Two studies of high-fat diets, one of the hunting-based Masai tribe of Africa and the other of Swiss dairy farmers, also indicated that untoward effects of high-consumption, high-fat diets are greatly mitigated by regular exercise. From these studies and others Cooper notes, ". . . activity that was forced on these three isolated groups was a major factor in their health and longevity and in breaking down these potentially troublesome fats and minimizing them as a health hazard" (1976).

Per-Olaf Astrand has described the practical implementation of a diet combined with regular exercise:

> In summary, increased physical activity during which neither intensity nor speed need to be high and a change from a diet rich in fat and sugar to one containing relatively more protein is the best regime for maintaining (or reducing down to) normal weight, which for most middle-aged or older people is what they weighed when they were about 20 years of age. It is a mistake to avoid carbohydrates (for instance in potatoes, bread or rice) completely, as muscles and nerve cells need carbohydrates in their metabolism. This is particularly important for anyone who is physically active (1979).

In sum, an individual can choose between being habitually inactive but often hungry, or being fairly active and eating larger quantities of food with greater diversity.

Periodic fasting is another subject of considerable debate since some athletes consider the practice to be beneficial in the course of training to induce relaxation. Recently, James B. Young and Lewis Landsberg of the Department of Medicine of the Harvard Medical School explored the effects of fasting as a therapeutic practice. Their research consisted of measuring norepinephrine levels in the hearts of laboratory rats during two days of fasting. Norepinephrine levels are mediated by the sympathetic branch of the central nervous system and are a sensitive indicator of stress. From their research, it is clear that fasting does lead to a temporary decrease in sympathetic activity as indicated by reduced norepinephrine levels in the heart. Their research contained clear indications that periodic fasting may induce relaxation. There were two other noteworthy findings: "(1) Since the sympathetic nervous system is important in the body's 'fight or flight' response to stress, individuals who are suffering from caloric deprivation may have an impairment in this survival response, especially as it pertains to cardiovascular reflexes. (2) Since hypertension probably involves the sympathetic nervous system, dietary factors may be important in the pathogenesis and treatment of some patients with high blood pressure" (Young & Landsberg, 1977). Research such as this indicates that both greatly enhanced and greatly diminished levels of food consumption interact significantly with physical activity to produce variations in central nervous system responses to stress. Regular physical activity in conjunction with choice of diet are the variables, and the volition of the individual is the pivotal point.

All too often exercise books and articles, including most of those cited in this chapter, are written as though the body were a machine devoid of consciousness. Yet the ultimate contribution of a regular exercise program to optimum health emerges not solely in the body but in the mind as well. Athletic competition in the Western world has tended to reinforce the concept of consciousness separate from its agent of action, the body. That dualistic perspective has created a quality of competition and conquest unique to Western sports, yet these are not necessarily inherent to any sport or exercise. Throughout all systems of meditation and relaxation-based therapies such as Autogenic Training and Progressive Relaxation there is the unequivocal message that mind and body are in inextricable interaction. Fortunately, there is an increased recognition of the role of exercise promoting a harmonious integration of body and mind (Roth, 1974). Among the innovating books that advocate such an orientation are Tim Gallwey's *The Inner Game of Tennis* (1976), Mike Spino's *Beyond Jogging* (1976), Ken Dychtwald's *Bodymind* (1977), and George Leonard's *The Ultimate Athlete* (1975). Each of these books addresses Western sports activity from an Eastern perspective; the process of participation and the wealth of inner experiences that accrue are the purpose of exercise, and the endpoint of victory is secondary. Winning is not abdicated; it remains an element of the exercise but the latter is not consumed by fevered competition. Actually, the attitude that is advocated during participation is one of "active passivity" or "detached involvement" as is so often paradoxically prescribed in meditation. Such an attitude was integral to the exercise described by Kostrubala: "Somehow in the running I find the way to let my natural body take over. 'It,' not me, begins to correct my excesses—'it' begins to demand quietness. I even find running at 5 A.M. a joy—dark and silent, even frightening. I am finding my soul in the middle of an insane asylum" (1976). Experiences such as these have been referred to as a "runner's high" by Mike Spino, and many other athletes also report peak experiences of a heightened consciousness strikingly parallel to those of adept meditators.

In exploring this realm, Esalen founder Michael Murphy has collected stories from athletes who have undergone such experiences. He found that athletes ranging from mountain climbers to long-distance runners have experienced sensations of detachment from their body or perceived a profound slowing down of time. Growing out of his book *Golf in the Kingdom* (1972), he collected these accounts and noted certain recurring patterns. Among these experiences were: "(1) extraordinary perception, as if the doors of perception were suddenly open; (2) extraordinary focus and concentration; (3) emptiness: a sense of nothingness or void; (4) de-autonomization: a breaking down of the perceptual constancies; (5) equality: a perception of oneness everywhere; (6) access to larger energies, insights, and behaviors; (7) communication with or perception of disembodied entities as reported by Charles Lindbergh during his historic flight and by Joshua Slocum, the first man to sail alone around the world; and (8) ecstacy, delight, supreme aesthetic enjoyment" (Murphy, 1976). As astounding as these observations are, they are thoroughly consistent with the vast research and anecdotal literature dealing with heightened states of consciousness (Pelletier & Garfield, 1976; Pelletier, 1978; Tart, 1975). All of these phenomena have been observed to occur following sustained physical exertion. They are noted here not as sensational experiences to be sought, but rather to point out that they need not be feared or denigrated. Since these phenomena are natural aspects of prolonged exercise, it is important to acknowledge them as such, since their occurrence could be disorienting or severely disturbing for the unprepared individual.

It is important to emphasize, however, that these are not experiences to be sought through sustained exercise or meditation, for that would radically violate the purpose of these practices. Recently, Harvard theologian Harvey Cox explored the upsurge of interest in such phenomena in his book *Turning East* (1978a). Commenting on our culture's renewed concern with human values, Cox also noted, "The other side of this turning movement is a pervasive gluttony, the obsessive need to acquire. Now, since we have almost all the things we want materially, we go to the acquisition of spiritual goodies: adding up groovy experiences, ecstatic experiences, wonderful teachers, all of that" (Cox, 1978b). Notwithstanding such justifiable cautions, involvement in physical exercise is an essential aspect of optimum health whose ultimate result may be a demonstration of humankind's highest potentials.

Related to the experience of heightened consciousness during prolonged exercise is the role of visualization in heightening athletic performance. Psychologist Richard M. Suinn of Colorado State University has trained Olympic athletes in a method he terms "visuomotor behavior rehearsal" (Suinn, 1976). His training proceeds in three steps, the first being relaxation through Jacobson's Progressive Relaxation. Second, the athletes practice visualization and imagery, which involves tactile, auditory, muscular, and emotional, as well as visual, imagery. Lastly, the athletes use their skills to practice a specific routine. Techniques similar to this have been noted by international champion skier Jean-Claude Killy, Grand Prix driver Jackie Stewart, and golf professional Jack Nicklaus (Lauck, 1978). Suinn cites the impressive records of the athletes he has trained as objective evidence of the value of this method and points out that athletes of the Soviet Union, Austria, and Great Britain employ similar techniques. These trials demonstrate the psychosomatic factors involved in eliciting states of optimum performance. During several experimental sessions Suinn recorded electromyographic activity from an Alpine skier as he rehearsed a downhill run. According to the record, "By the time he finished this psychological rehearsal of the downhill race his EMG recordings almost mirrored the course itself. There was even a final burst of muscle activity after he had passed the finish line, a mystery to me until I remembered how hard it is to come to a skidding stop after racing downhill at more than 40 miles an hour" (Suinn, 1976). Following Suinn's observations, Barbara Kolonay, a student at Hunter College in New York, applied these same methods in an experiment involving free throws with a basketball. For her experiment, Kolonay involved eight teams and conducted fifteen ten-minute sessions of free throws during the last half of the basketball season. According to her results, the two control teams dropped slightly in free throw percentages; the two using relaxation alone improved from 67.3 to 69.2 percent; the two using visual imagery only moved from 69 to 71.3 percent; however, the two groups using Suinn's technique of relaxation and visualization improved from 68.3 to 74.8 percent (Lauck, 1978).

Most recently, Arnold Schwarzenegger, five-time winner of the Mr. Universe competition, indicated that visualization was essential to his training. He also acknowledged that excessive, competitive physical training was physically destructive. During an interview Schwarzenegger stated, "When I train the biceps, I picture huge mountains, much bigger than the biceps can ever be—just these enormous things. You do something to the mind. . . . The mind is the limit. We know now that it's not the body. As long as the mind can envision the fact that you can do something, you can do it—as long as you really believe one hundred percent. It's all mind over matter" (1978). Schwarzenegger and many other successful athletes concur in lending to exercise the additional dimension of harmony of mind and body. While these concepts might seem too speculative for a discussion of health and exercise, it is important to point out that the

Eastern tradition behind such observations is much more ancient than that of Western sports. Zen Buddhism teaches that it is possible to act in a paradoxical state of controlled abandon wherein actions are free of anxiety and tension. For a few individuals, the experience of effortless endurance is a reality. A classic example of the attainment of that state is Eugen Herrigel's *Zen and the Art of Archery* (1953), which was widely read long before the "inner" dimensions of exercise became fashionable. Over the course of four years Herrigel practiced archery under a Zen master, the process involving the releasing of an arrow from the bow without a thought of the target. In all physical movement, labored concentration blocks relaxation and sheer enjoyment. This was the case with Herrigel who frequently experienced tension in shooting. When he finally challenged the Zen master, the words of his teacher contained a profound lesson.

> You only feel it because you haven't let go of yourself. It is all so simple. You can learn from an ordinary bamboo leaf what ought to happen. It bends lower and lower under the weight of the snow. Suddenly the snow slips to the ground without the leaf having stirred. Stay like that at the point of highest tension until the shot falls from you. So, indeed, it is: when the tension is fulfilled, the shot must fall, it must fall from the archer like snow from a bamboo leaf, before he even thinks of it (Herrigel, 1953).

In this state of harmony, acceptance, and a sense of profound detachment resides a glimpse of the ultimate exercise, to know thyself.

VIII

Longevity and Optimum Health

Sumerian legend proclaims that the god-king Larke lived to be 28,-800 years old. In the Bible are such lesser records of longevity as Methuselah who died at age 969, Noah who lived to be 950, and Abraham who was a virtual adolescent when he begat Sarah at the age of ninety and fathered Isaac at one hundred. Among more recent records is the unauthenticated report of an Englishman named Thomas Parr who was reputed to have died at the age of 152 and was buried in Westminster Abbey. From the post-mortem examination the English physician William Harvey concluded that Parr had died from the foul London air when he was brought from Shropshire County to be presented to Charles I (Favazza, 1977). Other unauthenticated claims include 145 years of age for Norway's Christian Drakenberg and 256 years for China's Li Ching-yun. Authenticated reports are even more remarkable. During the 1972 International Congress of Gerontology in the Soviet Union, Ramazan Alikishiyev, Master of Medicine and author of over sixty papers on gerontology, reported on several instances including the oldest man in Russia, Shirali Mislomov, 165 years, and the oldest woman, Ashura Omarova, 195 years (Novosti Press Agency, 1970). Alikishiyev also pointed out at that time that the oldest individuals whose ages could be authenticated were Said Musavi of Iran at 190 and a 203-year-old woman, Makarnajo, who still worked in her native Bolivia.

Throughout recorded history issues of immortality have been the central concern of virtually all major religions, and this concern extends into the present age with the renewed research interest focused upon centenarian communities. From the *Egyptian Book of the Dead* (Evans-Wentz, 1960) to Stanley Kubrick's epic film *2001: A Space Odyssey*, questions of death and immortality have intrigued humankind as much as the distant stars. Despite this pervasive concern, little progress has been made in understanding longevity until quite recently. At present there is a body of fascinating research into the biological limits of human life as well into the quality of health maintained during prolonged life. From this research, it appears that increasing the absolute lifespan beyond a certain point is unlikely at the present time but that it is clearly possible to extend life significantly beyond 100 years while maintaining a high quality of life. Perhaps even more intriguing than the quest for mere longevity is this very real possibility of vanquishing the afflictions of old age.

Authenticated instances of longevity demonstrate an untapped potential of the human species. There is extensive documentation from certain geographic regions of the planet of ethnic groups whose members uniformly live to a great age at optimum levels of health. Among these locales are the small kingdom of Hunza in northwestern Kashmir, the Vilcambaba in the Andes region of Ecuador, and the Abkhaz Republic lying between the Black Sea and the Caucasus Mountains in the Soviet Union (Leaf, 1977). Issues raised by such observations and research usually have been relegated to the status of idle curiosities but in fact they are among the most profound concerns of holistic medicine. Serious research into longevity pales before the crushing reality of dehumanizing nursing homes for the elderly, the inadequacies of gerontological medicine, and the marked increase of death immediately following retirement from employment. Holistic medicine replaces a focus upon pathology and life crisis with a vision of optimum health throughout extended life. The essential issues to be considered here are the lessons of research concerning long-lived people, aspects of the present medical care system which are in conflict with these lessons or prevent them from being implemented, and the effects upon aging of an optimum health orientation throughout life. Finally, this chapter will consider the implications of such an outlook upon the evolution of medicine.

It often comes as a surprise to Americans to learn that the United States ranks seventh in life expectancy, behind Sweden, Norway, Iceland, Denmark, Japan, and Canada. Men in Sweden have a life expectancy of 72 years as compared to 68.7 in the United States.

Women of Sweden live an average of 77.4 years as compared to 76.5 in this country. While the differences appear small, the fact that they represent years of life lends great significance.

Today it is certain, according to John Kurtzman and Phillip Gordon in *No More Dying,* that "we are without doubt—for good or bad —at the gate of a new era, when *Homo sapiens* will be medically transformed into *Homo longevus.* . . . If this is so, it demands an entirely new perception of life" (1976). A pervasive illusion of immortality seems to lie at the root of much of the self-destructive behavior evident in our culture's life-style. Statistics regarding increased mortality from the afflictions of civilization always seem to pertain to someone else; and even when the necessity of a positive life-style is recognized, it is relegated to a vanquishing tomorrow. Failure by individuals and institutions to exercise adequate health protection appears to be related to "living for the moment and maximizing profits with little evidence of concern for future health status. . . . there is also a sort of mystical belief (maybe even the illusion of immortality) that 'it won't happen to me' " (Saward & Sorenson, 1978). One of the few sobering realities that can shake a "fly now–pay later" orientation is a severe disorder such as cancer or a cardiovascular accident, which unequivocally demonstrates how precious life is. Once again we are back to the issue of individual motivation. It is possible for individuals to consciously choose a more optimal lifestyle, not out of the biological necessity of survival but out of the sheer enjoyment of living with intensity and involvement. "The concept of health also has highly subjective connotations, precisely because it is conditioned by the personal view of happiness. . . . Thus, medicine cannot by itself determine the quality of life. It can only help people to achieve the state of health that enables them to cultivate the art of life—but in their own way. This implies the ability to enjoy the fundamental satisfactions of the biological *joie de vivre"* (Dubos, 1976). Whereas the people of certain geographic regions live vigorously all their lives out of necessity, individuals in our culture must exercise a choice. For those who make that choice, and it is not an easy one, the life-styles of long-lived peoples in remote regions of the planet can serve as inspired examples.

Studies of centenarian populations bring the elements of stress management, nutrition, and exercise into sharp focus since they are the factors consistently cited as the basis of longevity and optimum health. Traditionally, research into longevity has concerned the processes responsible for the progressive decline in structure and function of the adult; the nature of the senile state as differentiated from other disease states; and the processes whereby progressive loss of structure and function become incompatible with continued life and lead to death. One of the outstanding researchers to study centenarian communities is Alexander Leaf of the Harvard Medical School. He has traveled the world to examine old people who are living in vigorous health, free from the infirmities and debility which plague so many of our elderly. Leaf sees in the study of centenarians the possibility of clues to the prevention of the main causes of premature death, heart disease, cancer, and stroke. Recently Leaf, as well as two other researchers, Richard B. Mazess of the University of Wisconsin and Sylvia H. Forman of the University of Massachusetts, have considerably lowered their estimates of the actual ages of the individuals studied in the Vilcambaba community. Systematic study of civil and church records indicated that ages were overestimated. Many Vilcambabians assume the identical names of their parents and "village elders gain esteem by exaggerating their age" (*Paradise Lost,* 1978; Leaf, 1979). While individuals of the Vilcambabian community are not as elderly as initially reported, they are still observed to be active into their late eighties and nineties. In any event, the primary concern in studying these individuals is not to establish a longevity goal or to add the "fountain of youth" to some achievements register. The main interest of studies is that individuals remain physically active and involved in the entire psychosocial matrix of their culture far beyond the point considered possible in our present culture.

Alexander Leaf studied villagers of the Vilcambaba in Ecuador, of the Hunza in West Pakistan, and of the Georgian highlands in the Soviet Caucasus. While the quality of the environment is very high in each of these areas, the actual living circumstances are highly varied. Vilcambaba is mountainous with rugged terrain, Hunza is an arid valley surrounded by 20,000-feet mountains with the soil under heavy irrigation, while the Caucasus communities range from humid and subtropical to to extremes of summer heat and winter cold. Although the high-quality environment is important, it appears that the life-style the people lead in harmony with that environment is even more important. Six factors are consistently cited as contributing to longevity and optimum health. First are the obvious genetic influences. All who have studied longevity concur that the offspring of long-lived parents also tend to live long. However, although this is undoubtedly a major contributor to longevity, it may not be the most significant. One of the foremost students of genetics and longevity who has made this observation is Irving S. Wright, Chairman of the New York Academy of Medicine's Section on Geriatric Medicine. From his wide-ranging research comes a means of assessing a person's "heredity longevity potential" based upon familial history. Wright believes that this should be included in any assessment of risk factors, such as in the Health Hazard Appraisal, since "unless the hereditary longevity potential is included the most important item will be missing" (1978). At the same time, he clearly recognizes the significance of life-style factors and has drawn the conclusion, "Nevertheless, the risk factors which we have discussed above, tobacco, obesity, untreated hypertension, hyperlipidemia, and excessive stress should be controlled if we wish to achieve our personal heredity longevity potential" (1978). Furthermore, for those of us who are already born, to be overly concerned about our genetic endowment is quite academic.

The second factor that contributes to longevity and continued health is nutrition. In all three of the above communities the inhabitants adhere to daily diets of about 1,700–1,900 calories, compared to 3,300 for the average American diet. Intake of animal protein and fats is low, comprising only 1.5 percent of the total diet. Vegetables, rough grains, low-fat cheese, whole-grain breads, and buttermilk are the staples. According to the research of S. Magsood Ali, a Pakistani nutritionist, the daily diet of the Hunza averages 1,923 calories; 50 grams are protein, 36 grams are fat, 354 grams are carbohydrate, while meat and dairy products account for only one percent of the total. Oil extracted from apricot seeds is used in cooking. Grains, leafy green vegetables, root vegetables, dried legumes, fresh milk and buttermilk, clarified butter and cheese, fresh and sun-dried apricots, mulberries, and grape wine comprise the usual diet. Many of the dietary practices and actual recipes of the Hunza have been adapted to ingredients readily available in the United States by Renee Taylor in *Hunza Health Secrets for Long Life and Happiness* (1964). Each of the communities had their own alcoholic drink with no evidence of alcoholism. The Vilcabambas imbibe a potent liquor made from sugar cane and the Abkhasian people drink two or three glasses of wine at each meal plus a moderate amount of vodka and brandy (Favazza, 1977). When members of the community were asked to what they attributed their long life, credit was most usually given to the local alcoholic beverage.

Low calorie consumption by these peoples is of special interest. As early as 1930, Clive M. McCay of Cornell University conducted classic studies indicating that the life expectancy of albino rats could be increased as much as forty percent by the restriction of caloric intake early in life. The most striking recent research to demonstrate this principle is the work of Paul E. Segall and his colleagues in the Department of Physiology and Anatomy at the University of California, Berkeley. His investigations have focused upon the involvement of specific neurotransmitters in the aging of the central nervous system (CNS), which affects the homeostatic functions of the entire organism. Maturation of the CNS and neuroendocrine system has been demonstrated to be drastically affected by various diets (Fernstrom & Wurtman, 1974; Kolata, 1976). Segall has found in a series of sophisticated experiments that "long-term feeding of rats with diets low in calories or deficient in tryptophan appears to increase the average and extreme lifespan and to delay the age of tumor onset, the age-related cessation of reproductive function, and the decline of homeostatic competence" (Segall et al., 1978). In another study, findings demonstrated that the "ability to reproduce" was present at 17–28 months of age in laboratory rats on the restricted diet, whereas "no controls over 17 months of age produced any offspring" (Segall & Timaras, 1976). Among the rats on a restricted caloric intake, the average lifespan was approximately 36.31 months while the control groups survived an average of 30.25 months. Also, the last rat of the experimental group lived to the astounding old age of 45.50 months while remaining in extremely good health (Segall, 1977). In accounting for these results, Segall has hypothesized that the controlled tryptophan deficiency in the restricted caloric diet is probably responsible for the delayed maturation and longevity. Tryptophan deficiency decreases the levels of the neurotransmitter serotonin for which tryptophan is the necessary precursor. These observations "suggest that diets deficient in tryptophan or restricted in calories can affect maturation and aging by interfering with CNS protein synthesis, or neurotransmitter metabolism, or both" (Segall & Timaras, 1976). There were some minor side effects of the calorie-restricted diet over a prolonged period of time but these were alleviated with supplements of endocrine hormones of the thyroid, adrenals, and gonads. Tryptophan and calorie restriction are thought to affect the hypothalamus, which induces an anterior pituitary deficiency which in turn affects neurotransmitter development resulting in a state of prolonged adolescence and healthy longevity. These regulatory mechanisms are virtually identical in laboratory animals and humans. An interesting note is that none of the diets of these centenarian communities meets the nutritional recommendations of the National Academy of Sciences, yet virtually none of the inhabitants have been found to be either malnourished or obese.

The third common factor found in studies of these communities is that the diets are all low in saturated fatty acids and cholesterol. Even in the Caucasus regions where the total fat intake is unusually high at forty to sixty grams, the local cheese is low in fat content. By contrast, the United States Department of Agriculture estimates the daily fat intake for Americans of all ages is 157 grams. According to Alexander Leaf, "The best-informed medical opinions today generally agree that the Americans' average daily intake of 3,300 calories, including substantial quantities of fat, is excessive and conducive neither to optimal health nor to longevity" (1973). In 1969, Miguel Salvador, one of Ecuador's leading cardiologists, received a grant from the government of Ecuador to research the village of Vilcambaba in the Loja Province. He wanted to confirm or refute the rumors that it was an "island of immunity" from cardiovascular disease. Not only were these people free of such disease, but he noted a marked absence of serious pathology of any kind among the 330 of the valley's 880 inhabitants who were examined. Furthermore, he confirmed the extraordinary longevity claims by noting that eleven percent of the natives were over seventy years old and one percent were in their hundreds. However, it is important to bear in mind that marked individual variability in tolerance to the quantity of fat and cholesterol in the diet makes it difficult to ascribe primary importance to this single factor. Another qualifying factor is that physical activity plays a pivotal role in mediating dietary factors.

Physical activity is the fourth and unequivocally the most important factor in the longevity and optimum health exhibited in these centenarian communities. Associated with it is the consistently very important fifth factor: active sexuality well into the hundreds. After extensive physical examinations of the people of the Caucasian village of Duripshi, Alexander Leaf concluded that physical activity was a potent preventive measure against cardiovascular disease such as myocardial infarction and atherosclerosis and other disorders such as osteoporosis. This latter condition, an increased porosity of the bones, is common among the elderly of the United States. When this condition is present, the calcium and salts which harden bones as well as the collagen and cartilage matrix for these components all begin to deteriorate and bones become thin, less dense, and fragile. Recent studies by the National Institutes of Health have found that astronauts experienced this condition under weightlessness since reduced stress on the skeletal system caused calcium and phosphate to pour out of the bones. Among the people of the centenarian communities, Leaf saw no evidence of osteoporosis and found the people to be consistently strong and active.

The value of physical activity is also confirmed by two classic studies in Great Britain and the U.S., cited by Leaf. J. N. Morris conducted studies which compared the incidence of heart attacks among postal workers in London who delivered mail versus those who had desk positions. From these data, Morris noted that only 51 of 171 postmen suffered myocardial infarctions while nearly half, or 70, of 143 office workers had heart attacks. Also, Morris conducted extensive post-mortem studies indicating that "men in physically active jobs have less coronary heart disease during middle age, what disease they have is less severe, and they develop it later than men in physically inactive jobs. The hearts of sedentary workers showed the pathology of the hearts of heavy workers ten to fifteen years older" (Leaf, 1977). The other study supporting the observation made among long-lived people was initiated by Curtis Harnes, an astute general physician in Evans County, Georgia. Harnes had observed a high incidence of coronary heart disease among his white male patients, but few cases of heart attacks among black male patients. A detailed survey of this observation was conducted by J. C. Cassel, who studied all adults over age forty and half of the males between the ages of fifteen and thirty-nine in Evans County between 1960 and 1962. From 1967 to 1968, ninety-one percent of this population was reexamined. Three groups were identified and it was clear that two groups of white sharecroppers and black men had less than half the incidence of coronary heart disease of the third group who were white nonfarmers. Most significant of the findings was that "analysis of the data revealed that it was the level of physical activity required by the blacks and white sharecroppers which largely protected these two groups from coronary artery disease. Most known risk factors were measured—namely blood pressure, serum cholesterol level, cigarette smoking, body weight, and diet—and could not account for the differences" (Leaf, 1977). These classic studies as well as others cited earlier make it clear that physical activity helps to burn excess calories and dispose of undigested fats, and appears to be a significant factor in preventing cardiovascular disease among centenarian people and other populations as well. Furthermore, exercise may well prove to be the most significant factor mediating nutrition and help to account for the great individual differences in tolerance for high-risk diets.

Among the centenarian communities, the evidence for the value of regular physical exercise is even more evident and confirms the research concerning the psychophysiological imperative of aerobic

activity. Of course, none of the dietary practices or exercise is deliberately planned, since it is a matter of biological survival from which
more modern cultures can learn a great deal. Leaf has drawn several
generalized conclusions regarding the role of exercise in optimum
health and longevity. The most beneficial pursuits are "repetitive
endurance exercises carried to the point of stressing the heart and
lungs mildly. Thus, long walks, jogging, slow swimming, bicycle riding, rowing are the kinds of exercises recommended. . . . Competitive, very strenuous exercises which place a sudden very large stress
on our hearts, on the other hand, may be harmful" (Leaf, 1977). From
his unique perspective, Leaf has underscored that the specific level
of exercise is the critical factor with respect to the heart and lungs
and that a competitive level or certain types of sport exercises may
even have "negative survival effects." All of these elements are identical to those recommended in Kenneth H. Cooper's aerobics and in
the fitness program of Per-Olaf Astrand—with the added dimension
of living proof gathered in the field. Research and field observation
clearly indicates that physical exercise increases the exercise tolerance and performance of individuals with coronary heart disease as
well as promoting a generally more efficient circulatory response.
Most important, demands on the heart muscle for any given level of
exercise decrease with physical fitness. This allows an increased level
of exercise decrease with physical fitness. This allows an increased
level of exertion before the supply of oxygen to the heart muscle
limits further activity.

   For the people of the long-lived regions of the world, regular
exercise derives largely from activities essential to survival: extensive
walking, climbing in rugged terrain, farming, and folk dancing. From
his research with these individuals, Leaf has established specific
beneficial effects of physical activity: (1) the physically trained person
has a slower heart rate at rest and experiences a lesser increase in
rate for a given level of exertion than an untrained individual. The
heart receives its nutrient blood supply during diastole, which is the
period of relaxation between contractions. Thus, a slower heart rate
allows a longer time for blood flow in the coronary arteries to supply
the heart muscle with oxygen and nutrients; (2) physical training
lowers blood pressure since exercise induces vasodilation of muscle
arteries. This means that circulating blood encounters less resistance
and less effort is required on the part of the heart. Among the elderly
people studied, continuous physical exertion contributed to a
marked absence of hypertension and cardiovascular disease; (3) exercise apparently increases the ability of the blood to dissolve clots.

According to the present thrombogenic theory of atherosclerosis, deposits of the protein fibrin adhere to the inner lining of diseased or injured arteries. Although the role of fibrin deposits in the development of atherosclerosis remains unclear, it is a regular constituent of atherosclerotic plaques. In light of his research, Leaf asserts that, "Exercise of a vigorous nature stimulates fibrinolytic activity—fibrin dissolving activity—and may in this manner also protect against the development of atherosclerosis" (1977); (4) exercise has a positive effect on the concentration of lipids in the blood. Leaf cites both basic research and the results of longitudinal studies in San Francisco, Albany, Hawaii, and Georgia in noting that "physical exercise increases the concentration of the protective high-density lipoproteins (HDL)" (1977), as was noted previously. There appears to be an inverse relationship between HDL levels and coronary heart disease in studies by C. J. Guleck of long-lived families, all of whom were found to have HDL levels at 75 mg/100 ml more than control groups. Summarizing his research concerning the relationship between exercise, optimum health, and longevity, Leaf states:

> In these, and possibly other ways, exercise seems to protect against the development of atheroslcerosis, that is, circumvent its delterious effects by increasing collateral circulation to an ischemic area of heart muscle, or actually promote the regression of the atheromatous process. . . . The beneficial effects of exercise on the development of coronary artery disease may even outweigh what are regarded as deleterious effects of diet (Leaf, 1977).

These observations are borne out among centenarian communities, where the people sustained a high level of vital organ function due to the conditioning effects of prolonged continuous exercise made necessary by farming rugged terrain and hillsides. For anyone, it is clear that exercise needs to be regular, frequent, and continued throughout life. Speed and strength are not of concern for endurance is the central factor.

Sexual activity is closely related to this last observation and comprises the fifth component noted by longevity researchers. Aging is generally associated with a gradual decrease in the number of cells in certain organs including the male testes. Cells that produce sperm are the first to be affected but later the cells producing testosterone may also diminish. For females the ovaries gradually cease functioning during the late forties or early fifties. Despite these tendencies,

sexual potency in the male and sexual interest in the female do
persist into advanced age. Sexual interest is even more evident in
females of advanced age than in males. According to the Kinsey
report, "There is little evidence of any aging in the sexual capacities
of the female until late in life" (1953). Later research has indicated
that "a longitudinal study of aged married couples in their sixties and
seventies [showed] that some women actually show an increase in
sexual interest and activity" (Fisher, 1973). Another demonstration
of continued sexual interest by both sexes is a report by Herman
Brotman of the Department of Health, Education, and Welfare that
each year "there are some 3,500 marriages among the twenty million
Americans over the age of sixty-five, and that sexual activity is cited
along with companionship as one reason for these late unions" (Leaf,
1973). Although there is no research concerning sexual activity in the
centenarian communities, it has been noted by several writers who
have visited these people. One person who has documented this fact
in both print and film is Gene Ayres, a Junior Fellow with the Metropolitan Applied Research Center of New York. Ayres studied the
Vilcambaba people primarily and reported that one Miguel Carpio
Mendieta was sexually active at 123 years of age. Ayres also pointed
out that the cardiologist Miguel Salvador observed that "in Vilcambaba there exist no stresses, including sexual hangups. Extramarital
children were the rule rather than the exception" (Ayres, 1973).
Other writers such as Grace Halsell, author of *Los Viejos—Secrets of
Long Life from the Sacred Valley* (1976), noted a clear sexual interest in one Vilcambaban male named Gabriel Brazo, aged 132. One
must take care not to overemphasize the factor of sexual activity
among centenarian people and certainly no direct causation has
been proved. Alexander Leaf puts the matter in perspective: "I returned from my three surveys convinced that a vigorous, active life
involving physical activity (sexual activity included) was possible for
at least 100 years and in some instances for even longer" (1973). All
too often, the small amount of information concerning long-lived
individuals is presented in a sensationalist manner or relegated to the
status of a curiosity and certainly their sexual attitudes and habits are
subject to such exploitation. Rather than seeing these magnificent
people as curiosities, it is more rewarding to look for the wisdom in
their life-styles, a living instance of optimum health. Whatever the
relationship between longevity and continued sexual activity, both
indicate a life of activity and fulfillment.

Actually this last observation points up the sixth and very important factor contributing to health and longevity, which is prolonged,

productive involvement in family and community affairs. Especially among the centenarians, as Alexander Leaf has noted, "It is characteristic of each of the areas I visited that the old people continue to be contributing, productive members of their society . . . people who no longer have a necessary role to play in the social and economic life of their society generally deteriorate rapidly" (1973). Among the Vilcambabans the elders are called "longevos" or "viejos," indicating persons who are either over 100 or soon to reach that age. Increased age is accompanied by increased social status, as in presiding over community councils. Meanwhile the elder remain active in the chores of farming and other natural labor. Retirement is unknown and daily hikes, swims, and horseback rides are common. None of the Vilcambabans live alone and unproductive idleness is unknown. Active participation and community involvement have been demonstrated to be of major significance in determining an elderly person's level of functioning in later years.

One innovative study, by physician Leslie S. Libow of the Mount Sinai Hospital Center in New York, was an eleven-year longitudinal study of twenty-seven "optimally healthy" men compared to twenty men of "average" health, with the mean age being seventy years old. His research sought to determine the interaction between medical, biologic, and behavioral factors in the aging, adaptation, and survival of these forty-seven individuals. In addition to finding the normal aging changes such as decreases in serum albumin, peak occipital EEG frequency, and cerebral metabolic utilization of glucose, this study confirmed the Framingham study indicating increased mortality with increased sytolic blood pressure. However, most significant in the findings was "the role of psychosocial factors in contributing to mortality, for example, the increased mortality related to environmental losses. . . . behavioral variables with the greatest accuracy in predicting mortality were the mental status test and organization and complexity of daily behavior" (Libow, 1974). Among the "optimally healthy elderly people" it was evident that "upward mobility and striving in midlife were related to better adaptation in late life . . . highly organized, purposeful, complex and variable daily behavior together with the absence of cigarette smoking were highly correlated with survival for these healthy elderly men" (Libow, 1974). Other studies have confirmed a high level of "life satisfaction" as a precondition of extended longevity "despite the usual declines of aging and approaching death" (Pamore & Cleveland, 1976; Bell, 1974). Research data also indicate that an active life-style allows "development, change and growth to continue through the later years of the lifespan in spite of the decrement of social, psychological and physiological functioning which typically accompanies the aging process" (Maddox & Douglass, 1974). Such observations are in direct opposition to the appalling practice of relegating elderly people to geriatric centers at an arbitrary retirement age. Only in a youth-fixated culture would the normal decrease in peak performance be viewed as pathological or as justification of enforced idleness and neglect of the elderly.

From the centenarian communities, it is evident that the elderly "viejos" remain active at a level of participation suited to their mental and physical abilities. Although they remain highly active, they also have the wisdom to recognize futile, stress-inducing striving and "have learned to accept things as they are, if they cannot change them" (Stanyan, 1976). When Alexander Leaf pressed 117-year-old Gabriel Chapnian of the Caucasus to say whether anything disturbed him, he responded cheerfully, "Oh, yes, there are a number of things that are not the way I would want them to be, but since I can't change them I don't worry about them" (1973). Perhaps that philosophy is at the heart of the prolonged optimum health and longevity sustained by these people. In 1969 Joshua Green, philanthropist and chairman of Seattle, Washington's People's National Bank, turned 100. Since he had been a friend of everyone from Rudyard Kipling to recent presidents of the United States, his birthday was a subject of national news coverage. From the enormous amount of mail he received, Green was prompted to formulate the seven great constants constituting the "syndrome of longevity" (Green, 1974). His philosophy consisted of a constant cheerfulness; good heredity; regular physical activity; maintaining good health especially in the "dangerous years" between fifty and seventy; self-imposed discipline such as no smoking; always working throughout life on something you enjoy; and high emotional stability. While there are individuals who violate all of these constants with impunity and also live beyond 100, these guidelines are in keeping with the observations of others. Throughout the research literature into the habits of centenarian people there are anecdotes and personal profiles that substantiate Green's philosophy. The objective data pale compared to the full spectrum of their lives. There are folk dancers, musicians at 142 who strum mandolins, their hands free of arthritis, eyes that are full of life and light, and mountain utopias farmed by people more than a hundred years old, in Alexander Leaf's *National Geographic* article, "Every Day Is a Gift when You Are Over 100." When all is researched about these people, an unknown magic will still remain. In the words of an old Abkhazian woman, "I can't explain it in scientific terms, but there just seems to be something special in the life here" (Strauss, 1973). That is most certainly true.

For people living outside of centenarian communities, the lifestyle of these long-lived individuals who remain disease-free until they die a peaceful death raises many important issues, many of which have implications for our present systems of health care. Alexander Leaf has noted that "if both arteriosclerosis and cancer could be prevented, it would be possible to extend man's life-span close to its as yet undetermined biological limit" (1973). In 1963 Robert Kohn calculated that if all diseases were eliminated the average lifespan would increase only to age ninety, given that other environmental and life-style conditions remain constant. Ninety years was also the figure mentioned by Alex Comfort, who noted that virtually the same proportion of people live to that age in populations dwelling under conditions ranging from the most primitive to the most developed. Given the longevity research which indicates that longer life is possible, it is necessary to delve further into both the biological and psychosomatic influences on aging, longevity, and death itself.

Biological limit is an imposing concept. Recent research has clearly indicated that there appears to be a genetically determined limit to life expectancy but that it is greatly in excess of the present average mortality ages for both men and women. Visions of immortality were given their first scientific impetus by the research of Nobel Laureate Alexis Carrell, who theorized that explants of embryo cells could be kept alive indefinitely. However, research by Leonard Hayflick, Professor of Medical Microbiology at Stanford University, indicated that such embryo fibroblasts do have a finite tissue culture lifespan. Variations ranged from eighteen passages, or divisions, for mice, twenty-eight for chickens, 100 passages for Galapagos turtles, and approximately fifty passages for humans. Under the best of conditions, normal human cells grown in laboratory culture plates do not divide indefinitely but eventually age and die (Hayflick, 1978). Human fibroblasts taken from four-month-old embryos replicated for those fifty passages but cells from mature adults over age twenty only survived for twenty passages. In accounting for this phenomenon, Hayflick has postulated that the deterioration may be genetic instability. Genetic "error theory" notes that when deoxyribonucleic acid (DNA) molecules replicate their genetic information there is a gradual blurring similar to copying one photography from another over many trials. Many of these errors are thought to be induced by environmental influences, and they are cumulative and inheritable.

Among the factors inducing these errors are certain to be the psychosomatic influences acting on a cellular level as noted in Chapters V and VII. The neuroendocrinological mechanisms behind these influences are detailed in Chapter 2 of *Mind as Healer, Mind as Slayer* (Pelletier, 1977). In a lengthy article in *Science*, Constance Holden gave an overview of the psychosomatic influences in cancer and noted, "Omitted from any of these studies is an attempt to identify mediating mechanisms—immunological or endocrinological —that might translate emotions into neoplasms" (1978). That same omission is evident in the biochemical research concerning cellular replication. Studies in centenarian communities clearly indicate that there are significant environmental, psychosomatic, and life-style variables which have a major influence upon longevity. The influence these variables have at a cellular level calls for extensive research. Under the reform model of medical research suggested in Chapter II, it would be not only possible but essential that these factors be considered, despite the fact that variables such as life satisfaction are not to be observed, even under a scanning electron microscope.

Attempts to rectify these errors in replication have led researchers to experiment with antioxidant chemicals such as butyl-hydroxytoluene (BHT), which is used by the food industry to preserve freshness. According to Armando R. Favazzo, Associate Editor of the professional journal *MD*, "Also under study is vitamin E, a natural antioxidant that has substantially increased the lifespan of fruit flies and roundworms as well as keeping human fibroblasts young and active until the 177th population doubling" (1977). An enormous variance in human tissue culture lifespan is evident in the fact that passages may range from 50 to 1,117 in the presence of the optimum nutrients noted in Chapter VI. Leonard Hayflick has also determined from his research that if all diseases were eliminated the average life expectancy would range somewhere between 96.5 and 100 years. Future research concerning aging and longevity will need to focus upon this cellular level to understand the factors which govern DNA replication.

Another aspect of such research is the theory of crosslinking, wherein molecules in aging organisms link together into dense knots and cease normal functioning. When these crosslinks form, they cannot be separated by the cell's normal repair process. Eventually they seem to interfere with the production of ribonucleic acid (RNA) by the DNA, resulting in impaired production of protein by the RNA and preventing the DNA from the proper cell division so that cells are not replaced. Collagen, the main protein of connective tissue, constitutes approximately thirty percent of all the protein in the human body and is adversely affected by crosslinking. From his research Alexander Leaf has hypothesized, "Such a stiffening of this important structural component of our bodies might underlie such classic features of aging as rigidity of blood vessels, resistance to blood flow, reduced delivery of blood through hardened arteries, and, as a final consequence, the loss of cells and of function" (1973). According to Hayflick, "Changes seen in the immune system and in the brain . . . may only be indirect effects of aging with the direct cause occurring at a more elementary level . . . fundamental triggers for age changes occur in individual cells that compose the brain, immune system, or perhaps some other system. . . . it seems that the root cause of age changes is contained within the genetic message of each cell. . . . the direct causes of death are most commonly seen as some form of vascular disease or cancer" (1978).

An immediate consequence of the error factor of genetic replication is its deleterious effects upon the immunological functions of the body. In addition to providing antibodies against bacteria and other foreign substances introduced into the body, the immunological system recognizes and destroys abnormal cells. Antibodies are protein molecules which kill or otherwise inactivate these foreign substances but their production is subject to error in a manner analogous to DNA replication errors. Leonard Hayflick has stated, "At least two important consequences of failures in the immune mechanism over time are possible. First, the immune system is less able to produce antibodies as we age; consequently, vulnerability to infections and cancer increases. Second, as we age the normal changes that occur in the chemistry of our cells may make the immune system recognize our own aging cells as foreign and produce antibodies against them" (1978). As a result, disturbances of the immune system coupled with the crosslinking of collagen could underlie the process recognized as aging.

Vital functions of the immunological system have been clearly demonstrated to be influenced by psychosomatic factors in both animal and human research (Solomon, 1969; Amkraut & Solomon, 1975; Stein, Schiavi & Camerino, 1976). New information on the effect of the hypothalamus on the immune system provides a possible link between specific emotions and specific biochemical events (Fox, 1976). To date, the evidence linking psychological and immunological states is sparse but very promising. Among the studies are findings such as: (1) levels of a certain adrenocortical hormone (17-hydroxy corticosteroid) were elevated in mothers of leukemic children (Mason, 1968); (2) high levels of corticosteroids lower immune functions, which are restored when corticosteroid antagonists are injected (Riley, 1975); and (3) functions of the T cells of the immune system were significantly depressed in twenty-six people, aged twenty to sixty-five, who were grieving over the loss of a spouse (Holden, 1978). Observations such as these suggest ways in which stress, emotional, and environmental factors influence longevity.

To consider any extension of the human lifespan or to undertake to change life-styles to extend the period of optimum health without planning for the impact of such measures would be irresponsible. One implication of such a reorientation would be the recognition that health is not a subspecialty of medicine. A revision in the role of the physician is anticipated by Franz J. Ingelfinger, the distinguished editor emeritus of the *New England Journal of Medicine:*

> The doctor should not be expected to play a major role in changing whatever lifestyle may be seriously detrimental. He has enough to do if he takes care of the crisis illnesses that do occur, and if he keeps up to date with the various scientific facts known about their nature and management. Hence, I would not consider the failure of the doctor to practice holistic medicine as substantive evidence of inferior medical practice (1978).

This acknowledgment is an affirmation that it is necessary to define both the applications and limitations of each segment of the present health care system. Most insidious among the range of attitudes expressed regarding holistic approaches is that they be subsumed under allopathic medicine as it is currently practiced. That would be a disaster, for a new approach is required when limits have been reached. Again, Ingelfinger articulates this necessity of acknowledging limits.

> Ironically, the present emphasis on eliminating 'bad' lifestyles and opting for the temperate life reflects the success of scientifically based medical practice in controlling acute illness and thus uncovering the importance of degenerative diseases and medicine's relative inability to do anything about them. . . . If the whole spectrum of medical care is included, ranging from a pat on the back to transplantation of the heart, it is doubtful that the benefit-harm ratio of personalized medical care has changed appreciably over the last 100 years (1978).

Diagnosis and treatment of pathology is clearly a medical concern, but the creation of a life-style conducive to optimum health and personal fulfillment is beyond the limited scope of pathology correction. Many prominent spokesmen such as Ernest Saward and Lewis Thomas have emphasized that the public needs to be better informed about "the limitations of medical care as well as its benefits" (Thomas, 1976) since "medicine is surely not in possession of special wisdom about how to live a life. . . ." (Thomas, 1977). In the absence of such public education the consequences will continue to be the "development of inappropriate expectations" (Saward & Sorenson, 1978). It is evident that the most effective means of disease prevention and improved health lie outside the medical care system and are related to reducing hazards in the environment, improving nutrition, exercising more frequently, and generally adopting appropriate personal practices.

Self-discipline and life-style change do not necessary mean austerity or puritanism. The active longevity evidenced in the centenarian communities indicates that an optimally healthy life-style is hardly one that is deprived in any manner. In fact, contrary to prevailing opinion, it appears that high achievers tend to live longer than others in the general population by thirty percent. This observation is based upon a twelve-year follow-up study of 6,239 men listed in the 1950–1951 edition of *Who's Who in America.* Compared with various other occupations, for instance, scientists had a twenty percent lower mortality rate (Quint & Cody, 1970). Individuals can lead highly productive lives while maintaining optimum health and extended longevity.

Patient education is the most powerful means available to achieve a system of holistic medicine based upon the maintenance of optimum health. By a margin of nearly two to one, a selected sample of 1,638 physicians responding to a nationwide survey by *Medical World News* concluded, "Medicine has already done all it can to reduce mortality and henceforth attention should shift to prevention" (1978). When these physicians were asked which single preventive program would promote health the most and therefore ought to receive top government priority, they uniformly put little faith in mass screening efforts while fifty-three percent favored "public education." This was four times the support won by any other preventive measure. As one general practitioner from Virginia responded, "The only effective way to reduce health care costs is for people to take better care of themselves." Many of the reasons for the relatively poor health status of millions of people in the United States lie in their adherence to self-destructive life-styles. These self-destructive habits are generally not the result of negative economic pressures. Among the more innovative inquiries is research by M. Harvey Brenner, a Johns Hopkins University sociologist. Much to his surprise, Brenner's research confirmed that positive events can be as precipitous to illness as negative occurrences. Brenner, one of the country's leading epidemiological authorities, examined economic change and determined that upward economic trends induce pathology. Analysis of the data based upon a five-year period between 1970 and 1975 "shows that rapid economic growth that follows directly on the heels of an economic downturn, has a deleterious effect . . . even though good things are happening" (Brenner, 1978). Aside from the impact of the economic pressures themselves, Brenner notes that the economy constantly interacts with positive and negative personal stresses such as marriage, moving to a new house, or a death in the family. By understanding such stresses and altering habits which aggravate them, the individual can prevent serious illness.

The responsibility of the health care professions lies in patient education. During an annual meeting of the Association of American Physicians, President Kurt J. Isselbacher noted that "we must learn to respond more humanely to patients' distress and break down the barriers that sophisticated instruments have erected between us and our patients. . . . the process must be one to demystify medical procedures so that the patient can assume some responsibility for his own management. . . . while in the past it was frowned upon for physicians to 'go public,' we need no longer be apologetic or defensive. 'Going public' is now a necessity—to inform, to educate, to guide and to help shape our own destinies" (1978). While the motivation for Kurt J. Isselbacher is humanitarian, the greatest impetus for medicine as a whole to undertake such objectives is likely to be economic. Many assessors of the current status of health care have consistently noted that the reason why there has not been a great deal of resistance or hostility between traditional and holistic approaches is that medical-care budget allocations have grown in proportion to demand. However, that period is ending rapidly. According to Ernest Saward, "Health planners now anticipate that at some time in the near future the resource allocation to health will be limited in its rate of expansion to that of the productivity of society in general. As this process occurs, the emphasis will shift from continuing to expand the share for health care to establishing limits to it and then to setting priorities within the resources available" (Saward & Sorenson, 1978). When that occurs, expansion of the right to health care to equality of care for all will be curtailed by judgmental decisions about how to best allocate finite resources. If this allocation can be wisely undertaken "without expecting that this goal can be achieved through investing in the medical care system" (Saward & Sorensen, 1978), then it can be possible to direct considerable economic and human energies toward the enhancement of optimum health.

After an extensive study of the health utilization patterns in six countries of Europe, F. L. Logan, who is Director of Medical Care Research at the University of Manchester in England, stated that it was clear to the research teams that psychosocial variables and patient education were key determinants of health status. "Despite the free and equal availability of resources, the use of medical services is influenced more by the personal factors in the patient, the general practitioner and the specialist at the point of translation of need into demand, and less by the clinical situation" (1963). The need for patient education was also underscored by the Stanford Heart Disease Prevention Program mentioned earlier in this book and in two others currently under way, the Multiple Risk Factor Intervention Trial (MRFIT) of the National Heart and Lung Institute and the North Karelia Project in Finland. Data from the Stanford program demonstrated that a community-focused multimedia campaign over a two-year period substantially improved knowledge of cardiovascular disease and reduced the incidence (Farquhar et al., 1977). Findings at the end of four and one-half years of the six-year study in North Karelia, where residents were determined to have the highest rate of coronary heart disease of any geographic area in the world, are also encouraging and impressive. Results indicate good cooperation and participation by the people and applications are already being planned nationwide in Finland. To date the data indicate:

A decline in cigarette smoking among middle-aged males (from 54 percent of the population smoking to 43 percent); an increase in the use of low-fat milk by from 17 to 50 percent of the population; an increase from 3 to 11 percent of the male population under hypertensive therapy, and among females from 9 to 13 percent; and a decrease in systolic blood pressure of 10 mm-Hg or more among 53 percent of the 1,799 persons on the hyptertension register, with 40 percent showing a decrease of 10 mm-Hg in diastolic blood pressure. Results have also included a considerable decline in the annual incidence of strokes: from 3.6 per 1,000 males in 1972 to 1.9 in 1975 and from 2.8 per 1,000 females to 1.8. Myocardial infarction rates slightly declined (Breslow, 1978).

Thus far, the evidence indicates that efforts to prevent disease and maintain health will probably focus increasingly on risk factor education. According to Lester Breslow, "It is these factors that now largely predict and apparently determine the extent of chronic disease and premature death; they should receive higher priority in health efforts than the diseases themselves" (1978). To date, the MRFIT program has not produced enough data to permit full evaluation of its results. If it is as successful as these other two programs, and preliminary indications are that it is, it will have considerable impact in channeling the future course of health-care resource allocations toward patient education and a holistic approach.

Ultimately, the final point of reckoning resides within each individual. Philosophers of medicine from Sir William Osler, in his 1901 classic *Aequanimitas*, to Jerome D. Frank and Rene Dubos in the present era, have emphasized the factor of patient volition in determining the balance between health and illness, life and death. Mutual cooperation between patients and practitioners is a two-edged sword, for freedom of choice is no guarantee that optimum health will ensue, nor will the vital choices of life be diminished to any degree. Writing in the *Western Journal of Medicine,* Rene Dubos observed:

> The day has passed when we can declaim with thunder from Olympus, "I *know* what is best for you." On what basis do we judge a patient who opts for a short, pain-free, joyful (for him) life—rather than a longer road of discipline and discomfort. (I realize the options are rarely black or white, but I must confess I am not sure of my own reaction where I given the choice of an additional year or two of life with palliative cancer chemotherapy and its sequelae, or a trip to see the Taj Mahal by moonlight and the wonders of the Nile and other untasted delights, while aided by morphia.) Certainly full disclosure measured to the intellectual and emotional capacity of the patient, with forthright recommendations is the obligation of every physician. But we must respect the judgment of a patient who still elects to place priority on something other than health or longevity or even freedom from discomfort. I feel this philosophy represents a new plane in the evolution of the healing art (1976).

Underlying the healing process is a phenomenon variously referred to as the "faith that heals" (Frank, 1975), the "will to live" (Hutschnecker, 1953), or the "very powerful belief" factor noted by Bernard H. Fox to be common to cases of spontaneous remission from cancer. One thought-provoking case history is often cited as evidencing the paradoxical strength and delicacy of this force. Reported in Bruno Klopfer's classic article, "Psychological Variables in Human Cancer" (1957), is the case study of a man with advanced lymphosarcoma. He was included in an experimental study of the now discredited chemotherapeutic agent Krebiozen. After one dosage, his tumors disappeared. However, when reports were publicized that the drug was ineffective, he again became bedridden. In an attempt to save his patient, the man's physician told him not to believe what he read and that he was going to be administered "double strength" Krebiozen, which was actually an injection of distilled water. Following this, the man again went into rapid remission. Later, however, when both the AMA and the FDA pronounced the drug worthless, the man died within a few days.

Other studies have explored the effect of involvement and participation. In an ingenious experiment, Judith Rodin and Ellen J. Langer of Harvard University explored the variable of patient responsibility in a nursing-home setting. Ninety-one elderly patients were randomly divided into two groups and each patient was given a small plant. Patients in the "responsibility-induced group" were told that they would be responsible for caring for and watering their plants. Patients in the second control group were told that the staff would take care of their plants. As simple as this involvement was, the results were astounding. From the data collected eighteen months later Rodin and Langer noted, "Patients in the responsibility-induced group showed a significant improvement in alertness and increased behavioral involvement in many different kinds of activities, such as movie attendance, active socializing with staff and friends, and contest participation" (1977). These findings were based upon both nurses' and physicians' independent ratings. Even more striking was the general improvement in the "responsibility group's" physical health, averaging twenty-five percent over an eighteen-month period in the nursing home. After eighteen months of caring for their plants the responsibility group evidenced a fifteen percent mortality rate while the control group suffered a thirty percent mortality rate. In interpreting these data, Rodin and Langer noted that the nurses played a vital role in this outcome: "Once the patients began to change, the nurses must have responded favorably to improved behavior, sociability, and self-reliance. . . . nurses' evaluations of the patients and not the overall health ratings were more closely related to subsequent life and death" (1977). Finally, these two sensitive researchers acknowledged that such findings reflected a holistic approach to patient responsibility and noted, "The long-term beneficial effects observed in the present study probably were obtained because the original treatment was not directed toward a single behavior. . . . [It] instead fostered generalized feelings of increased competence in day-to-day decision-making where it was potentially available" (1977). Giving responsibility for a single plant to elderly patients had a profound effect upon them and their entire psychosocial system. A heightened sense of efficacy and participation ensued from this task and appeared to slow and even reverse degenerative disorders and lessen mortality.

Further evidence of the necessity of active involvement in a supportive psychosocial matrix is found in a follow-up study undertaken in the Italian-American town of Roseto, Pennsylvania. During the early 1960s, Stewart Wolf of St. Luke's Hospital in Bethlehem, Pennsylvania, studied the people of Roseto and found they had an unusually low death rate from cardiovascular disease despite the fact that they were not significantly different from their neighbors in risk factors such as obesity, smoking, fat consumption, lack of exercise, and serum cholesterol levels. From his findings Wolf speculated that the difference was due to psychosocial factors since Rosetans supported each other in crisis, were involved in each other's lives, and respected the elderly. According to Wolf, "This was more than ethnicity—they developed such a cohesive, mutually supportive society that no one was ever abandoned" (Wolf, 1978). Recent data in this longitudinal study have indicated that there has been a marked increase in mortality from myocardial infarction over the last fifteen years as the Rosetans assumed a more typical life-style. As analyzed by Wolf, "By the mid-1960s younger Rosetans had begun to resent social isolation and clannishness. They began to marry non-Italians, joined country clubs, bought Cadillacs and ranch houses, changed churches, or quit going to church. Tradition and community closeness declined" (1978). Research data from this community are a mirror image of those from the nursing home in that the Rosetans lost the sense of community participation which was rejuvenated in the elderly people of the nursing home. In both cases, the intangible factors of support, involvement, and community were demonstrated to have profound effects upon health status. Simple measures which acknowledge an individual's sense of being needed, of efficacy and vitality, can swing the balance between health and illness, life and death.

Effects such as that of the plant in the nursing home are often dismissed as "placebo," which literally translates from Latin as "I shall please." Before the 1960s, placebos were commonly defined as "pharmacologically inactive medications such as salt water or starch, given primarily to satisfy patients that something is being done for them" (Bok, 1974). More recently, it has become clear that any medical or psychological procedure has an implicit placebo effect. Placebo has now come to be defined as "any therapy (or component of therapy) that is deliberately or knowingly used for its nonspecific, psychologic, or psychosphysiologic effect, or that . . . unknown to the patient or therapist, is without specific activity for the condition being treated" (Bok, 1974). Fifty percent of patients with minor emotional difficulties seen in general practice display a response to a placebo in various drug studies, compared to an active drug response of approximately seventy-five percent of the patients (Wheatley, 1972). "Placebo" has come to connote any aspect of the healing process which cannot be attributed to physical or pharmacological effects. Included in this category are the patient's volition, doctor-patient interaction, life-style changes, and a host of other variables that are essential features of a holistic model.

Disdain for "placebo effects" is not justified even in traditional medicine, since the existence of curative placebo effects is well substantiated in the treatment of a wide variety of diseases ranging from hay fever to rheumatoid arthritis (Beecher, 1955). Writing in the *Journal of the American Medical Association,* Herbert Benson and Mark D. Epstein of Harvard Medical School noted, "Patient and physician attitudes that create a sound doctor-patient relationship contribute to the production of the placebo effect. The placebo effect in most instances enhances the well-being of the patient, and this is an essential aspect of medicine. . . . More emphasis on the potency of the placebo and its positive effects is needed" (Benson & Epstein, 1975). Other types of placebo effects can be seen when the patient becomes an active participant in the healing process. As long as "placebo" remains a perjorative term, clinicians and researchers will continue to ignore the subtle and complex factors which enhance healing. Serious consideration of placebo effects would require the coordinated efforts of researchers in such divergent areas as anthropology and molecular biology. A holistic model of optimum health would provide a framework for such research.

Clinicians are now devising means to deliberately enhance

placebo effects. Through methods of clinical biofeedback, meditation, hypnosis, Jacobson's Progressive Relaxation, Autogenic Training and related approaches, patients have learned to self-regulate previously autonomic functions as well as experience the efficacy of the psychosomatic system in restoring its own homeostatic equilibrium. Pharmaceutical-free approaches to deep relaxation are of particular importance in the light of recent research indicating that diazepam, the primary constituent of muscle relaxants such as the ubiquitous Valium, may interfere with proper protein synthesis by muscle tissues. Research by Everett Bandman and his colleagues at the University of California, Berkeley, indicates "the presence of diazepam in cultures of chick embryos arrests normal muscle cell differentiation" (Bandman et al., 1978). Although further research is required, these results indicate that diazepam may induce muscular atrophy rather than muscular relaxation. If this proves to be the case, then methods of voluntary stress reduction will require development even more pressingly.

Of all these methods, clinical biofeedback has been most amenable to bridging the evolutionary gap between the existing medical care system and the evolving holistic model. Writing in the *Journal of the American Medical Association,* Julius Segal, Director of the Division of Scientific and Public Information of the National Institute of Mental Health, has noted, "Although researchers in the field are rightly cautious, they regard biofeedback as an avenue for returning to a more holistic kind of medicine in which the patient is taught to acquire more responsibility over his own health. . . . researchers see their techniques as related to other, older approaches such as meditation, yoga. . . . Such approaches share an emphasis on providing the patient with a new perception of himself and his body by teaching him techniques he can use for himself. Biofeedback shifts some of the responsibility for health onto the patient. More important, perhaps, it encourages attention to the relationship between health and life patterns—and away from the expectation of an instant pharmaceutical cure" (1975). Considering the source, this is quite a radical statement. Although oriented toward biofeedback, it is equally applicable to the range of holistic modalities including stress management, diet, and particularly exercise.

Clinical efficacy with biofeedback and relaxation procedures has prompted reevaluation of cancer therapy, as noted in *Science* by Constance Holden: "If all this is possible, it seems reasonable to some people that cancer patients can also regain control over endocrine functions that affect the immune system, or whatever other physiological processes that govern the course of the disease" (1978). At the present time, biofeedback research has focused upon bioelectrical parameters of musculature, cardiovascular processes, and the central nervous system, primarily the brain. Future research of biochemical variables such as insulin levels and white blood cell count, and deep tissue circulation as evidenced in thermography (Jöbsis, 1977) may provide a means of monitoring immunological processes for voluntary regulation.

At the core of any of these methods will be the use of imagery since imagery has been demonstrated to be a sensitive reflection of a patient's emotional state as well as the means by which psychophysiological regulation is achieved. Among the most impressive pioneering efforts are those mentioned earlier of oncologist O. Carl Simonton and Stephanie Matthews-Simonton in their recent book *Getting Well Again* (Simonton, Matthews-Simonton & Creighton, 1978). Throughout the book is powerful evidence of the efficacy of psychotherapy and visualization in the management of terminal cancer. Over the past four years the Simontons have worked with 159 patients with "medically incurable" malignancies and average life expectancies of one year or less. From their data, they note that the average survival time of these people turned out to be 20.3 months. Of the sixty-three people still surviving after four years, 22.2 percent had "no evidence of disease" and tumors were regressing in 19 percent. Their impressive results have been given significant empirical validation by the extensive research of Jeanne Achterberg and her husband G. Frank Lawliss of the University of Texas Health Science Center. They administered a battery of psychological tests, kept records of patient imagery as indicated by drawings and structured interviews, and conducted related inquiries with 126 patients who elected to follow the Simonton approach. Among these patients, ninety percent had widely metastisized cancers. From their research, Achterberg and Lawliss determined that the psychosocial variables were more predictive of survival time and course of the disease than the standard hematological analyses. Based on these results they noted, "Blood chemistries are merely reflective of the body's current status. . . . Psychological factors, on the other hand, seem to foretell or precede certain physiological response patterns" (Achterberg & Lawliss, 1978). Extending their research, they developed the IMAGE-CA test, which was described in Chapter V. Their research is applicable to the wide range of psychosomatic disorders and provides one of the first empirical methods for assessing and predicting both the positive and negative aspects of subjective imagery. Furthermore, their research underscores the major reason for focusing upon psychosocial variables in primary prevention since these predictable life-style predispositions to various diseases predate the occurrence of the organic disorder. Subtle alterations occurring within the psychophysiological and neuroendocrine systems of the body while under unabated stress eventually manifest as severe psychosomatic disorders (Pelletier, 1978). Potential research in this area has been greatly hampered by to the simple fact that "biochemists don't know about psychology and psychologists don't know about biochemistry" (Holden, 1978). This deficiency can be rectified through team research.

All of these holistic approaches are complementary to, not a substitute for, orthodox medical treatment. Fundamental to the former system is an acceptance of the premise that a patient's life-style and willingness to participate in the healing process can significantly affect the course of his or her health. Such a premise can actually expand the role of health-care professionals beyond purely biomedical concerns into psychological, psychosocial, environmental, and spiritual domains. An ironic danger in such an extension is that it might further erode each individual's sense of personal responsibility. That would be true if it were not for the fact that holistic approaches simply cannot be imposed upon any given patient. In addition to the therapies already mentioned, there needs to be further consideration of noninvasive therapeutic methods such as acupuncture (Melzack, 1973; Bresler, 1973), homeopathy (Vithoulkas, 1971), and electromagnetic effects in inducing limb regeneration (Adey, 1975; Cohen, 1975; Becker, 1977) as well as potentially destructive genetic aberrations (Malinin et al., 1976). All of these innovative approaches demonstrate that subtle processes which are subject to subtle interventions are just as potent determinants of disease and health as such gross influences as bacterial infection or traumatic injury.

While the goal of optimum health is given high priority by both individuals and society, our current understanding of the concept of health has not been conducive to establishing useful attitudes and practices that lead toward health. Writing in *Science*, Philip H. Abelson has examined the same evidence and concluded, "Because treatment of degenerative disease is not uniformly successful and since the course of some of them can be altered by changes in the patient's behavior, there is increasing interest in preventive medicine. . . . substantially better health cannot be bought with 118.5 billion dollars. Isn't it time the nation began to pay more attention to approaches that promise great improvement at little cost?" (1976). Improvement in general health is dependent upon lessening environmental hazards, improved nutrition, genetic selection, population control, stress management, and regular exercise, all outside the realm of traditional medicine.

Although there is a wide distribution of degrees of health in any human population, the tendency in making generalizations about normal health expectations for people has been to average and combine data to the point where normality is reduced to a statistical abstraction based upon the absence of disease. If this deficiency-oriented paradigm is taken literally, the end-product of being symptom-free is a state of passive waiting for unwelcome symptoms to arise and to be dispelled in their turn. There is little or no framework for change, development, or positive movement toward levels of greater and greater health. In contrast, the Institute of Humanistic Medicine has advocated an "aspirationally oriented health paradigm" emphasizing those life-style qualities which would maximize the quality and length of life. "Healthy individuals use whatever physical capacity they have available to achieve purpose in the world. They do not establish the boundaries of their potential on the basis of their physical capacity. They have an awareness of the body as that dimension of their being which acts in the world as a colleague and collaborator in the joys, goals, and purposes of life. Healthy individuals recognize and respect the body's needs and rhythms. . . . the whole being is greater than the sum of its parts. Body, emotions, mind, will, and spirit are elements of the human system which is an ever-evolving dynamic process. It is the synthesis of these elements which results in optimal health and indeed defines humanity itself. Health is an innate ability which can be evoked and developed by choice" (Garrell & Carlson, 1979). A change in philosophical outlook such as this must underlie any new system of health care.

Drawing the circle to a close, it is clear that optimum health extends out from the individual into the psychosocial and physical environment yet returns finally to the individual. In the seventeenth century the Japanese poet Basho wrote, "I do not seek to follow in the footsteps of the men of old; I seek the things they sought" (Lewis, 1970). Jungian psychiatrist R. James Yandell elaborates upon Basho's statement: "One who walks in another's footsteps engages in the most concrete and literal kind of imitation and also the most shallow, since one can follow footprints without purpose or destination of his own" (1978). Among the great teachers, Krishnamurti has always been one of the most outspoken in advocating that individuals attend to their own inner directives. In a 1928 lecture he stated, "The time has come when you must no longer subject yourself to anything. . . . I hope you will not listen to anyone, but will listen only to your own intuition, your own understanding, and give a public refusal to those who would be your interpreters. . . . Do not quote me afterwards as an authority. I refuse to be your crutch. I am not going to be brought into a cage for your worship" (Lutyens, 1975). Although it is a Cretan paradox to quote Krishnamurti advocating self-reliance, it is precisely this paradoxical prescription that the great religious and secular teachers have always advocated. In a 1929 talk Krishnamurti emphasized this point again: "Truth, being limitless, unconditioned, unapproachable by any path whatsoever, cannot be organized; nor should any organization be formed along any particular path. If you first understand that, then you will see how impossible it is to organize a belief. A belief is purely an individual matter, and you cannot and must not organize it. If you do, it becomes dead, crystallized; it becomes a creed, a sect, a religion, to be imposed on others" (Lutyens, 1975).

At this point in time there are numerous political, social, religious, and economic dogmas vying for dominance. Groups such as the worldwide organization of guru cults, followers of the latest fads in psychotherapy such as Primal Therapy, advocates of the newest pharmaceutical or surgical panaceas such as coronary bypass procedures—all such vested interests vie for numbers of followers, conversion of the savages, money, power, and hierarchies of authority. Perhaps at the base of the search for a comprehensive system of health care is a movement of individuals seeking the ideals missing from these petrified modern religions. If that is the case, then hopefully it can remain a viable and constantly evolving process of discovery rather than one more set of rigid prescriptions dispensed by a hierarchy of New Age politicians.

Behind the goals of holistic health is one of inner peace and harmony, of individuals free of all fears and all cages, a state of unconditional freedom based upon a profound inner equilibrium. This has been termed "samadhi," or a state of consciousness characterized by a sense of unity with all animate and inanimate beings and an end to the fear of death. In the American Indian tradition, the same thought is echoed by Sioux medicine man Lame Deer: "I believe that being a medicine man, more than anything else, is a state of mind, a way of looking at and understanding this earth, a sense of what it is all about. . . . I've been up to the hilltop, got my vision and my power; the rest is just trimmings" (Lame Deer & Erdoes, 1976).

Clearly, this is not a state with which to establish new dogmas or movements.

With the exception of John W. Farquhar's book *The American Way of Life Need Not Be Hazardous to Your Health* (1978), this dimension of optimum health has usually been overlooked. Norman Cousins expressed it eloquently: "But labels are unimportant; what is important is the knowledge that human beings are not locked into fixed limitations. The quest for perfectability is not a presumption or a blasphemy but the highest manifestation of a great design" (1977). Twentieth-century science has permitted humankind to peer with electron microscopes into the intercellular space and chart the helical coils of amino acid molecules at the very heart of all life. Arcane Buddhist scriptures formulated a thousand years ago have advocated the journey inward toward wisdom and enlightenment. Together they remain inviolate reminders of awe and humility.

Appendix A
Nutrition, Health, and Activity Profile

NOTE: Both lay people and doctors can take advantage of the Nutrition, Health, and Activity Profile which follows. Lay people are advised to take the analysis to their doctor for best results. Doctors should write for the special Doctor packet on their letterheads.

NUTRITION, HEALTH, AND ACTIVITY PROFILE

INTRODUCTION

Over the past ten years, researchers in the health field have discovered and re-discovered numerous factors which relate to physical and mental performance, sexual functioning, and aging.

The importance of nutrition has been emphasized. At the same time, however, it has been shown that nutrition alone is just not enough to attain the best possible health. To keep the body functioning at peak performance and to increase resistance to diseases like heart attack and possibly cancer, several other aspects of life-style must be considered as well. Exercise, financial security, general health habits, exposure to pollution, stress, etc., are among these other important factors.

Even if you had all this information for yourself, it would be extremely difficult to evaluate and determine where to start a personal program for better health. As an aid to you and your doctor in overcoming these difficulties, this computerized Nutrition, Health, and Activity Profile was developed. Experts in nutrition, biochemistry, statistics, and exercise collaborated in the design and development of this test to bring you the very latest findings in these areas as they apply to you personally. Your doctor can review the results together with your case history to develop a comprehensive personal health program for you.

This computerized profile will determine your dietary intake of proteins, carbohydrates, fats, vitamins, minerals, fibers, calories, etc., compare them to established requirements, and discuss their meaning and interpretation for your particular case. In fact, each major area of life-style critical to health and longevity will be contrasted with essential requirements for a healthier and longer life. Suggestions will be made for supplemental reading, where necessary, to further clarify important points. For those concerned with losing weight, a safe and sane approach will be discussed for losing extra pounds sensibly and keeping them off permanently. These recommendations can be carefully reviewed by your doctor and modified, as necessary, to suit your life-style.

The knowledge you will gain about your life and your health from the results of this test can play a significant role in your future health and longevity. So please be sure to answer all the questions to the best of your ability.

Doctor's
Name: _____

Phone
Number: (   ) _____

Doctor's
Address: _____
     Number   Street   City   State   Zip

Name of
Patient: _____

Date of Birth: _____ Sex: _____
             Month   Day   Year

Pregnant? _____ Lactating? _____

Occupation: _____

Height: _____ft._____ins. Weight: _____ Ideal Weight: _____

Number of pounds   Frame
you want to lose: _____ Size: small (   ) medium (   ) large (   )

Are you currently
losing weight (   ), gaining weight, (   )
or staying about the same (   )?

+-----------------------------+
| For Doctor's |
| Use Only |
| |
| [ ] [ ] [ ] |
+-----------------------------+

There are five sections to complete, each provided with instructions and examples where necessary.

    —Nutrition I: Important Nutritional Factors
    —Nutrition II: Food Consumption
    —Vitamin and Mineral Supplementation
    —Health Factors
    —Physical Activities

Be certain to answer the questions as they appear—please do not change any questions and then answer. You may find that this questionnaire does not cover some food or activity that is an important part of your everyday living. You will find spaces provided in each section to write in your additions.

PACIFIC RESEARCH SYSTEMS, P.O. BOX 64218, LOS ANGELES, CA. 90064

©COPYRIGHT 1976 PACIFIC RESEARCH SYSTEMS

NUTRITION I: IMPORTANT NUTRITIONAL FACTORS

Please answer the questions below as follows:

A) Complete each square with a numerical response. If you do not know the answer or the question does not apply to you, leave it blank.

B) Complete each parenthesis with a check ( ) for a "Yes" response. If the answer is "No" or if you do not know the answer, leave it blank.

1. How many cups of the following beverages do you drink per week?

Regular Coffee ☐   Decaf ☐   Regular Tea ☐   Low Calorie Soft Drinks ☐   Regular Soft Drinks ☐

2. Do you use cream with your. . .

Coffee? ( )   Decaf? ( )   Tea? ( )

3. Fill in the number of teaspoons of sugar used with each cup of. . .

Coffee ☐   Decaf ☐   Tea ☐

4. How many teaspoons of sugar do you use with each serving of cereal? ☐

5. Beyond beverages or cereal, how many teaspoons of sugar do you add to your food per week? ☐

6. Do you use any artificial sweeteners? (i.e., saccharine, sucaryl, etc.)   ( )

7. How many times per week do you eat:

convenience foods like TV dinners? ☐   fried foods? ☐   at hamburger or taco stands? ☐   in restaurants? ☐

8. Are you a regular meat eater? ( )   If yes, how is it prepared?

medium to well done ( )   rare ( )   very lean ( )   with gravy ( )

9. Do you eat:

less than average? ( )   more than average? ( )   foods with extra salt? ( )   breakfast 5 or more days per week? ( )

10. Do you drink tap water? ( )

11. Do you use iodized salt? ( )

In percentage (%) terms, what form of the following two food groups do you consume? The percentage must total 100%.

Example:
If one quarter of your vegetables are frozen, just under three quarters are fresh-cooked, very little are fresh-raw, and none are canned, your numerical response should be:

What percentage of the vegetables that you consume are . . .

Fresh-raw   Fresh-cooked   Frozen   Canned

☐ % + ☐ % + ☐ % + ☐ % = 100%

---

12. What percentage of the vegetables that you consume are . . .

Fresh-raw   Fresh-cooked   Frozen   Canned

☐ % + ☐ % + ☐ % + ☐ % = 100%

13. What percentage of the fruits that you consume are . . .

Fresh-raw   Fresh-cooked   Frozen   Canned

☐ % + ☐ % + ☐ % + ☐ % = 100%

NUTRITION II: FOOD CONSUMPTION

Nutrition II lists foods or groups of foods together with serving sizes in parentheses:

Please: 1) For each food you consume, fill in how often you eat the specified serving size under one of the columns: "daily," "weekly," or "monthly." **Do not change the specified serving sizes. Fill in only one box under "daily," "weekly," or "monthly" for each food.**

2) Leave the line entirely **blank** if you **do not consume** the food or **foods listed** (do not use zeros). Remember, your answers are to represent your nutrition as of now. **Do not include any foods which have not been consumed over the past month.**

3) If you are certain about how often you eat a given food, just ask yourself how frequently you have eaten it over the last week to two weeks, to a month at most, and answer accordingly. It may be helpful to discuss your answers with someone familiar with your eating habits.

4) Be sure to enter all your snacks as well as regular meals.

To make sure that you don't forget any foods, it may be helpful to write down your intake of food and drink for a week and then check the list again.

Example 1: If you drink 2 cups of whole milk per day, the correct response is:

Daily   Weekly Monthly

Whole milk
(1 cup)   ☐   ☐   ☐

IMPORTANT: Do not fill in unused boxes with zeros.

Example 2: If you have 3 waffles (3 servings) and six pancakes (2 servings) per week, your answer will be:

Daily   Weekly Monthly

Waffle (3),
pancakes (2)   ☐   ☐   ☐

IMPORTANT: Fill in one box only - leave the other two blank.

	Daily	Weekly	Monthly
1) Whole milk (1 cup, 8 oz.)	☐	☐	☐
2) Skim/nonfat milk (1 cup, 8 oz.)	☐	☐	☐
3) Low-fat milk (1 cup, 8 oz.)	☐	☐	☐
4) Yogurt (1 cup, 8 oz.)	☐	☐	☐
5) Yogurt, low-fat (1 cup, 8 oz.)	☐	☐	☐
6) Regular cottage cheese (1/2 cup, 4 oz.)	☐	☐	☐
7) Low-fat cottage cheese (1/2 cup, 4 oz.)	☐	☐	☐
8) Cream cheese (1 oz.)	☐	☐	☐
9) Sour cream (1 Tbsp., 1/2 oz.)	☐	☐	☐
10) Other cheeses (1 oz.)	☐	☐	☐
11) Milk shake (16 oz.)	☐	☐	☐
12) Egg (one)	☐	☐	☐
13) Protein powder (1 Tbsp.)	☐	☐	☐

	Daily	Weekly	Monthly
14) White bread (1 slice)	☐	☐	☐
15) Whole wheat bread (1 slice)	☐	☐	☐
16) Corn bread (1 square, 2 oz.)	☐	☐	☐
17) Oatmeal (1 cup)	☐	☐	☐
18) Cereal, wheat germ (1/2 cup), whole grain (1 cup)	☐	☐	☐
19) Bran (2 Tbsp.)	☐	☐	☐
20) Cereal, hi vitamin (1 cup)	☐	☐	☐
21) Cereals without sugar (1 cup)	☐	☐	☐
22) Cereals, sugared or frosted (1 cup)	☐	☐	☐
23) Waffle (1), pancakes (3, 2 1/2 oz.)	☐	☐	☐
24) French toast (2 slices, 1 1/2 oz.)	☐	☐	☐
25) Sweet roll (one, 1 3/4 oz.)	☐	☐	☐
26) Muffin or roll (one, 1 3/4 oz.)	☐	☐	☐

	Daily	Weekly	Monthly
27) Bagel (3" diam., 2 oz.)	☐	☐	☐
28) Spaghetti with meat sauce (1 cup)	☐	☐	☐
29) Spaghetti or macaroni with cheese (1 cup)	☐	☐	☐
30) Macaroni, plain (1 cup)	☐	☐	☐
31) Noodles, egg enriched (1 cup)	☐	☐	☐
32) Pizza (1 slice, 2½ oz.)	☐	☐	☐
33) Brown rice (1 cup)	☐	☐	☐
34) White rice (1 cup)	☐	☐	☐
35) Doughnut, or cupcake (one, 1 oz.)	☐	☐	☐
36) Cake with icing (1 slice, 4 oz.)	☐	☐	☐
37) Cake without icing (1 slice, 4 oz.)	☐	☐	☐
38) Fudge (1 square, 3 oz.)	☐	☐	☐
39) Brownies (1 square, 2 oz.)	☐	☐	☐
40) Pumpkin or custard pie (1 slice, 4 oz.)	☐	☐	☐
41) Any other pie (1 slice, 4 oz.)	☐	☐	☐
42) Ice cream (½ cup)	☐	☐	☐
43) Cookie (one, 3" diam., ½ oz.)	☐	☐	☐
44) Butter (1 Tbsp., ½ oz.)	☐	☐	☐
45) Margarine (1 Tbsp., ½ oz.)	☐	☐	☐
46) Vegetable oil (1 Tbsp., ½ oz.)	☐	☐	☐
47) Salad dressing Thousand/French (2 Tbsp., 1 oz.)	☐	☐	☐

	Daily	Weekly	Monthly
48) Italian dressing (2 Tbsp., 1 oz.)	☐	☐	☐
49) Roquefort/Blue cheese (2 Tbsp., 1 oz.)	☐	☐	☐
50) Steak (6 oz.)	☐	☐	☐
51) Hamburger (one, 3 oz.)	☐	☐	☐
52) Hot dog (one regular size)	☐	☐	☐
53) Taco, tamale, tostada (one)	☐	☐	☐
54) Chicken, duck, fowl (6 oz.)	☐	☐	☐
55) Lamb, beef (6 oz.)	☐	☐	☐
56) Pork, ham (5 oz.)	☐	☐	☐
57) Pork sausage (3 oz.)	☐	☐	☐
58) Bacon (2 slices, ½ oz.)	☐	☐	☐
59) Veal (4 oz.)	☐	☐	☐
60) Corned beef (4 oz.)	☐	☐	☐
61) Beef liver (3½ oz.)	☐	☐	☐
62) Chicken liver (3½ oz.)	☐	☐	☐
63) Organ meat, kidney, heart etc. (3½ oz.)	☐	☐	☐
64) Liverwurst, liver pate (2 oz.)	☐	☐	☐
65) Other luncheon meats or sausages (2 oz.)	☐	☐	☐
66) Chicken, beef pot pie (1, 8 oz.)	☐	☐	☐
67) Oysters, clams (6 oz.)	☐	☐	☐
68) Shrimp, crab, lobster (3 oz.)	☐	☐	☐

	Daily	Weekly	Monthly
69) Salmon (3 oz.)	☐	☐	☐
70) Sardines (3 oz.)	☐	☐	☐
71) Tuna, swordfish (3 oz.)	☐	☐	☐
72) Other fish (3 oz.)	☐	☐	☐
73) Soybeans (½ cup)	☐	☐	☐
74) Tofu (½ cup)	☐	☐	☐
75) Lima, kidney, navy beans (½ cup)	☐	☐	☐
76) Green beans (½ cup)	☐	☐	☐
77) Bean sprouts (1 cup)	☐	☐	☐
78) Avocado (½ large, 4 oz.)	☐	☐	☐
79) Olives, ripe (10, 2 oz.)	☐	☐	☐
80) Asparagus (6 spears, 3½ oz.)	☐	☐	☐
81) Broccoli (½ cup)	☐	☐	☐
82) Beets (½ cup)	☐	☐	☐
83) Cabbage (½ cup)	☐	☐	☐
84) Peas, brussels sprouts, rutabagas (½ cup)	☐	☐	☐
85) Sauerkraut, eggplant (½ cup)	☐	☐	☐
86) Spinach, chard, mustard greens (½ cup)	☐	☐	☐
87) Cucumbers radishes (½ cup)	☐	☐	☐
88) Kale, carrot-pea mix (½ cup)	☐	☐	☐
89) Turnips, kohlrabi (½ cup)	☐	☐	☐
90) Carrots (½ cup)	☐	☐	☐

	Daily	Weekly	Monthly
91) Celery (1 stalk)	☐	☐	☐
92) Corn (1 ear or ½ cup)	☐	☐	☐
93) Mushrooms (¼ cup)	☐	☐	☐
94) Tomatoes (½ cup)	☐	☐	☐
95) Tomato juice (1 cup)	☐	☐	☐
96) V-8 juice (1 cup)	☐	☐	☐
97) Squash (½ cup)	☐	☐	☐
98) Artichoke (1 large)	☐	☐	☐
99) Cauliflower (½ cup)	☐	☐	☐
100) Green pepper (½ large)	☐	☐	☐
101) Onions, raw (¼ cup, 2 oz.)	☐	☐	☐
102) Lettuce (⅛ head)	☐	☐	☐
103) Potato (1 med.) mashed (½ cup)	☐	☐	☐
104) French fries (10 pieces, 2 oz.)	☐	☐	☐
105) Coleslaw (½ cup)	☐	☐	☐
106) Bean soup (1 cup)	☐	☐	☐
107) Chicken soup (1 cup)	☐	☐	☐
108) Vegetable soup (1 cup)	☐	☐	☐
109) Beef & vegetable soup (1 cup)	☐	☐	☐
110) Clam chowder (1 cup)	☐	☐	☐
111) Tomato soup (1 cup)	☐	☐	☐
112) Split pea soup (1 cup)	☐	☐	☐

	Daily	Weekly	Monthly
113) Other creamed soup (1 cup)	☐	☐	☐
114) Crackers (2 med.)	☐	☐	☐
115) Popcorn, popped (1 cup)	☐	☐	☐
116) Peanuts (⅓ cup), peanut butter (5 Tbsp.)	☐	☐	☐
117) Sunflower seeds (½ cup)	☐	☐	☐
118) Pecans, walnuts (½ cup)	☐	☐	☐
119) Almonds, other nuts (½ cup)	☐	☐	☐
120) Milk chocolate, candy bar (2 oz.)	☐	☐	☐
121) Jam, jelly, honey, syrup (2 Tbsp.)	☐	☐	☐
122) Potato chips (10 2" Diam.)	☐	☐	☐
123) Wine (1 glass, 4 oz.)	☐	☐	☐
124) Scotch, whiskey, gin, etc. (1 oz.)	☐	☐	☐
125) Drink mixer, sweet (1 glass, 8 oz.)	☐	☐	☐
126) Cola drink (12 oz.) Not low calorie	☐	☐	☐
127) Other soft drink (12 oz.) Not low calorie	☐	☐	☐
128) Beer (12 oz.)	☐	☐	☐
129) Orange or grapefruit juice (½ cup, 4 oz.)	☐	☐	☐
130) Orange (1 med.) grapefruit (½ med.)	☐	☐	☐
131) Peaches, canned (½ cup)	☐	☐	☐
132) Peach, fresh (1 med.)	☐	☐	☐
133) Apricot, canned (½ cup)	☐	☐	☐
134) Apricot, fresh (3 med.)	☐	☐	☐
135) Applesauce (½ cup)	☐	☐	☐
136) Apple juice (½ cup, 4 oz.)	☐	☐	☐
137) Apple, pear canned (½ cup)	☐	☐	☐
138) Apple, pear, fresh (1 med.)	☐	☐	☐
139) Pineapple (½ cup)	☐	☐	☐
140) Strawberries, fresh (½ cup)	☐	☐	☐
141) Other berries, fresh (½ cup)	☐	☐	☐
142) Berries, canned (½ cup)	☐	☐	☐
143) Banana (1 med.)	☐	☐	☐
144) Cantaloupe (½ med.)	☐	☐	☐
145) Dates, dried (½ cup)	☐	☐	☐
146) Papaya, fresh (½ med.)	☐	☐	☐
147) Raisins (¼ cup)	☐	☐	☐
148) Grapes (½ cup)	☐	☐	☐
149) Lecithin granules (1 Tbsp.)	☐	☐	☐
150) Brewers yeast (1 Tbsp.)	☐	☐	☐
151) Bone meal (½ Tsp.)	☐	☐	☐

Additional Foods

Please write in the names and serving sizes of any additional foods that you eat at least twice monthly

Food	Serving size	Daily	Weekly	Monthly
152) _____ _____		☐	☐	☐
153) _____ _____		☐	☐	☐
154) _____ _____		☐	☐	☐
155) _____ _____		☐	☐	☐
156) _____ _____		☐	☐	☐
157) _____ _____		☐	☐	☐
158) _____ _____		☐	☐	☐
159) _____ _____		☐	☐	☐
160) _____ _____		☐	☐	☐

Vitamin and Mineral Supplementation

Check (✓) the supplements that you presently use.

Blank spaces are provided for your additions.

(1)	Multivitamin with minerals	( )
(2)	Multivitamin (only)	( )
(3)	Multimineral (only)	( )
(4)	Vitamin B-complex	( )
(5)	Vitamin A	( )
(6)	Vitamin C	( )
(7)	Vitamin E	( )
(8)	Calcium	( )
(9)	Magnesium	( )

_____   _____

_____   _____

(10) How long have you been taking the supplements checked above?
more than 1 year ( )
more than 3 mos. ( )
less than 3 mos. ( )

HEALTH FACTORS

Please answer the questions below with the usual check (✓) for a "Yes" response. If the answer is "No" or you do not know the answer, leave it blank.

1) Have you had a medical examination in the past 6 months? ( )

2) Do you have high blood pressure? ( )

3) Do you know your blood triglyceride level? ( )

4) Do you know your blood cholesterol level? ( )

5) Do you have a tendency to get ulcers? ( )

6) Is there a history of diabetes in your family? ( )

7) Is there a history of cancer in your family? ( )

8) Is there a history of heart disease in your family? ( )

9) Is there a history of respiratory ailments in your family? ( )

10) In your personal life, are you often under stress? ( )

11) At work, are you often under stress? ( )

12) Do you take a drink before you do something important? ( )

13) Do you often go 3 or more days without alcohol? ( )

14) Do you take any form of tranquilizers? ( )

15) Have you had a dental check-up in the past year? ( )

16) Do you drink diet beverages regularly? ( )

17) Will you or do you have a monthly income for retirement other than social security? ( )

18) Physically, are you often tired, sluggish? ( )

19) Physically, do you feel average, could be better? ( )

20) Physically, do you feel full of energy? ( )

21) Is your stamina poor? ( )

22) Is your stamina average? ( )

23) Is your stamina excellent? ( )

24) Do you get enough sleep (7-8 hours)? ( )

25) Are you most often in a good mood and at ease with the world? ( )

26) Are you often depressed and moody? ( )

27) Is your mood mostly average? ( )

28) Do you smoke cigarettes? ( )

29) Do you often spend time in closed rooms with cigarette smokers? ( )

30) Do you live in highly polluted air? ( )

31) Do you work in highly polluted air? ( )

32) Do you use air purifiers where needed? ( )

33) Do you take any drugs on a regular basis? ( )

PHYSICAL ACTIVITIES
PART A

The profile is designed to provide information on the calories burned during physical activity. Those activities you are now doing are to be entered in part A below. Part B provides spaces for activities you are not doing but would like to do. **If you indicated a desire to lose weight** on page one of this questionnaire, **the calories burned from the activities of both parts A and B will be properly combined to help meet your goal. But you must specify at least two physical activities.**

From the Activity Table below, please select physical activities in which you are now (this season) participating. Select only those which you are doing at least twice a month and place their numbers in the squares provided after the example. Be sure to complete each line for the selected activity indicating, in the appropriate square provided, how many minutes you spend each day, week, or month at that activity. Please do not include any activities which are part of your daily work routine. A few spaces are provided for you to add more entries in the Activity Table, if necessary.

For example, if you jog for 15 minutes a week and practice yoga 15 minutes each morning, your response should be:

Activity Number   Daily   Weekly   Monthly

In Minutes

☐   ☐   ☐   ☐

☐   ☐   ☐   ☐

IMPORTANT: On each line, fill in an activity number plus the time spent. Use only one box from the "daily", "weekly" or "monthly" columns.

Activity Number   Daily   Weekly In Minutes   Monthly

1. ☐   ☐ ☐ ☐   6. ☐   ☐ ☐ ☐

2. ☐   ☐ ☐ ☐   7. ☐   ☐ ☐ ☐

3. ☐   ☐ ☐ ☐   8. ☐   ☐ ☐ ☐

4. ☐   ☐ ☐ ☐   9. ☐   ☐ ☐ ☐

5. ☐   ☐ ☐ ☐   10. ☐   ☐ ☐ ☐

ACTIVITY TABLE

1. Back packing with heavy pack
2. Baseball
3. Basketball
4. Bicycling, slow
5. Bicycling, fast
6. Bowling
7. Boxing
8. Boxing (punching bag)
9. Calisthenics/Tai Chi
10. Canoeing, slow
11. Canoeing, fast
12. Climbing stairs
13. Dancing, slow
14. Dancing, vigorous
15. Fencing
16. Football, tackle
17. Football, touch
18. Gardening
19. Golf
20. Handball
21. Hockey, ice
22. Hockey, field
23. Horseback riding
24. Horse vaulting
25. Horseshoes
26. Housework
27. Hunting
28. Isometrics
29. Jai Alai
30. Jogging (over eight minutes per mile)

31. Karate
32. Motorcycling
33. Mountain climbing
34. Parallel bars
35. Polo
36. Racquetball
37. Rugby
38. Running (under eight minutes per mile)
39. Shuffleboard
40. Skating, ice
41. Skating, roller
42. Skiing, snow
43. Skiing, cross country
44. Skiing, water
45. Skin diving
46. Soccer
47. Softball
48. Squash

49. Surfing
50. Swimming, competitive
51. Swimming, recreational
52. Tennis, singles
53. Tennis, doubles
54. Volleyball
55. Walking, slow
56. Walking, moderate
57. Walking, fast
58. Water polo
59. Weight lifting
60. Yoga/Akido
61. Working out in a gym or spa with varied equipment
62. _____
63. _____
64. _____

PART B

Referring again to the Activity Table, please select physical activities that meet all of the following requirements:

—you are not now doing them
—the activities are currently in season
—you would enjoy doing these activities and could do them in your present state of health
—the activities are both practical and convenient for your personal circumstances and environment.

Place the numbers which correspond to the selected activities in the squares provided below. Do not include any activities listed above in Section A.

1. ☐   2. ☐   3. ☐   4. ☐

5. ☐   6. ☐   7. ☐   8. ☐

NUTRITION HEALTH AND ACTIVITY PROFILE

OF MR AMERICAN ANY STREET   7/16/78

THIS PROFILE IS DESIGNED FOR YOU PERSONALLY AND
IS MEANT TO BE YOUR GUIDE TO MUCH IMPROVED
HEALTH. THOUSANDS OF ERROR FREE CALCULATIONS
HAVE BEEN MADE TO DETERMINE THE AVERAGE DAILY
LEVEL OF KEY NUTRIENTS IN YOUR DIET. THESE RE-
SULTS ALONG WITH YOUR HEALTH HABITS HAVE BEEN
COMPARED WITH STANDARDS ADJUSTED FOR YOUR OWN
PERSONAL CHARACTERISTICS. WHEREVER APPROPRIATE,
EASY TO UNDERSTAND EXPLANATIONS AND SUGGESTIONS
ARE OFFERED TO HELP YOU MAKE THE CHANGES NECES-
SARY TO AVOID DISEASE AND TO ATTAIN YOUR BEST
POSSIBLE HEALTH.

THE CONTENTS OF YOUR PROFILE

I. PROTEIN

THERE ARE TWO STANDARDS AGAINST WHICH YOUR IN-
TAKE OF PROTEIN CAN BE COMPARED. THE FIRST STAN-
DARD, THE RDA(RECOMMENDED DAILY ALLOWANCE), SUG-
GESTS 109.1 GRAMS PER DAY FOR YOU. IT IS BASED
SOLELY ON YOUR WEIGHT AND DOES NOT TAKE INTO AC-
COUNT WHETHER YOU ARE OVER OR UNDER WEIGHT, VERY
ACTIVE OR SEDENTARY. THE SECOND STANDARD, A MORE
PRECISE METHOD OF ESTIMATING YOUR PROTEIN RE-

QUIREMENT, IS BASED ON CALORIC EXPENDITURE AND RECOMMENDS THAT YOUR INTAKE BE BETWEEN 68.6 AND 87.0 GRAMS PER DAY.*(SCRIMSHAW—THE NEW ENGLAND JL. OF MEDICINE, JAN. 22, 1976)

EVEN SLIGHTLY MORE PROTEIN MAY BE NEEDED IF YOU ARE VERY ACTIVE OR HAVE LOW ABSORPTION OR WHEN DISORDERS LIKE HYPOGLYCEMIA EXIST. JUST BE SURE YOUR INTAKE OF COMPLEX CARBOHYDRATES ARE NOT SACRIFICED FOR INCREASED PROTEIN (FOR A DETAILED DISCUSSION OF THE RELATIVE IMPORTANCE OF ALL THE NUTRIENTS AND HEALTH FACTORS READ DR KUGLERS SEVEN KEYS TO A LONGER LIFE—H. KUGLER PH.D.).

YOUR TOTAL PROTEIN FROM ALL FOOD SOURCES AVER-AGES 95.6 GRAMS PER DAY.

PROTEIN IS ONE OF THE MOST IMPORTANT NUTRIENTS THE BODY REQUIRES FOR MAINTAINING GOOD HEALTH. PROTEIN FROM DIFFERENT SOURCES IS COMPRISED OF VARYING AMOUNTS OF DIFFERENT AMINO ACIDS. THERE ARE ABOUT 22 DIFFERENT AMINO ACIDS WHICH CAN FORM A PROTEIN. THEY HAVE BEEN CLASSIFIED AS ES-SENTIAL AND NON—ESSENTIAL.

FOODS RICH IN ALL THE ESSENTIAL AMINO ACIDS ARE EGGS, CHEESE, MEAT, POULTRY AND FISH. WHEN ONE OR MORE OF THESE FOODS ARE PRESENT AT EACH MEAL AND COMPRISE MORE THAN 50 PCT OF YOUR PROTEIN INTAKE, SPECIFIC AMINO ACID DEFICIENCIES ARE MUCH LESS LIKELY. EACH MEAL SHOULD BE COMPRISED OF FOODS THAT INDIVIDUALLY OR TAKEN TOGETHER ARE RICH IN ALL THE ESSENTIAL AMINO ACIDS TO ASSURE GOOD NUTRITION. THIS TASK IS PARTICULARLY DIF-FICULT IF YOUR DIET IS RESTRICTED TO VEGETABLES AND GRAINS ONLY.

*CALCULATIONS INCLUDE A 20% EXCESS.

FATS

THE AVERAGE AMERICAN DIET DERIVES ABOUT 40% OF ITS CALORIES OR ENERGY FROM FAT. EXPERTS IN HEART DISEASE AND DISEASES OF THE ARTERIES AGREE THAT AN ACROSS THE BOARD RECOMMENDATION TO LOWER FAT INTAKE WOULD BENEFIT THE MAJORITY OF PEOPLE. SOME EXPERTS FEEL FAT SHOULD BE ABOUT 34% WHILE OTHERS FEEL IT SHOULD BE AS LOW AS 10%. A RANGE

OF 20 TO 34% SEEMS REASONABLE (ATHEROSCLEROSIS, MEDCOM).

53.5% OF THE CALORIES IN YOUR DIET COME FROM FATS.

REDUCED CONSUMPTION OF ANIMAL SOURCE FATS SUCH AS GRAVIES, FATTY SAUCES, FRIED FOODS, WHOLE MILK, BUTTER, OILS AND FATS IS ADVISABLE WHEN YOUR OVERALL FAT INTAKE IS HIGH.

FAT INTAKE CAN INFLUENCE SERUM CHOLESTEROL AND TRIGLYCERIDES, THE FAT IN THE BLOOD. STUDIES HAVE SHOWN A HIGH CORRELATION BETWEEN CORONARY HEART DISEASE AND INCREASED TRIGLYCERIDE LEVELS. THIS IS ONE IMPORTANT REASON FOR SEEING YOUR DOCTOR REGULARLY AND HAVING THESE FACTORS CHECKED. YOUR DOCTOR CAN INTERPRET THE RESULTS AND/OR YOU CAN READ RICHARD PASSWATERS BOOK—SUPERNUTRITION FOR HEALTHY HEARTS—FOR A DE-TAILED EXPLANATION.

WITH RESPECT TO HEART DISEASE, THERE ARE TWO IM-PORTANT FRACTIONS OF CHOLESTEROL IN THE BLOOD, HDL AND LDL. THE HDL FRACTION SHOULD BE HIGH AND THE LDL FRACTION SHOULD BE LOW. GOOD EXERCISE, ESPECIALLY OF THE ENDURANCE TYPE, LIKE RUNNING, CAN CHANGE THESE VALUES FOR THE BETTER.

LEARN YOUR PRESENT CHOLESTEROL AND TRIGLYCERIDE LEVELS, CHECK THEM ON A REGULAR BASIS, KEEP A RUNNING WRITTEN RECORD AND WATCH FOR ANY CHANGES.

SERUM CHOLESTEROL LEVELS OF ABOUT 170 TO 190 OR LOWER AND TRIGLYCERIDE LEVELS OF ABOUT 100 OR LOWER ARE DESIRABLE. SOME EXPERTS ACCEPT VALUES SLIGHTLY HIGHER; OTHERS FEEL EVEN LOWER LEVELS ARE DESIRABLE. OFTEN IF ONE IS HIGH SO IS THE OTHER. SHOULD THESE VALUES BE HIGH, ACHIEVING NORMAL VALUES IS VERY IMPORTANT. SOME OF THE FACTORS THAT CAN GREATLY HELP TO NORMALIZE THESE IMPORTANT INDICATORS OF HEART DISEASE RISK ARE: ACHIEVING NORMAL WEIGHT, CAREFULLY INCREASED EX-ERCISE, LOWERING FAT INTAKE, AND BEING SURE YOU HAVE NO VITAMIN/MINERAL DEFICIENCIES. FIBER (DISCUSSED LATER ON) ALSO HELPS IN LOWERING CHO-LESTEROL LEVELS(TROWELL, H. C. AMER JOURNAL OF CLINICAL NUTRITION 25:464, 1972).

IT IS POSSIBLE FOR A PERSON WITH A HIGH FAT IN-
TAKE TO HAVE NORMAL TRIGLYCERIDES. IN MOST CASES
THIS WILL NOT BE SO. IN ANY EVENT DO NOT GO TO
EXTREMES, YOU MAY HAVE A DISORDER REQUIRING MED-
ICAL TREATMENT.

THERE IS, OF COURSE, A NEED FOR SOME ESSENTIAL
FATTY ACIDS. THE MOST IMPORTANT OF THESE IS
LINOLEIC ACID. IT PLAYS A VERY IMPORTANT ROLE IN
MAINTAINING PROPER CHOLESTEROL METABOLISM, HOR-
MONAL CONTROL, THE DEVELOPMENT OF NEW CELLS AND
THE MAINTENANCE OF HEALTHY BODY TISSUES, PARTIC-
ULARLY OF THE SKIN, LIVER AND KIDNEYS. YOUR AV-
ERAGE DAILY LINOLEIC ACID INTAKE IS 9.5 GRAMS.

ACCORDING TO THE LATEST STUDIES, A DAILY INTAKE
OF 3 TO 5 GRAMS IS DESIRABLE. YOU MAY FULFILL
THIS NEED BY TAKING ONLY 1 TEASPOON TO 1 TABLE-
SPOON DAILY OF A RICH SOURCE OF UNSATURATED
FATTY ACIDS SUCH AS SUNFLOWER SEED OIL, SAF-
FLOWER OIL OR CORN OIL. SUNFLOWER SEED OIL IS
ALSO RICHER IN VITAMIN E THAN SAFFLOWER OIL OR
CORN OIL, WHICH GIVES IT AN ADDED PLUS. SUCH
OILS SHOULD BE REFRIGERATED AND SEALED TIGHTLY,
WHEN NOT IN USE, TO PROTECT FROM RANCIDITY.

NOTE: INCREASED EXERCISE, ESPECIALLY ENDURANCE
TYPE EXERCISES, INCREASES THE NEED FOR POLYUN-
SATURATES.

FIBER

FIBERS ARE RECOGNIZED AS IMPORTANT SUBSTANCES IN
THE DAILY DIET. RESEARCHERS HAVE SHOWN THAT A
DIET HIGH IN FIBER HELPS PREVENT CANCER OF THE
COLON AND DISORDERS OF THE DIGESTIVE TRACT(BUR-
KITT). NO MINIMUM DAILY REQUIREMENTS HAVE BEEN
ESTABLISHED. EXPERTS CONSULTED ON THE ISSUE HAVE
INDICATED THAT 6 GRAMS PER DAY IS A MINIMAL
AMOUNT FOR YOUR WEIGHT RANGE. YOUR AVERAGE DAILY
FIBER INTAKE WAS 2.5 GRAMS WHICH IS TOO LOW.
CONSIDER DIETARY CHANGES GEARED TO INCREASING
YOUR FIBER INTAKE.

FOODS RICH IN NATURAL FIBERS ARE BRAN, WHOLE
WHEAT, OTHER WHOLE GRAIN PRODUCTS, FRUITS AND
VEGETABLES, ESPECIALLY IN THE RAW STATE.

CARBOHYDRATES

NUTRITIONISTS OFTEN REFER TO CARBOHYDRATES AS REFINED (SUGAR, WHITE FLOUR, ETC.) AND COMPLEX (CARBOHYDRATES IN THE NATURAL STATE AS FOUND IN VEGETABLES, WHOLE GRAIN PRODUCTS, ETC.). FOODS WHICH ARE USUALLY HIGH IN REFINED CARBOHYDRATES ARE ICE CREAM, CANDY, WHITE FLOUR, CAKES, SOFT DRINKS, ETC. THE RATIO OF REFINED CARBOHYDRATES TO TOTAL CARBOHYDRATES SHOULD BE KEPT AS LOW AS POSSIBLE.

REFINED CARBOHYDRATES, IN EXCESSIVE QUANTITIES, MAY HAVE DRUG-LIKE ACTIVITY, CAUSE TOOTH DECAY, LOWER BLOOD SUGAR, CAUSE OVERWEIGHT AND TAKE THE PLACE OF IMPORTANT NUTRIENTS. THEY ARE ALSO SUSPECT IN A HOST OF OTHER DISORDERS. HOWEVER, THESE FOODS IN VERY SMALL QUANTITIES ARE NOT CONSIDERED TO BE HARMFUL AS LONG AS ALL OTHER NUTRITIONAL REQUIREMENTS ARE FULFILLED.

EVEN THOUGH EXPERTS HAVE NOT YET ESTABLISHED GUIDELINES FOR REFINED CARBOHYDRATES, AN INTAKE GREATER THAN 30% SUCH AS YOUR INTAKE OF 80% SEEMS TOO HIGH. IN FACT YOUR DAILY INTAKE IS EQUAL TO THE CALORIES FROM 43 TEASPOONS OF SUGAR. INCLUDING ALCOHOL, IT IS 54 TEASPOONS OF SUGAR DAILY ON AVERAGE.

EXPERTS RECOMMEND MODERATION IN CARBOHYDRATE CONSUMPTION FOR PEOPLE, SUCH AS YOURSELF, WHO SHOW A HISTORY OF DIABETES IN THEIR FAMILY. BE SURE AND FOLLOW THE DOCTORS ADVICE ON THIS TOPIC.

REFINED CARBOHYDRATES YOU
EAT AT LEAST ONCE PER WEEK

	SERVINGS/WEEK
SCOTCH,GIN,VODKA,ETC(1 OZ)	12
DRINK MIXERS,SWEET(8 OZ)	12
WHITE BREAD(1 SLICE)	14
ICE CREAM(½ CUP)	2
POTATO CHIPS(10)	1
COLA DRINK(12 OZ)	14
BEER(12 OZ)	3
DOUGHNUT,CUPCAKE(ONE, 1 OZ)	1
COOKIE(ONE,3INS, DIAM)	4
PIZZA(1SLICE,2.5 OZ)	2

II. UNDERSTANDING YOUR NEEDS
FOR VITAMINS, MINERALS
AND OTHER NUTRIENTS

LISTED IN THE TABLE BELOW ARE THE LATEST RECOM-
MENDED DAILY ALLOWANCES(RDA) SET FORTH ON CER-
TAIN NUTRIENTS BY THE UNITED STATES FOOD AND
DRUG ADMINISTRATION(FDA) IN 1976. ASTERISKS, AP-
PEARING IN THE RDA COLUMN ABOVE, MEAN THAT NO
RDA HAS YET BEEN ESTABLISHED FOR THAT NUTRIENT.
THE RDA REPRESENTS WHAT THE FDA CONSIDERS TO BE
AN ESTIMATED APPROXIMATE NEED FOR A HEALTHY POP-
ULATION.

THE RDA VALUES HAVE BEEN REVISED OVER THE YEARS
TO TRY TO KEEP ABREAST OF THE LATEST NUTRITIONAL
KNOWLEDGE. MANY NUTRITIONISTS RECOMMEND HIGHER
DAILY INTAKE FOR MANY OF THESE NUTRIENTS WHEN A
PERSON HAS NOT BEEN GETTING COMPLETE NUTRITION
ON A REGULAR BASIS. DIFFERENCES IN METABOLISM,
WEIGHT, LIFESTYLE AND OTHER FACTORS ALSO HAVE AN
EFFECT ON VITAMIN AND MINERAL REQUIREMENTS.
THEREFORE YOU MIGHT REQUIRE MORE OF SOME OF
THESE NUTRIENTS. THE RDA SHOULD ONLY SERVE AS A
YARDSTICK AGAINST WHICH YOUR DAILY NUTRITION MAY
BE CONTRASTED FOR ABOUT ONE HALF OF THE KNOWN
ESSENTIAL NUTRIENTS. REMEMBER, A VERY LARGE EX-
CESS OF FAT SOLUBLE VITAMINS, LIKE VITAMIN A,
MAY CAUSE TOXICITY EFFECTS.

THERE ARE SEVERAL CIRCUMSTANCES WHICH MAY
GREATLY ELEVATE THE NEED FOR ONE OR MORE OF
THESE OR OTHER ESSENTIAL NUTRIENTS. SOME OF
THESE CIRCUMSTANCES ARE:

1. ENVIRONMENTAL FACTORS—AIR POLLUTION, ALCOHOL
INTAKE, CIGARETTE SMOKING, STRESS, POLLUTED
WATER, FOOD CONTAMINANTS, TAKING BIRTH CONTROL
PILLS, ETC., ARE BUT A FEW ENVIRONMENTAL FACTORS
THAT CAN GREATLY CHANGE AND/OR ELEVATE MANY OF
YOUR NUTRITIONAL REQUIREMENTS.

2. DECLINE IN FOOD QUALITY—THE NUTRITIONAL
QUALITY OF FOOD HAS DECLINED SUBSTANTIALLY IN
THIS CENTURY, WITH THE ADVENT OF WHITE FLOUR,
REFINED SUGAR AND EXTRACTED OILS, ACCORDING TO
DR. H. ROSENBERG M.D., AND A.N. FELDZAMEN, PH.D.
WRITING IN THEIR TEXT, THE DOCTORS BOOK OF VITA-
MIN THERAPY.

WHITE FLOUR WAS FIRST PRODUCED TO PREVENT SPOIL-AGE AND INCREASE SHELF LIFE WITHOUT REALIZING THE NUTRITIONAL RAMIFICATIONS. YEARS LATER, ALARMED BY THE SAD STATE OF OUR NATIONAL HEALTH, THE GOVERNMENT INSTITUTED A MANDATORY ENRICHMENT PROGRAM FOR THE FLOUR USED IN BREAD. REFINING FLOUR REMOVES AT LEAST 22 KNOWN NUTRIENTS IN-CLUDING VITAMIN E AND MOST OF THE B COMPLEX VITAMINS AS WELL AS IMPORTANT OILS AND MINERALS. ENRICHMENT, ON THE OTHER HAND, REPLACES ONLY FOUR NUTRIENTS: VITAMIN B1(THIAMINE), VITAMIN B2(RIBOFLAVIN), VITAMIN B3(NIACIN) AND IRON.

CONSUMPTION OF LARGE QUANTITIES OF REFINED FOODS CAN SUBSTANTIALLY INCREASE THE NEED FOR MANY ES-SENTIAL NUTRIENTS TO MAINTAIN HEALTH. OBVIOUSLY, WHOLE GRAIN PRODUCTS SHOULD BE EATEN IN PREFER-ENCE TO ONES MADE OF REFINED FLOUR AND FRESH VEGETABLES SHOULD BE USED INSTEAD OF CANNED ONES. NOTE THAT WHOLE GRAIN PRODUCTS HAVE A SHORTER SHELF LIFE AND CAN BE MORE HARMFUL WHEN STALE OR RANCID THAN PRODUCTS MADE FROM REFINED FLOUR, SO BE SURE THEY ARE FRESH BEFORE YOU EAT THEM.

3. ATTAINMENT OF YOUR BEST STATE OF HEALTH
TO ATTAIN YOUR BEST POSSIBLE STATE OF HEALTH FREQUENTLY REQUIRES HIGHER LEVELS THAN THE RDA VALUES FOR SEVERAL NUTRIENTS, ESPECIALLY AFTER AN ILLNESS, AN EXTENDED PERIOD OF STRESS OR FOR PHYSICALLY VERY ACTIVE PEOPLE.

THE VITAMIN QUESTION IS FAR FROM BEING COM-PLETELY RESOLVED. WHILE SOME NUTRITIONISTS FEEL A BALANCED DIET WILL SUPPLY ALL THE VITAMINS AND MINERALS NEEDED, OTHERS LIKE PROF. CHERASKIN CHAIRMAN OF THE DEPARTMENT OF ORAL MEDICINE AT ALABAMA SCHOOL OF MEDICINE, TELL US OUR NEEDS MIGHT BE MUCH HIGHER. PROF. CHERASKIN, RECENTLY CONDUCTED A STUDY ON HUMANS AND CONCLUDED THAT THE AMOUNTS OF VITAMIN A, C AND NIACIN NEEDED BY THE AVERAGE PERSON FOR BEST HEALTH MAY BE 4 TO 6 TIMES THE RDA (MEETING OF THE INTERNATIONAL ACADEMY OF PREVENTIVE MEDICINE, LOS ANGELES, SEPTEMBER 1975).

III. YOUR FOOD VITAMIN AND MINERAL CONTENT VERSUS RDA

(DAILY INTAKE BELOW DOES NOT INCLUDE
VITAMIN/MINERAL SUPPLEMENTS)

VITAMINS	DAILY INTAKE	U.S. RDA	PCT OF RDA	CURRENTLY TAKES THIS VITAMIN
VITAMIN A				
(INT UNITS)	11407.0	5000.0	228.1	YES
VITAMIN C(MGS)	34.0	60.0	56.7	YES
VITAMIN E				
(INT UNITS)	4.7	30.0	15.6	NO
VITAMIN B1(MGS)				
THIAMINE	0.4	1.5	29.0	NO
VITAMIN B2(MGS)				
RIBOFLAVIN	1.2	1.7	72.1	NO
VITAMIN B3(MGS)				
NIACIN	21.1	20.0	105.6	NO
VITAMIN B6(MGS)				
PYRIDOXINE	1.0	2.0	49.5	NO
FOLACIN(MCGS)				
FOLIC ACID	91.0	400.0	23.0	NO
VITAMIN B12(MCG)	9.0	6.0	150.8	NO
PANTOTHENIC				
ACID(MGS)	4.5	10.0	45.2	NO
BIOTIN(MCGS)	38.7	300.0	12.9	NO
CHOLINE(MGS)	388.0	*****	*****	—
INOSITOL(MGS)	149.0	*****	*****	—

MINERALS	DAILY INTAKE	U.S. RDA	PCT OF RDA	CURRENTLY TAKES THIS MINERAL
CALCIUM(MGS)	629.0	1000.0	62.9	NO
PHOSPHORUS(MGS)	1848.0	1000.0	184.9	NO
**CALCIUM AND PHOSPHORUS ARE OUT OF BALANCE.				
MAGNESIUM(MGS)	98.0	400.0	24.7	NO
IRON(MGS)	12.4	18.0	68.9	NO
COPPER(MGS)	0.3	2.0	13.3	NO
ZINC(MGS)	8.4	15.0	55.7	NO
IODINE(MCGS)				
IN FOOD ONLY	11.0	150.0	7.9	NO
MANGANESE(MGS)	0.3	*****		

```
POTASSIUM(MGS)     1879    * * * * * * * * * * *
SODIUM(MGS)
  IN FOOD ONLY     3434    * * * * * * * * * * *
FLUORINE(MCG)       520    * * * * * * * * * * *
```

IODINE CONCENTRATION IN FOODS VARIES WIDELY DE-
PENDING ON THEIR ORIGIN. WE HAVE BEEN CONSERVA-
TIVE IN ESTABLISHING YOUR INTAKE FROM FOODS. IT
IS IMPORTANT TO PROVIDE SOME DIETARY INSURANCE
AGAINST A POSSIBLE DEFICIENCY BY USING KELP OR
BY USING IODIZED SALT SPARINGLY.

** YOUR DIETARY INTAKE OF PHOSPHORUS IS MORE
THAN TWICE THAT OF CALCIUM WHICH CAN LEAD TO
MINERAL LOSS, MUSCLE SPASMS, AND EVEN HYPERPARA-
THYROIDISM.

SINCE YOUR CALCIUM INTAKE IS BELOW THE RECOM-
MENDED DAILY ALLOWANCE, CONSIDER INCREASING YOUR
INTAKE OF FOODS RICHER IN CALCIUM THAN PHOSPHO-
RUS SUCH AS SWISS CHEESE, CHEDDAR CHEESE, AMERI-
CAN CHEESE, MILK(PREFERABLY NON-FAT MILK), KALE,
MUSTARD OR DANDELION GREENS AND WATERCRESS.

PHOSPHORUS INTAKE SHOULD BE REDUCED. THE FOODS
CONTAINING LARGE AMOUNTS OF PHOSPHORUS AND LIT-
TLE OR NO CALCIUM ARE GRAINS AND MEATS.

NOTE: INCREASED PHYSICAL ACTIVITY ALSO SLIGHTLY
INCREASES YOUR VITAMIN AND MINERAL NEEDS.

IV. YOUR VITAMINS / MINERALS
BELOW THE RDA

YOUR DIETARY INTAKE OF THE FOLLOWING NUTRIENTS
IS BELOW THE RDA, HOWEVER, YOU ARE SUPPLEMENTING
THESE NUTRIENTS. SUPPLEMENTS CAN BE A FORM OF
DIETARY INSURANCE BUT YOU SHOULD FIX YOUR DIET
SO IT PROVIDES ADEQUATE AMOUNTS OF THESE ESSEN-
TIAL NUTRIENTS FROM FOODS. TO HELP YOU BOLSTER
THOSE NUTRIENTS IN YOUR DIET THAT ARE BELOW THE
RDA, RICH FOOD SOURCES HAVE BEEN LISTED BELOW.

IF YOU HAVE ANY FOOD ALLERGIES OR OTHER NUTRI-
TION-RELATED DISORDERS, YOU MIGHT WANT TO CHECK
WITH YOUR DOCTOR BEFORE USING ANY NEW FOODS IN
YOUR DIET.

GOOD FOOD SOURCES

NUTRIENT
BELOW RDA

VITAMIN C   BRUSSEL SPROUTS, BROCCOLI,
CANTALOUPE, STRAWBERRIES, GREEN
VEGETABLES, AND CITRUS FRUIT OR
JUICE

ADDING IODIZED SALT TO FOOD, AS YOU DO, PROVIDES
INSURANCE AGAINST A DEFICIENCY OF IODINE.

YOUR DIETARY INTAKE OF THE FOLLOWING NUTRIENTS
IS BELOW THE RDA AND YOU HAVE NOT INDICATED YOU
ARE TAKING FOOD SUPPLEMENTS WHICH COULD COMPEN-
SATE FOR THESE NEEDS. CONTINUED LONG TERM INTAKE
BELOW THE RDA MAY LEAD TO ILLNESSES. BE SURE TO
WORK AT BOLSTERING YOUR INTAKE OF THESE NUTRI-
ENTS. STUDY THE TABLE BELOW AND THE CORRESPOND-
ING LIST OF FOODS RICH IN THAT NUTRIENT.

REMEMBER, IF YOU HAVE ANY FOOD ALLERGIES OR
OTHER NUTRITION-RELATED DISORDERS, YOU MIGHT
WANT TO CHECK WITH YOUR DOCTOR BEFORE USING ANY
NEW FOODS IN YOUR DIET.

GOOD FOOD SOURCES

NUTRIENT
BELOW RDA

VITAMIN E   SUNFLOWER SEED OIL, WHEAT GERM OIL,
WHEAT GERM
VITAMIN B1   BREWERS YEAST, SPLIT PEAS,
SUNFLOWER SEEDS
VITAMIN B2   LIVER, ORGAN MEATS, MUSHROOMS,
MILK(PREFERABLY NON-HOMOGENIZED),
BREWERS YEAST
VITAMIN B6   BREWERS YEAST, MOLASSES, SALMON,
LIVER, WHEAT BRAN
FOLIC ACID   LIVER, LIMA BEANS, CANTALOUPE,
CHICKEN, BEEF, WHOLE WHEAT BREAD,
ASPARAGUS, BREWERS YEAST
PANTOTHENIC
  ACID   ORGAN MEATS, EGGS, PEANUTS, WHEAT
BRAN, WHEAT GERM, MUSHROOMS,
BROCCOLI, BEEF AND BREWERS YEAST
BIOTIN   ORGAN MEATS, PEANUTS, EGGS,
CAULIFLOWER, MUSHROOMS, AND
MOLASSES

```
CALCIUM AND
  PHOSPHORUS   ARE PLENTIFUL AND IN GOOD BALANCE
               IN MILK(PREFERABLY
               NON-HOMOGENIZED), CHEESE, DARK
               GREEN LEAFY VEGETABLES
MAGNESIUM      WHEAT GERM, ALMONDS, PEANUTS, GREEN
               VEGETABLES, EGGS, BRAN(IN SMALL
               AMTS, LARGE AMTS CAN INCREASE
               CALCIUM REQD)
IRON           LIVER, MEATS, EGGS, LENTILS,
               MUSHROOMS, SUNFLOWER SEEDS
COPPER         OYSTERS, LIVER, WHOLE WHEAT, OATS,
               DRY BEANS, AVOCADO, MOLASSES AND
               APRICOTS
ZINC           OYSTERS, HERRING, OATMEAL,
               SUNFLOWER AND PUMPKIN SEEDS,
               BREWERS YEAST, LIVER, EGGS
```

WHILE THERE ARE MANY OTHER FOODS WHICH MAY BE
GOOD OR EVEN BETTER DIETARY SOURCES OF ONE OR
MORE ISOLATED NUTRIENTS, WE HAVE ATTEMPTED TO
SELECT FOODS WHICH ARE READILY AVAILABLE, BAL-
ANCED WITH RESPECT TO OTHER NUTRIENTS, FREE FROM
SPECIAL PREPARATION REQUIREMENTS AND HAVE A REA-
SONABLE STORAGE LIFE.

YOU MAY ALSO WISH TO TAKE A GOOD VITAMIN AND
MINERAL SUPPLEMENT TO BOLSTER THESE NUTRIENTS.
IF SO, BE SURE TO DISCUSS THE QUANTITIES WITH
YOUR DOCTOR.

V. FURTHER NUTRITIONAL CONSIDERATIONS

AN INTAKE OF 1 OR 2 CUPS OF COFFEE AND OR TEA
PER DAY OR EVEN LESS IS ADVISED BY EXPERTS. TEN-
TATIVE RESEARCH FINDINGS HAVE LINKED CAFFEINE TO
SEVERAL DISORDERS. CONSIDER REDUCING YOUR INTAKE
OF 70 CUPS PER WEEK(PROFESSOR JEAN MAYER, HAR-
VARD, LOS ANGELES TIMES, JUNE 10, 1976).

ONE THIRD OR MORE OF YOUR MEALS ARE EATEN AWAY
FROM HOME OR ARE CONVENIENCE FOODS. THE FRESH-
NESS AND NUTRITIONAL QUALITY OF THESE FOODS IS
NOT COMPARABLE TO THAT OF A FRESHLY PREPARED
MEAL AT HOME. IF YOU MUST EAT OUT FREQUENTLY, OR
REALLY HATE TO COOK, TRY TO FIND RESTAURANTS

THAT SERVE FRESH RAW VEGETABLES AND/OR BEGIN TO
FIX THEM YOURSELF. IT TAKES LESS TIME THAN COOK-
ING AND PROVIDES MANY NUTRIENTS VITAL TO YOUR
HEALTH AND WELL BEING.

O PERCENT OF YOUR VEGETABLES ARE CONSUMED IN THE
FRESH, RAW STATE. USING FRESH RAW VEGETABLES IN-
CREASES ROUGHAGE AND PROMOTES HEALTHY ELIMINA-
TION OF WASTE PRODUCTS (SEE DISCUSSION OF FIBERS
ABOVE).

95 PERCENT OF THE FRUIT YOU CONSUME IS FRESH
WHICH IS IMPORTANT SINCE LARGE AMOUNTS OF SUGAR
HAVE BEEN ADDED TO CANNED AND FROZEN FRUIT. KEEP
IT UP.

DRINKING TAP WATER, AS YOU DO, MAY BE A HEALTH
HAZARD. IMPURITIES IN TAP WATER ARE UNDER INVES-
TIGATION AS POSSIBLE CONTRIBUTING FACTORS TOWARD
CANCER AND HEART DISEASE. EVEN THOUGH THIS IS
NOT 100% ESTABLISHED, SOME CAUTION SEEMS ADVISA-
BLE. CONSIDER PURCHASING GOOD WELL WATER OR AT-
TACHING A FILTER TO YOUR WATER FAUCET.

IT IS IMPORTANT TO BE SURE YOU GET AN ADEQUATE
SUPPLY OF IODINE DAILY. THIS CAN EASILY BE AC-
COMPLISHED THROUGH SPARING USE OF IODIZED SALT.
BE SURE TO USE SALT IN MODERATION SINCE TOO MUCH
CAN CAUSE HIGH BLOOD PRESSURE AND OTHER PROB-
LEMS.

VI. OTHER CRITICAL HEALTH FACTORS

NUTRITION IS IMPORTANT BUT IT ALONE IS NOT
ENOUGH TO ACHIEVE A HEALTHIER AND LONGER LIFE;
SEVERAL GOOD HEALTH HABITS MUST BE CONSIDERED.
AT THE UCLA SCHOOL OF PUBLIC HEALTH SEVEN GOOD
HEALTH HABITS WERE STUDIED WITH RESPECT TO AVER-
AGE LIFE SPANS AND IT WAS FOUND THAT THERE COULD
BE A DIFFERENCE OF AT LEAST 12.5 YEARS BETWEEN
DOING THINGS RIGHT OR WRONG.

WHEN APPROXIMATELY THE SAME 7 MAJOR GOOD HEALTH
HABITS WERE INVESTIGATED IN ANOTHER STUDY, IT
WAS FOUND THAT ONLY ABOUT 3 TO 5% OF ALL PEOPLE
CAME REASONABLY CLOSE TO DOING THINGS RIGHT IN

ALL THESE MAJOR HEALTH HABITS (H. KUGLER, PH.D.,
MEETING OF THE INTERNATIONAL ACADEMY OF PREVEN-
TIVE MEDICINE, DENVER, MARCH 1976).

TO PROTECT YOUR HEALTH, A CHECK UP AT LEAST ONCE
A YEAR IS ADVISABLE. BE SURE TO HAVE YOUR BLOOD
SERUM CHOLESTEROL AND TRIGLYCERIDES TESTED, AS
DISCUSSED ABOVE IN THE SECTION ON FATS. RECORD
THESE VALUES TOGETHER WITH YOUR BLOOD PRESSURE
EACH TIME YOU HAVE THEM MEASURED. WATCH FOR ANY
CHANGES THAT MAY OCCUR. SHOULD THERE BE A
CHANGE, BE SURE TO DISCUSS IT WITH YOUR DOCTOR.

IT IS ALSO IMPORTANT TO HAVE REGULAR DENTAL
CHECKUPS EVERY SIX MONTHS OR AT LEAST ONCE PER
YEAR.

STRESS CAN ADVERSELY AFFECT YOUR HEALTH AND YOUR
DAILY LIFE. HOWEVER, YOU CAN LEARN TO DEAL WITH
IT MORE EFFECTIVELY THROUGH CONSULTATION AND IM-
PROVED NUTRITION.

DISCUSS YOUR WORK STRESS SITUATION WITH YOUR
FELLOW WORKERS. ANALYZE THE SITUATION CAREFULLY
AND TRY TO RESOLVE IT.

IT IS VERY IMPORTANT TO BE AWARE OF THE ADVERSE
EFFECTS OF STRESS ON YOUR HEALTH AND LIFE. IF
YOU CAN NOT RESOLVE YOUR STRESS SITUATION OR
WOULD LIKE TO KNOW MORE ABOUT THIS SUBJECT,
THERE IS AN EXCELLENT PAPERBACK BOOK BY THE AU-
THORITY ON STRESS, DR. HANS SELYE, CALLED STRESS
WITHOUT DISTRESS.

SINCE THERE IS A HISTORY OF HEART DISEASE IN
YOUR FAMILY, IT IS VERY IMPORTANT TO CORRECT
FAULTY HEALTH HABITS, INCLUDING ENVIRONMENTAL
FACTORS. THESE ASPECTS OF LIFE ARE BELIEVED TO
BE MAJOR CONTRIBUTORS TO CANCER AND HEART DIS-
EASE.

SMOKING CIGARETTES, AS YOU DO, IS CONSIDERED, BY
MOST EXPERTS, TO HAVE A VERY HIGH RISK OF TRIG-
GERING CANCER OR HEART DISEASE. FURTHER, IT HAS
BEEN ASSOCIATED WITH PREMATURE AGING, I. E., IN-
CREASED WRINKLE FORMATION AND, IN SOME CASES,
IMPOTENCE IN MEN DUE TO THE POTENTIAL HORMONE
LOWERING EFFECT. FOR YOUR LONG TERM HEALTH AND
WELL BEING, IT IS OF GREAT IMPORTANCE TO STOP
SMOKING. IF YOU TRY OR HAVE TRIED AND HAVE DIF-

FICULTY STOPPING, SEEK OUT ONE OF THE SEVERAL
ORGANIZATIONS THAT HELP PEOPLE BREAK THE HABIT.

THE EFFECT OF AIR POLLUTION IS WELL ESTABLISHED.
IT CONTRIBUTES TO CANCER, HEART DISEASE AND EM-
PHYSEMA. CONSIDER INSTALLING AIR PURIFIERS WHERE
THE POLLUTION IS VERY HIGH TO PROTECT YOURSELF.

LACK OF MONEY HAS PROVEN TO BE A MAJOR OBSTACLE
IN THE SUCCESSFUL AGING OF THE AVERAGE AMERICAN.
LOOK INTO SETTING UP AN INDEPENDENT RETIREMENT
ACCOUNT TO BE SURE YOU DO NOT FACE YOUR ADVANCED
YEARS WITH FINANCIAL PRESSURE.

IMPROVED HEALTH HABITS OF NUTRITION AND EXERCISE
MAY SIGNIFICANTLY IMPROVE YOUR PHYSICAL WELL
BEING AND YOUR MOOD TOO.

THE ROLE OF FOOD, EXERCISE AND OTHER KEY HEALTH
FACTORS IS EXPLAINED IN MORE DETAIL BY DR. KU-
GLER IN HIS NEW BOOK—DR KUGLERS SEVEN KEYS TO A
LONGER LIFE.

VII. THE IMPORTANCE OF EXERCISE

YOU CONSUME 3230 CALORIES DAILY, ON AVERAGE.
CALORIES, AS YOU MAY KNOW, ARE A MEASURE OF EN-
ERGY. FOODS PROVIDE THIS ENERGY WHICH THE BODY
BURNS THROUGH PERFORMANCE OF ROUTINE TASKS AND
ESPECIALLY THROUGH VIGOROUS EXERCISE. BY DE-
CREASING CALORIC INTAKE AND ALSO INCREASING
PHYSICAL ACTIVITIES, THE BODY CAN SHED UNWANTED
EXTRA POUNDS. IN FACT, IF SUGAR OR REFINED CAR-
BOHYDRATE INTAKE WERE REDUCED 1 TABLESPOONFUL
PER DAY AND FAT INTAKE ALSO REDUCED 1 TABLE-
SPOONFUL, YOU COULD LOSE APPROXIMATELY A HALF
POUND PER WEEK.

EXPERTS HAVE SHOWN REGULAR EXERCISE TO BE A KEY
LINK TO LONGEVITY AND ESSENTIAL TO THE ATTAIN-
MENT OF YOUR BEST POSSIBLE STATE OF HEALTH. SO,
IT MAKES SENSE, IN PLANNING ANY WEIGHT REDUCTION
PROGRAM TO COUPLE A REGULAR EXERCISE REGIMEN
WITH CALORIC FOOD RESTRICTIONS.

NO RECOMMENDED LEVEL OF CALORIC INTAKE IS PRO-
VIDED SINCE YOUR INDIVIDUAL REQUIREMENTS DEPEND
ON FACTORS SUCH AS STRESS, ENVIRONMENT, UNIQUE
BIOCHEMICAL NEEDS, ETC. FURTHER, IT IS NOT USU-
ALLY ADVISABLE THAT ANYONE TRY TO LOSE MORE THAN
2 POUNDS PER WEEK OR LOWER THEIR CALORIC INTAKE
BELOW 1200 CALORIES PER DAY WITHOUT FIRST CON-
SULTING A DOCTOR.

YOUR CURRENT EXERCISES PLUS THE EXERCISES YOU
WANT TO ADD, IF ANY, ARE LISTED BELOW TOGETHER
WITH THEIR CORRESPONDING CALORIC EXPENDITURE IN-
FORMATION.

PHYSICAL ACTIVITIES

EXERCISE	CURRENT WEEKLY ACTIVITY IN MIN.	CALORIES BURNED IN 10 MIN. EXERCISE	CALORIC EXPENDITURE PER WEEK
1 JOGGING (OVER 8 MIN./MILE)	60	113	680
2 TENNIS, SINGLES	60	71	425
3 HANDBALL	0	129	0
4 WORKING OUT W. VARIED EQPT	0	50	0
		WEEKLY TOTAL	1105

VIII. SUGGESTED WEIGHT LOSS PROGRAM

A WEIGHT LOSS GOAL OF 1.4 POUNDS PER WEEK IS
SUGGESTED. AT THIS RATE, YOU SHOULD LOSE YOUR
UNWANTED 45 POUND(S) IN 32 WEEK(S), PROVIDED YOU
ARE A NORMALLY HEALTHY PERSON. REMEMBER THAT
3500 CALORIES LESS PER WEEK COMING FROM RE-
STRICTED FOOD INTAKE AND/OR INCREASED PHYSICAL
ACTIVITY WILL RESULT IN LOSING ONE MORE POUND
EACH WEEK.

YOUR GOAL CAN BE ACHIEVED THROUGH CALORIC RE-
STRICTION AND INCREASED PHYSICAL ACTIVITY EQUAL
TO A TOTAL OF 4886 CALORIES PER WEEK.

EATING HALF AS MUCH OF THE REFINED CARBOHYDRATE
FOODS LISTED IN THE TABLE BELOW WILL CONTRIBUTE
3263 CALORIES TO YOUR TOTAL WEEKLY GOAL. THE
BALANCE OF 1623 CALORIES MUST BE BURNED UP BY
YOUR EXERCISE PROGRAM. ONE SUCH PROGRAM IS PRE-
SENTED IN THE SUGGESTED PHYSICAL ACTIVITIES
TABLE DISPLAYED FOLLOWING THE FOODS TABLE.

	FOODS FOR YOU TO AVOID	NO. OF SERVINGS YOU NOW EAT PER WEEK	CALORIES SAVED IF YOU EAT HALF AS MUCH
1	SCOTCH, GIN, VODKA, ETC(1 OZ)	12	420
2	COLA DRINK(12 OZ)	14	959
3	DRINK MIXERS, SWEET(8 OZ)	12	420
4	BEER(12 OZ)	3	257
5	WHITE BREAD (1 SLICE)	14	427
6	DOUGHNUT, CUPCAKE(ONE, 1 OZ)	1	68
7	ICE CREAM(½ CUP)	2	150
8	COOKIE (ONE, 3INS, DIAM)	4	288
9	POTATO CHIPS(10)	1	64
10	PIZZA (1 SLICE,2.5 OZ)	2	210
		WEEKLY TOTAL	3263

SUGGESTED PHYSICAL ACTIVITIES PROGRAM

	EXERCISE	INCREASE IN WEEKLY ACTIVITY (MIN.)	INCREASE IN CALORIC EXPENDITURE (CALORIES)
1	JOGGING (OVER 8 MIN./MILE)	30	339
2	TENNIS, SINGLES	30	210
3	HANDBALL	60	774
4	WORKING OUT W. VARIED EQPT	60	300
	WEEKLY TOTALS:	180	1623

THIS PROGRAM MAY NOT BE PRACTICAL. INSTEAD YOU MAY
PREFER TO DO MORE OF SOME EXERCISES AND LESS OF

OTHERS. BE SURE THE TOTAL CALORIES BURNED FROM
INCREASED EXERCISE IS AT LEAST 1623 OR MORE SO YOU
CAN ACHIEVE YOUR WEIGHT LOSS GOAL OF 1.4 POUNDS
PER WEEK. THE CALORIC EXPENDITURE INFORMATION,
PROVIDED IN THE PHYSICAL ACTIVITIES TABLE
ABOVE, HAS BEEN PREPARED TO SERVE AS AN AID IN
COMPUTING THE NEEDED ADDITIONAL MINUTES IF YOU
CHOOSE TO BUILD A PLAN OF YOUR OWN DESIGN.

YOU CAN AID YOUR CALORIC RESTRICTION BY CONSUM-
ING NEGATIVE CALORIE FOODS INSTEAD OF REFINED
CARBOHYDRATE AND ANIMAL FAT. IN THE PROCESS OF
DIGESTING THE NEGATIVE CALORIE VEGETABLES AND
FRUITS LISTED BELOW, THE BODY USES AN EQUAL OR
GREATER AMOUNT OF CALORIES THAN THEY CONTAIN.
THE VEGETABLES(STEAMED OR EATEN RAW) ARE: BROC-
COLI, BEAN SPROUTS, BEETS, CELERY, CARROTS, AS-
PARAGUS, CUCUMBERS, EGGPLANT, LETTUCE, MUSH-
ROOMS, GREEN PEPPER, SUMMER SQUASH AND TOMATOES.
THE FRUITS ARE: GRAPEFRUIT, STRAWBERRIES, HONEY-
DEW, CANTALOUPE AND WATERMELON.

WEIGHT CONTROL AND/OR MAINTAINING CARDIOVASCULAR
FITNESS SHOULD BE EVERYONES GOAL. A GOOD PAPER-
BACK BOOK ON THE SUBJECT IS THE NEW AEROBICS BY
KENNETH COOPER M.D. ANOTHER GOOD TEXT IS ACTE-
VITICS BY CHARLES T. KUNTZLEMAN. REMEMBER THAT
ANY EXERCISE PROGRAM SHOULD BE STARTED SLOWLY
AND CAREFULLY. OFTEN, PEOPLE OVER-DO THE FIRST
FEW DAYS OF EXERCISE WHICH CAN BE HARMFUL.

IF YOU ARE A MEMBER OF A HEALTH CLUB, BE SURE TO
FOLLOW THE INSTRUCTORS ADVICE. AFTER YOU HAVE
BUILT UP TO A CERTAIN LEVEL OF EXERCISE, YOUR
EXERCISE SHOULD BE VIGOROUS. IT SHOULD BE DONE
AT LEAST 3 TIMES PER WEEK AND FOR A MINIMUM OF
30 MINUTES AT A STRETCH.

IX. CONCLUSIONS

OF ALL THE FACTORS CONSIDERED IN YOUR PROFILE,
THE MOST CRITICAL PROBLEM AREAS ARE SUMMARIZED
BELOW IN ORDER OF IMPORTANCE:

1 STOP SMOKING.
2 REDUCE YOUR PERCENT CALORIES FROM FAT TO
   HELP PROTECT YOU FROM CANCER AND POSSIBLE
   HEART DISEASE.

3 INCREASE YOUR INTAKE OF ALL VITAMINS AND
  MINERALS BELOW THE RDA SEE PAGE 6.
4 CORRECT YOUR CALCIUM/PHOSPHOROUS IMBALANCE
  SEE PAGE 5.
5 EATING LESS REFINED CARBOHYDRATES AND MORE
  VEGETABLES AND WHOLE GRAINS IS ESPECIALLY
  IMPORTANT DUE TO YOUR FAMILY HISTORY OF
  DIABETES SEE PAGE 3.
6 CORRECT YOUR STRESS SITUATIONS.
7 REDUCE YOUR INTAKE OF REGULAR COFFEE AND
  OR TEA.

THIS CONCLUDES YOUR NUTRITION, HEALTH AND ACTIV-
ITY PROFILE. WE ENJOYED HAVING THE OPPORTUNITY
OF BRINGING YOU THE LATEST DIETARY AND LIFESTYLE
FINDINGS THAT PERTAIN TO YOU. IT WOULD BE A GOOD
IDEA FOR YOU TO RETAKE THIS TEST AGAIN IN 3 TO 6
MONTHS SO WE CAN APPRAISE THE CHANGES YOU MAY
MAKE BETWEEN NOW AND THEN. KEEP IN MIND THAT
THIS TEST WILL BE REVISED TO INCORPORATE NEW IN-
FORMATION AND WILL REMAIN AN UP TO THE MINUTE
MEDIUM OF LIFESTYLE EVALUATION.

IN PARTING, WE HAVE THREE FINAL NOTES OF **CAUT-
ION**:

1. THIS PROGRAM IS DESIGNED TO BE EDUCATIONAL,
TO POINT OUT RISK FACTORS, TO TEACH GOOD HEALTH
HABITS AND NUTRITION AND IS NOT MEANT TO DETECT
MEDICAL DISORDERS OR DISEASES.

2. REMEMBER YOUR ANALYSIS WAS BASED ON STANDARDS
FOR NORMAL HEALTHY PEOPLE OF YOUR AGE AND MAY
NOT APPLY IN SOME INSTANCES, ESPECIALLY WHEN A
MEDICAL CONDITION SUCH AS HEART DISEASE, ULCERS,
ETC. IS PRESENT. SEE YOUR DOCTOR TO DETERMINE IF
YOU MAY HAVE A MEDICAL CONDITION DIFFERENTIATING
YOU FROM THE NORMAL HEALTHY INDIVIDUAL.

3. THROUGHOUT THIS EVALUATION OF YOUR LIFESTYLE,
SUGGESTIONS FOR SUPPLEMENTAL READING HAVE BEEN
MADE. WE FEEL, OVERALL, THAT EACH OF THE RECOM-
MENDATIONS ARE VERY WORTHWHILE. HOWEVER, WE DO
NOT NECESSARILY ENDORSE ALL THEIR CONTENTS.

FOOD INTAKE AMINO ACID COMPOSITION IS LISTED
BELOW FOR REFERENCE ONLY, SINCE SOME DOCTORS RE-
QUIRE THIS INFORMATION.

AMINO ACID COMPOSITION
(IN MILLIGRAMS,MGS APPROXIMATE)

AMINO ACID	YOUR INTAKE	AMINO ACID	YOUR INTAKE
ARGININE	5968	HISTIDINE	2459
THREONINE	4467	VALINE	5544
LEUCINE	8374	ISOLEUCINE	5241
LYSINE	6917	METHIONINE	2718
PHENYLALANINE	4688	TRYPTOPHAN	1156

NUTRITION, HEALTH, AND ACTIVITY PROFILE
OF MR AMERICAN ANY STREET

X. DOCTORS
    SUMMARY OF 7/16/78   AGE 38; WT 240; SEX M

(SEE TEXT FOR EXPLANATION)	DAILY INTAKE	RECOMMENDED INTAKE
		24740
WEEKLY EXERCISE CALORIES 1105		
TOTAL CALORIES	3230	
PROTEIN(GRAMS)	95.6	109.1 ; 68.6 TO 87.0
FAT(GRAMS	191.9	
CALORIES FROM FAT	1727	
PCT CALORIES FROM FAT	53.5	20% TO 34%
LINOLEIC ACID(GRAMS)	9.5	3 TO 5
FIBER(GRAMS)	2.5	6
CARBOHYDRATES (GRAMS)	198.4	(CALORIES 896; PCT CALORIES 28)
REFINED(GRAMS)	159.0	(EQUALS 43 TSPS SUGAR)
PCT REFINED	80	(INCLUDING ALCOHOL 83 PCT)

REGULAR COFFEE / TEA 70 CUPS/WK

VITAMINS	DAILY INTAKE	U.S. RDA	PCT OF RDA	CURRENTLY TAKES THIS VITAMIN
VITAMIN A (INT UNITS)	11407.0	5000.0	228.1	YES
VITAMIN C(MGS)	34.0	60.0	56.7	YES
VITAMIN E (INT UNITS)	4.7	30.0	15.6	NO
VITAMIN B1(MGS) THIAMINE	0.4	1.5	29.0	NO
VITAMIN B2(MGS) RIBOFLAVIN	1.2	1.7	72.1	NO
VITAMIN B3(MGS) NIACIN	21.1	20.0	105.6	NO
VITAMIN B6(MGS) PYRIDOXINE	1.0	2.0	49.5	NO
FOLACIN(MCGS) FOLIC ACID	91.0	400.0	23.0	NO
VITAMIN B12(MCGS)	9.0	6.0	150.8	NO
PANTOTHENIC ACID(MGS)	4.5	10.0	45.2	NO
BIOTIN(MCGS)	38.7	300.0	12.9	NO
CHOLINE(MGS)	388.0	*****	******	
INOSITOL(MGS)	149.0	*****	******	

MINERALS	DAILY INTAKE	U.S. RDA	PCT OF RDA	CURRENTLY TAKES THIS MINERAL
CALCIUM(MGS)	629.0	1000.0	62.9	NO
PHOSPHORUS(MGS)	1848.0	1000.0	184.9	NO

** CALCIUM AND PHOSPHORUS ARE OUT OF BALANCE.

	DAILY INTAKE	U.S. RDA	PCT OF RDA	
MAGNESIUM(MGS)	98.0	400.0	24.7	NO
IRON(MGS)	12.4	18.0	68.9	NO
COPPER(MGS)	0.3	2.0	13.3	NO
ZINC(MGS)	8.4	15.0	55.7	NO
IODINE(MCGS) IN FOOD ONLY	11.0	150.0	7.9	NO
MANGANESE(MGS)	0.3	*****	******	
POTASSIUM(MGS)	1879.0	*****	******	
SODIUM(MGS) IN FOOD ONLY	3434.0	*****	******	
FLUORINE(MCGS)	520.0	*****	******	

HAS TAKEN SUPPLEMENTS ABOVE MORE THAN 1 YEAR.

HEALTH FACTORS

1 DIABETES IN   2 HEART DISEASE   3 LIVES/WORKS IN
  FAMILY   IN FAMILY   POLLUTION
4 UNDER STRESS   5 PHYSICALLY   6 STAMINA POOR
                      SLUGGISH
7 SMOKES   8 NO RETIREMENT   9 DRINKS TAP
  CIGARETTES   SECURITY   WATER

Appendix B

Exercise Testing Facilities

Prepared by Juhani Seppa

(As coaches and athletes look for new tools to help them in their coaching and training, there has been an upsurge of interest in physiological testing and testing centers. All of the following medical health/physical training centers conduct electrocardiogram stress testing while the subject is running at various speeds on a treadmill. Reprinted by permission of the National Jogging Association, 1910 K Street, N.W., #202, Washington, D.C. Any additions or corrections should be sent to Mr. Seppa, c/o the NJA.) *Physician referral centers are indicated with *.*

ALABAMA

L. Thomas Sheffield, M.D.
Allison Laborabory of Exercise
    Electrophysiology
School of Medicine
The University of Alabama in
    Birmingham
Birmingham, Ala. 35233
(205)934-2274

ARIZONA

William J. Stone, Ph.D.
Research Lab., Dept of HPER
Arizona State University
Tempe, Az. 85281
(602)965-3647

ARKANSAS

Barry S. Brown, Ph.D.
Dept. of HPER

University of Arkansas
Fayetteville, Ar. 72701
(501)575-2859

Harry Olree, Ed.D.
Performance Physiology Lab.
Harding College
Searey, Ar. 72143
(501)268-6161

CALIFORNIA

Forrest Smith, M.D.
Total Health Medical Center
690 40th Street
Oakland, Ca. 94609
(415)655-8730

Fred Kasch, Ed. D.
Physical Fitness Research Lab.
San Diego State University
San Diego, Ca. 82115
(714)286-5560

William L. Haskell, Ph.D.
Division of Cardiology
Stanford University Medical
  School
Palo Alto, Ca.
(415)321-1200
X6256

Albert A. Kattus, M.D.
Division of Cardiology
The Ctr. of Health Sciences
  UCLA
Los Angeles, Ca. 90024
(213)525-5236

Ronald Selvester, M.D.
Rancho Los Amigos Hospital
7601 East Imperial Highway
Downey, Ca. 90242
(213)242-9535

Jack H. Wilmore, Ph.D.
Dept. of Physical Education

University of California
Davis, Ca.
(916)756-3115

Bruce H. McFadden, M.D.
Cardiovascular Medical Group,
  Inc.
5333 Hollister Ave.
Santa Barbara, Ca. 93105

Norman H. Mellor, M.D.
Cardiovascular Stress Test &
  Work Eval. Unit
Circle City Hospital
730 Old Magnolia Ave.
Corona, Ca. 91720
(714)735-1211

Koshore S. Ambe, M.D.
Health Enhancement Institute
Leisure World Medical Center
Paseo de la Valencia
Laguna Hills, Ca. 93561
(714)830-0350

Alan J. Rice, M.P.H.
Director, Health Ctr. Programs
St. Helena Hospital & Health
  Center
Deer Park, Ca. 94576
(707)963-3611

John L. Boyer, M.D.
California State University
Physical Fitness Research Lab.
San Diego, Ca.
(714)286-5560

John L. Boyer, M.D.
Thomas B. Rice, M.A.
Cardio-Pulmonary Rehabilitation
  Inst.
6501 Linda Vista Rd. POB 11284
San Diego, Ca. 92111
(714)298-5300

J. Douglas McNair, M.D.
Arcadia CPR Center
The Mutual Savings Bldg.

660 W. Duarte Road
Arcadia, Ca. 91006
(213)446-6607

Robert Oblath, M.D.
Burbank CPR Center
2727 W. Alameda Avenue
Burbank, Ca. 91505
(213)843-6595

Donald D. Mahoney, M.D.
Fullerton CPR Center
1937 Sunny Crest Drive
Fullerton, Ca. 92632
(714)870-9577

Robert Astone, M.D.
South Bay CPR Center
22352 Hawthorne Blvd.
Torrance, Ca. 90505
(213)373-6769

James Dooley, M.D.
Glendale CPR Center
1134 N. Brand Blvd.
Glendale, Ca. 91202
(213)247-5001

Morton Futterman, M.D.
Whittier CPR Center
9210 S. Colima Road
Whittier, Ca. 90605
(213)696-2800

George Griffith, M.D.
Wilshire Metropolitan CPR
  Center
1111 Wilshire Blvd., Suite 300
Los Angeles, Ca. 90017
(213)481-1410

COLORADO

L. Loring Brock, M.D.
Spalding Rehabilitation Ctr.
1919 Odgen Street
Denver, Colo.
(303)222-8951

CONNECTICUT

C. Goldenthal, M.D.
Alfredo F. Nino, M.D.
Cardiatrics, P.C.
132 Jefferson St.
Hartford, Ct. 06106
(203)249-7579*

DISTRICT OF COLUMBIA

Samuel M. Fox, M.D.
School of Medicine, Div. of
  Cardiology
George Washington University
2150 Pennsylvania Ave., N.W.
Washington, D.C. 20037
(202)331-6286

James R. Snyder, M.D.
Washington Cardiovascular
  Evaluation Center
916 19th St., 8th floor
Washington, D.C. 20006
(202)223-5015

FLORIDA

C.W. Zauner, Ph.D.
Research Laboratory
College of Phys. Ed.
University of Florida
Gainesville, Fl. 32601
(305)392-0584

Dr. Albert F. Robbins
Weight Control & Physical
  Fitness Medical Clinic
51 S.E. 3rd Street
Boca Raton, Fl. 33432
(305)395-3282

Hugh R. Gilmore III M.D.
The L.D. Pankey Institute for
  Advanced Dental Education

300 Biscayne Boulevard
  Way, Suite 304
Miami, Fl.
                  (305)371-8711

Elwyn Evans, M.D.
Central Florida CPR Center
500 E. Colonial Drive
Orlando, Fl. 32803
                  (305)843-5142

Edward St. Mary, M.D.
Mercy CPR Center
Professional Office Bldg.
Mercy Hospital
3661 S. Miami Ave., Suite 2
Miami, Fl. 33133
                  (305)854-0982

GEORGIA

Nanette K. Wegner, M.D.
Charles Gilbert, M.D.
Dept. of Cardiology
Emory Univ. School of Medicine
69 Butler St., S.E.
Atlanta, Ga. 30303
                  (404)623-4711

Frank H. Ramsey, Ph.D.
Dept. of Physical Education
Georgia Southern College
Statesboro, Ga. 30458
                  (912)764-6611

John D. Cantwell, M.D.
Preventive Cardiology Clinic
615 Peachtree St., N.E., Suite
  1100
Atlanta, Ga. 30308

Fred I. Allman, M.D.
Spts. Medicine Rehabilitation
  Clinic
77 E. Andrews Dr., No. 109
Atlanta, Ga. 30309

HAWAII

J.H. Scaff, Jr., M.D.
Cardiology Section
Honolulu Medical Grp.
1133 Punchbowl Street
Honolulu, Ha. 96813
                  (808)537-2211

ILLINOIS

Benjamin Massey, Ph.D.
Physical Fitness Research Lab.
305 Huff Gymnasium
University of Illinois
Champaign, Ill. 61820
                  (217)333-4932

Roland G. Knowiton, Ph.D.
Physical Ed. Research Lab
Southern Illinois University
Carbondale, Ill. 62801
                  (618)453-2575

Jeremiah Stamler, M.D.
Chicago Board of Health
Heart Disease Control Program
Chicago, Ill. 60602
                  (312)744-4281

INDIANA

David Costill, Ph.D.
Human Performance Lab.
Ball State University
Muncie, Ind. 47306
                  (317)289-1241

IOWA

C.V. Gisolfi, Ph.D.
Human Exercise Physiology Lab.
Dept. of Physical Education
University of Iowa
Iowa City, Iowa 52240
                  (319)353-2121

Neal Tremble, Ph.D.
Cardiovascular Fitness Clinic
Department of Physical
    Education
Drake University
Des Moines, Iowa 50311
                    (515)271-2866

KANSAS

Wayne H. Osness, Ph.D.
Department of Physical
    Education
University of Kansas
Lawrence, Ks. 66044
                    (913)864-2700

KENTUCKY

Pentti Teraslinna, Ph.D.
Dept. of HPER
University of Kentucky
Lexington, Ky. 40501
                    (606)258-8675

Jack Baker, Ed. D.
Human Performance Lab.
Murray State University
Murray, Ky. 42071
                    (502)753-8732

LOUISIANA

Robert W. Patton, Ph.D.
Northwestern State College
Natchitoches, La. 71457
                    (318)857-5461

MARYLAND

Drs. Segal, Silverberg, Ari &
    Waters
Cardiovascular Associates
5530 Wisconsin Ave.
Chevy Chase, Md. 20015
                    (301)656-9070

David Clarke, Ph.D.
Dept. of Physical Education
University of Maryland
College Park, Md. 20705

Donald Dembo, M.D.
Daniel Lindenstruth, M.D.
Mt. Vernon CPR Center
701 St. Paul Street
Mt. Vernon Bldg., Suite 413-414
Baltimore, Md. 21202
                    (301)539-6508

MASSACHUSETTS

Howard G. Knuttgen, Ph.D.
Dept. of Biology
Boston University
2 Cummington St.
Boston, Mass. 02215
                    (617)353-2477

Benjamin Ricci, Ph.D.
Laboratory of Applied
    Physiology
University of Massachusetts
Amherst, Mass. 01022
                    (413)545-2480

MICHIGAN

Merel L. Foss, Ph.D.
Physical Performance Research
    Lab.
University of Michigan
Ann Arbor, Mi. 48103

Ronald J. Stewart, D.O., P.C.
Practice of Internal Medicine
Cardiology
11474 15 Mile Road
Sterling Heights, Mi. 48077

John Faulkner, Ph.D.
Department of Physiology
School of Medicine
University of Michigan
Ann Arbor, Mi. 48104

Heart Station
Ingham Medical Hospital
401 W. Greenlawn
Lansing, Mi. 48910

J. Ardens, M.D.
Medical Square of Troy*
Suite D 14
1551 West Big Beaver Rd.
Troy, Mi. 48084
                    (313)643-7770

Jeffrey L. Roitman, M.D.
Richard B. Parr, M.D.
Gordon W. Schultz, M.D.
Central Michigan University
Mount Pleasant, Mi. 48858

MINNESOTA

Clem W. Thompson, Ph.D.
Physiology of Exercise Lab.
Mankato, Mn. 56001
                    (507)389-2463

MISSISSIPPI

Chief of Cardiology
St. Dominics Hospital
615 Medical Arts
Jackson, Ms. 39201
                    (601)352-3361

Harold B. Falls, Ph.D.
Kinetoenergetics Laboratory
Dept. of Health and Physical
    Education
Southwest Missouri State
    University
Springfield, Mo. 65802
                    (417)831-1561
                             X330

MONTANA

Brian Sharkey, Ph.D.
Dept. of Health, Physical

Education and Recreation
University of Montana
Missoula, Mt. 59801
                    (406)243-4211

NEBRASKA

Kenneth D. Rose, M.D.
Physical Fitness Research Lab.
University Health Center
University of Nebraska
Lincoln, Ne. 68508
                    (502)472-2297

NEW JERSEY

Gerald Crousnore, Ex. Sec.
Society for Coronary
    Rehabilitation & Research
135 Madison Avenue
Elizabeth, N.J. 07201
                    (201)352-0850

George Sheehan, M.D.
Brookdale Community Col-
    lege
Newman Springs Road
Lincroft, N.J. 07738
                    (201)842-1900

David J. Henderson, Ph.D.
Anthropometrics
Cherry Hill Plaza
1415 Rt. 70 East
Cherry Hill, N.J. 08034
                    (609)795-2220

NEW MEXICO

Hemming A. Atterborn, Ph.D.
Human Performance Lab.
University of New Mexico
Albuquerque, N.M. 87106
                    (605)211-2603

NEW YORK

Murray Low
Health & Physical Education
 York College of the City
University of New York
150-14 Jamaica Avenue
Jamaica, N.Y. 11432
(212)780-4059

Vojin Smodlaka, M.D.
Dept. of Rehabilitation Medicine
Methodist Hospital of Brooklyn
506 Sixth Street
Brooklyn, N.Y. 11215
(212)780-3393

William D. McArdle, Ph.D.
Lab. of Applied Physiology
Queens College
Queens, N.Y. 11829
(212)445-7500

William J. Tomik, Ph.D.
School of Physical Education
Cortland State College
Cortland, N.Y. 13045
(607)753-2011

William Gualtiere, Ph.D.
Cardiometrics
295 Madison Avenue
New York, N.Y. 10017
(212)889-6123

Robert Kohn, M.D.
50 High Street
Buffalo, N.Y. 14203

F. Suarez, M.D.
John Addriozzo, M.D.
Richmond CPR Center
530 Narrows Road South
Staten Island, N.Y.

NORTH CAROLINA

Henry S. Miller, M.D.
N.C. Baptist Hospital

300 S. Hawthorne Blvd.
Winston-Salem, N.C. 27103
(919)725-7251

Andrew G. Wallace, M.D.
Dept. of Medicine
Cardiovascular Division
Duke University Medical Center
Box 3022
Durham, N.C. 27710
(919)684-8111

William P. Marley, Ph.D.
Physical Fitness Laboratory
Dept. of Physical Education
North Carolina State University
Raleigh, N.C. 27607

OHIO

Herman K. Hellerstein, M.D.
Case Western Reserve University
2065 Albellert Road
Cleveland, Ohio 44106
(216)791-7300

Lawrence A. Golding, Ph.D.
Applied Physiology Research
 Lab.
Kent State University
Kent, Ohio 44240
(216)672-2859

Edward L. Fox, Ph.D.
Ohio State University
337 W. 17th Ave.
Columbus, Ohio 43210
(614)442-6887

William J. Rowe, M.D.
St. Vincent Hospital
2213 Cherry Street
Toledo, Ohio 43608

OKLAHOMA

David Hodges
Downtown YMCA
Tulsa, Ok.

OREGON

Michael Tichy, Ph.D.
Dept. of Physical Ed.
Portland State University
Portland, Or. 97207
                              (503)226-7271

E. Evonuk, Ph.D.
Human Performance Lab.
University of Oregon
Eugene, Or. 97403

PENNSYLVANIA

E.R. Buskirk, Ph.D.
Noll Laboratory for Human Perf.
  Research
Pennsylvania State University
University Park, Pa. 16802
                              (814)865-3453

Alan J. Barry, Ph.D.
Division of Research
Lankenau Hospital
Lancaster & City Line Ave.
Philadelphia, Pa. 19151
                              (215)649-1400

Bruce J. Noble, Ph.D.
Human Energy Research Lab.
University of Pittsburgh
242 Trees Hall
Pittsburgh, Pa. 15213
                              (412)624-4387

Thomas M. McGuigan, D.P.M.
Pennsylvania College of
  Podiatric Medicine
804 Pine St.
Philadelphia, Pa. 19140
                              (215)922-5420

Ralph H. Kapilian, Ph.D.
Research Laboratory
School of Health and Physical
  Education
West Chester, Pa. 19380
                              (215)436-2764

Stanley Zeeman, M.D.
Allentown CPR Center
1730 Chew Street
Allentown, Pa. 18104
                              (215)433-1101

Gilbert Hoffman, M.D.
Bethlehem CPR Center
35 E. Elizabeth Avenue
Bethlehem, Pa. 18018
                              (215)694-0595

F. Thomas Hopkins, M.D.
Harold Robinson, M.D.
John Strang, M.D.
Bryn Mawr CPR Center
958 County Line Road
Conestoga Medical Bldg., Suite
  201
Bryn Mawr, Pa. 19010
                              (215)LA5-4037

Morris Kramer, M.D.
Easton CPR Center
2024 Lehigh Street
Easton, Pa. 18042
                              (215)252-0301

Gilbert Grossman, M.D.
Elkins Park CPR Center
One Abbington Plaza
Old York Road and Twp. Line
  Road
Jenkintown, Pa. 19046
                              (215)TU7-1519

Charles Joy, M.D.
William Underhill, M.D.
Erie CPR Center
155 W. Eight Street
Summer Nichols Bldg.
Erie, Pa. 16501
                              (814)453-5485

Robert Sagin, M.D.
Northeast Phila. CPR Cen-
  ter
8220 Castor Avenue
Philadelphia, Pa. 19152

Sandy Furey, M.D.
Scranton CPR Center
Moses Taylor Hospital
748 Quincy Avenue
Scranton, Pa. 18501
(717)961-3090

Raymond Grandon, M.D.
Frank Jackson, M.D.
Harrisburg CPR Center
1625 N. Front Street
Harrisburg, Pa. 17102
(717)232-7091

Herman Auerbach, M.D.
Leo Corazzo, M.D.
Peter Saras, M.D.
Hazleton CPR Center
Northeastern Bldg.
Suite 1108-1110
Hazleton, Pa. 18201
(717)455-9070

Raymond Grandon, M.D.
Frank Jackson, M.D.
Mechanicsburg CPR Center
4950 Wilson Lane
Mechanicsburg, Pa. 17055
(717)697-8350

Benjamin Hoover, III, M.D.
York CPR Center
924C Colonial Avenue
York, Pa. 17403
(717)854-4698

SOUTH CAROLINA

Peter G. Gazes, M.D.
Medical University of S.C.
80 Barre Street
Charleston, S.C. 20401
(803)792-3953

Steven N. Blair, PED.
Human Performance Lab.
University of S.C.
Columbia, S.C. 29208
(803)777-3815

SOUTH DAKOTA

Paul Brynteson, Ph.D.
Dept. of HPER
South Dakota State University
Brookings, S.D. 57006
(605)688-4151

TENNESSEE

Joseph E. Acker, Jr., M.D.
Cardiac Rehabilitation Unit
St. Mary's Memorial Hospital
Knoxville, Tn. 37920
(615)971-6011

Hugh E. Welch, Ph.D.
Human Performance Lab.
University of Tennessee
Knoxville, Tn. 37916
(615)974-5111

Irvin S. Perry, M.D.
Veterans Administration Ctr.
Mountain Home, Tn. 37684

TEXAS

Jere Mitchell, M.D.
University of Texas
Southwestern Medical School
5323 Harry Hines Blvd.
Dallas, Tx. 75235
(214)ME1-3220

Kenneth H. Cooper, M.D.
The Aerobics Center
12100 Preston Road
Dallas, Tx. 75230
(214)239-7223

UTAH

Phil Allsen, Ph.D.
269 SFJ
Brigham Young University
Provo, Utah 84601

VIRGINIA

Leif O. Torkelson, M.D.
Rockingham Memorial Hospital
South Mason Street
Harrisonburg
Office: 635 South Main Street
Harrisonburg, Va. 22801
(703)434-8105

WASHINGTON

Robert A. Bruce, M.D.
Div. of Cardiology
School of Medicine
University of Washington
Seattle, Wa. 98195
(206)543-3265

Howard R. Pyfer, M.D.
Universal Testing Services, Inc.
8118 Greenlake Dr. No.
Seattle, Wa. 98103
(206)523-4700

Cardio-Pulmonary Res. Inst.
(CAPRI)*
914 East Jefferson Street
Seattle, Wa. 98122
(206)523-7550

WISCONSIN

Robert J. Corliss, M.D.
Dept. of Physical Exercise
Laboratories
University of Wisconsin
Madison, Wi. 53705

Bibliography

ABELSON, P. H. "Cost effective health care." *Science,* 1976, *192,* 3.

ABESHOUSE, B. S., & SCHERLIS, I. "Spontaneous disappearance of retrogression of bladder neoplasm: Review of the literature and report of three cases." *Urol. Cutan. Rev.,* 1951, *55*(1).

ACHTERBERG, J., & LAWLISS, G. F. *Imagery of cancer.* Champaign, Ill.: Institute for Personality and Ability Testing, 1978.

ACHTERBERG, J., LAWLISS, G. F., SIMONTON, O. C., & SIMONTON, S. "Psychological factors and blood chemistries as disease outcome predictors for cancer patients." *Multivariate Clinical Experimental Research,* December 1977.

ACHTERBERG, J., SIMONTON, O.C., & MATTHEWS-SIMONTON, S. *Stress, psychological factors, and cancer.* Fort Worth, TX: New Medicine Press, 1976.

ADEY, W. R. "Introduction: Effects of electromagnetic radiation on the nervous system." *Annals of the New York Academy of Sciences,* 1975, *247,* 15–20.

AGRADI, E., et al. "Diet, lipids, and lipoproteins in patients with peripheral vascular disease." *American Journal of the Medical Sciences,* 1974, *268*(6), 325–332.

AIROLA, P. *How to get well.* Phoenix, AZ: Health Plus Publishers, 1974.

AIROLA, P. *Are you confused?* Phoenix, AZ: Health Plus Publishers, 1977.

AKISHIGE, Y., ed. *Psychological studies on Zen.* Tokyo: Zen Institute of Komazawa University, 1970.

ALEXANDER, F. *Psychosomatic medicine.* New York: Norton, 1950.

ALIKISHIEU, R. "Very old people in the USSR." *The Gerontologist,* Summer 1970, 151–152.

ALLEN, E. P. "Malignant melanoma, spontaneous regression after pregnancy." *British Medical Journal,* 1955, *2,* 1955.

ALLEN, J. *As a man thinketh.* New York: National Colorgraphics, 1970.

ALLISON, J. "Respiration changes during transcendental meditation." *Lancet,* 1970, *1,* 833–834.

ALTSCHULE, M.D. "Is it true what they say about cholesterol?" *Executive Health,* August 1976, *12*(11).

ALVAREZ, W. C. *Minds that came back.* New York: J. B. Lippincott, 1961.

ALVAREZ, W. C. "The spontaneous regression of cancer." *Geriatrics,* 1967, *22,* 89–90.

AMERICAN CANCER SOCIETY. *Cancer facts and figures.* New York: American Cancer Society, 1976.

"American death rates at a record low in 1976." *Behavior Today,* October 10, 1977, 2.

AMKRAUT, A. E., & SOLOMON, G. F. "From the symbolic stimulus to the pathophysiologic response: Immune mechanisms." *International Journal of Psychiatry in Medicine,* 1975, *5*(4), 1.

ANAND, B. K., CHHINA, G. S., & SINGH, B. "Some aspects of electro-encephalographic studies in yogis." *Electroencephalography and Clinical Neurophysiology,* 1961, *13,* 452–456. (Reprinted in Tart, C., ed. *Altered states of consciousness.* New York: Wiley, 1969, 503–506.

ANAND, B. K. et al. "Studies on Shri Ramananda Yogi during his stay in an air-tight box." *Indian Journal of Medical Research,* 1961, *49,* 82–89.

ANDERSON, T. W. *Magnesium, soft water, and heart disease.* Second International Symposium on Magnesium, Montreal, 1976.

ANDERVONT, H.B. "Influence of environment on mammary cancer in mice." *Journal of National Cancer Institute,* 1944, *4,* 579–581.

"Anxiety over anti-anxiety drugs." *Behavior Today,* May 27, 1974, 149.

APPLE, D. How laymen define illness. *Journal of Health and Human Behavior,* 1960, *1*(3), 219–225.

APPLEY, M. H. E., & TRUMBULL, R. *Psychological stress.* New York: Appleton-Century-Crofts, 1967.

ARMS, S. *Immaculate deception.* Boston: Houghton Mifflin, 1975.

ARROW, K. "Limited knowledge and economic analysis." *American Economic Review,* March 1974, *64,* 1.

ASHLEY, R., & DUGGAL. *Dictionary of nutrition.* New York: St. Martin's Press, 1975.

ASSAGIOLI, R. *Psychosynthesis.* New York: Viking, 1965.

ASTALDI, G., & LISIEWICZ, J. *Lymphocytes: Structure, production, function.* Naples: Idelson, 1971.

ASTRAND, P., & RODAHL, K. *Textbook of work physiology.* New York: McGraw-Hill, 1970.

ASTRAND, P. O., & RODAHL, K. *Manuel de physiologie de l'exercise musculaire.* Paris: Masson et Cie., 1972.

ASTRAND, P. O. *Health and fitness.* Canada: Minister of Health and Welfare, 1979.

AUGENER, W., COHNEN, G., REUTER, A., & BRILLINGER, G. "Decrease of T lymphocytes during aging." *Lancet,* 1974, *1,* 1164.

AX, A. *Electic therapy.* Paper presented at the Biofeedback Research Society, October 25, 1971, Clayton, Missouri.

AYRES, G. "Vilcambaba." *Harper's,* June 1973, 6–7.

BACON, C. L., RENNECKER, R., & CUTLER, M. "A psychosomatic survey of cancer of the breast." *Psychosomatic Medicine,* 1952, *14,* 453–460.

BADGLEY, C. E., & BATTS, M., JR. "Osteogenic sarcoma: An analysis of eighty cases." *Archives of Surgery,* 1941, *43,* 541.

BAEKELAND, F. "Exercise deprivation." *Archives of General Psychiatry,* April 1970, *22,* 265–369.

BAHNSON, B., & BAHNSON, M. B. "The role of ego defenses: Denial and repression in the etiology of malignant neoplasm." *Annals of New York Academy of Science,* 1966, *125*(3), 827.

BAHNSON, M. B., & BAHNSON, C. B. "Ego defenses in cancer patients." *Annals of New York Academy of Science,* 1969, *164,* 546–559.

BAKER, H. W. "Spontaneous regression of malignant melanoma." *American Surgeon,* 1964, *30,* 825–831.

BAKKER, G. B., & LEVENSON, R. M. "Determinants of angina pectoris." *Psychosomatic Medicine,* 1967, *29,* 621–633.

BANDMAN, E., WALKER, C. R., & STROHMAN, R. C. "Diazepam inhibits myblast fusion and expression of muscle specific protein synthesis." *Science,* May 5, 1978, *200,* 559–561.

BARBER, T., et al, eds. *Biofeedback and self-control, An Aldine reader.* Chicago: Aldine, 1971. (Contains 75 selected articles on Biofeedback, prior to 1970.)

BARDAWIL, W. A., & TOY, B. L. "The natural history of choriocarcinoma: Problems of immunity and spontaneous regression." *Annals of New York Academy of Sciences,* 1959, *80,* 197.

BARLOW, W. *The Alexander technique.* New York: Knopf, 1973.

BARTLEY, O., & HULTQUIST, G. T. "Spontaneous regression of hypernephromas." *Acta Pathology of Microbiology, Scandinavia,* 1950, *27,* 448.

BASMAJIAN, J. V. "Control and training of individual motor units." *Science,* 1963, *141,* 440–441.

BASMAJIAN, J. V. *More on EMG and biofeedback. Muscles alive: Their functions revealed by electromyography, 3rd ed.* Baltimore: Williams & Wilkins, 1974.

BASMAJIAN, J. V., KUKLKA, C. G., NARAYAN, M. G., & TAKEBE, K. "Biofeedback treatment of foot-drop after stroke compared with standard rehabilitation technique: Effects on voluntary control and strength." *Archives of Physical Medicine and Rehabilitation,* 1975, *56,* 231–236.

BASOLWITZ, H., PERSKY, H., KORCHIN, S. J., GRINKLER, R. R. *Anxiety and stress.* New York: McGraw-Hill, 1955.

BAUM, J. "Rheumatoid arthritis linked to broken homes." *Medical World News,* April 17, 1978, 70.

BAUMANN, B. "Diversities in conceptions of health and physical fitness." *Journal of Health and Human Behavior,* 1961, *3,* 34–46.

BECK, A., & CASSELL, H. "Role inconsistency and health status." *Social Science and Medicine,* 1972, *6*(6), 737–749.

BECKMAN, B. L. "Life stress and psychological well being." *Journal of Health and Social Behavior,* 1971, *12*–35-45.

BEECHER, H. K. "The powerful placebo." *Journal of American Medical Association,* 1955, *159,* 1602–1606.

BELL, B. D. "Cognitive dissonance and life satisfaction of older adults." *Journal of Gerontology,* September 1974, *29*(5), 564–571.

BENSON, H. *The relaxation response.* New York: Morrow, 1975.

BENSON, H., BEARY, J. F., & CAROL, M. P. "The relaxation response." *Psychiatry,* 1974, *37,* 37–46.

BENSON, H., & EPSTEIN, H. D. "The placebo effects: A neglected asset in the care of patients." *Journal of the American Medical Association,* 1975, *232*(12).

BENSON, H., ROSNER, B. A., & MARZETTA, B. R. "Decreased systolic

blood pressure in hypertensive subjects who practice meditation."
Journal of Clinical Investigation, 1973, *52,* 8a.

BENSON, H., SHAPIRO, D., TURSKY, B., & SCHWARTZ, G. E. "Decreased systolic blood pressure through operant conditioning techniques in patients with essential hypertension." *Science,* 1971, *173,* 740–742.

BENSON, H., & WALLACE, R. K. "Decreased drug abuse with transcendental medication—A study of 1,862 subjects." In C. J. D. Zarafonetis, ed., *Drug abuse—proceedings of the international conference.* Lea & Febiger, 1972, 369–376.

BERKMAN, L. "News roundup." *Behavior Today,* December 26, 1977, 7.

BERNARD, C. *Leçons sur les phénomènes de la vie commune aux animaux et aux vegetaux.* Paris: J. B. Baillière et Fils, Vol. 1, 1878; Vol. 2, 1879.

BERNARD, C. *An introduction to the study of experimental medicine.* New York: Dover, 1957.

BERNSTEIN, D. A., & BORKOVEC, T. D. *Progressive relaxation training: A manual for helping professions.* Champaign, IL: Research Press, 1973.

BESWICK, I. P., & QVIST, G. "Spontaneous regression of cancer." *British Medical Journal,* 1963, *2,* 930.

BETTELHEIM, B. *The informed heart.* New York: Free Press of Glencoe, 1960.

BEYER, R. T., & WILLIAMS, A. O., JR. *College physics.* Englewood Cliffs, NJ: Prentice-Hall, 1957.

BIERMAN, E. O. "Spontaneous regression of malignant disease." *Journal of the American Medical Association,* 1959, *170,* 1842.

BIOFEEDBACK SOCIETY OF CALIFORNIA. *Handbook and directory,* 1976.

BIRK, L., ed. *Biofeedback: Behavioral medicine.* New York: Grune & Stratton, 1973.

BIRREN, J. E., et al. *Human aging: A biological and behavioral study.* DHEW Publication No. (HSM) 71-9051, 1974.

BLACKWELL, B. "Minor tranquilizers, misuse or overuse?" *Psychosomatics,* January-February 1975, *16,* 28–31.

BLADES, B., & MCCORKE, R. G., JR. "A case of spontaneous regression of an untreated bronchiogenic carcinoma." *Journal of Thoracic and Cardiovascular Surgery,* 1954, *27,* 415.

BLAKESLEE, S. "Study of Japanese-Americans indicates stress can be a major factor in heart disease." *New York Times,* August 5, 1975, 8.

BLATT, S. J. "An attempt to define mental health." *Journal of Consulting Psychology,* 1964, *28*(2), 146–153.

BLISS, E. L., MIGEON, C. J., BRANCH, C. H. H., & SAMUELS, L. T. "Reaction of the adrenocortical and thyroid hormones in acutely disturbed patients." *Psychosomatic Medicine,* 1956, *18,* 324–333.

BLOOM, H. J. G. "The natural history of untreated breast cancer." *Annals of New York Academy of Science,* 1964, *114,* 747.

BLOOMFIELD, H., CAIN, M., & JAFFE, R. *TM: Discovering inner energy and overcoming stress.* New York: Delacorte Press, 1975.

BLOOMFIELD, H. H., & KORY, R. *The holistic way to health and happiness.* New York: Simon & Schuster, 1978.

BLUM, R. *The management of the doctor-patient relationship.* New York: McGraw-Hill, 1960.

BLUMBERG, E. T., WEST, P. M., & ELLIS. F. W. "A possible relationship between psychological factors and human cancer." *Psychosomatic Medicine,* 1954, *16,* 277–290.

BOHR, N. *Atomic physics and the description of nature.* London: Cambridge University Press, 1934.

BOK, S. "The ethics of giving placebos." *Scientific American,* November 1974, *231*(5), 17–23.

BONIUK, M., & GIRARD, L. J. "Spontaneous regression of bilateral retinoblastoma." *Trans. Amer. Acad. Ophthal. Otolaryng.,* 1969, *73,* 194–198.

BOOKER, H. E., RUBOW, R. T., & COLEMAN, P. J. "Simplified feedback in neuromuscular retraining: An automated approach using electromyographic signals." *Archives of Physical Medicine and Rehabilitation,* 1969, *2,* 615–621.

BOUDREAU, L. "Transcendental meditation and yoga as reciprocal inhibitors." *Journal of Behavior, Therapy and Experimental Psychiatry,* 1972, *3,* 97–98.

BOYD, W. "The spontaneous regression of cancer." *Journal of Canadian Association of Radiologists,* 1957, *8,* 45, 63.

BOYD, W. *The spontaneous regression of cancer.* Springfield, IL: Charles C Thomas, 1966.

BRENNER, B. "Quality of affect and self-evaluation of happiness." *Social Indicators Research,* 1975, *2*(3), 315–331.

BRENNER, M. H. "The stressful price of prosperity." *Science News,* March 18, 1978, *113*(11), 166.

BRESLER, D. E. *Electrophysiological and behavioral correlates of acupuncture therapy.* International Symposium on Pain, Seattle, Washington, 1973.

BRETTAUER, J. "Spontaneous cures of carcinoma." *American Journal of Obstetrics,* 1908, *57,* 405–406.

BRILL, N. Q. "Are psychiatrists physicians, too?" *Psychosomatics,* August 1977, 5–6.

BRINDLE, J. M. "Spontaneous regression of cancer." *British Medical Journal,* 1963, *2,* 1132.

BRODY, H. "The system's view of man: Implications for science, medicine and ethics." *Perspectives in Biology and Medicine,* Autumn 1973, 71–92.

BROWN, B. "Awareness of EEG-subjective activity relationships detected within a closed feedback system." *Psychophysiology,* 1970, *7,* 451–468.

BROWN, B. *New mind, new body.* New York: Harper & Row, 1975.

BROWN, B. *Stress and the art of biofeedback.* New York: Harper & Row, 1977.

BROWN, R. S. "Jogging may be therapeutic for psychiatric patient." *Clinical Psychiatry News,* May 1978, *6*(5), 1.

BROZEK, J., KEYS, A., & BLACKBURN, H. "Personality differences between potential coronary and noncoronary subjects." *Annals of the New York Academy of Sciences,* 1966, *134,* 1057–1064.

BRUDNY, H., GRYNBAUM, B. B., & KOREIN, J. "New therapeutic modality for treatment of spasmatic torticillis." *Archives of Physical Medicine and Rehabilitation,* 1973, *54,* 575.

BRUNSCHWIG, A. "Spontaneous regression of cancer." *Surgery,* 1963, *53,* 423.

BUDZYNSKI, T. H., & PEFFER, K. "Twilight state learning: The presentation of learning material during a biofeedback-produced altered state." *Proceedings of the Biofeedback Research Society.* Denver: Biofeedback Research Society, 1974.

BUDZYNSKI, T., STOYVA, J. M. "EMG biofeedback in generalized and specific anxiety disorders." In Legewie, H., ed., *Biofeedback-therapie: Lernmethoden in der Psychosomatick, Neurologie und Rehabilitation (Fortschritte der Klinischen Psycholgie,* Vol. 6). Muchen-Berlin-Wien: Urban & Schwarzenberg, 1975.

BUDZYNSKI, T. H., STOYVA, J. M., & ADLER, C. "Feedback-induced muscle relaxation: Application to tension headache." *Journal of Behavior Therapy and Experimental Psychiatry,* 1970, *1,* 205–211.

BUMSTEAD, C., CARTER, B., & FIELD, A. *Nutrition: How much can government help?* Washington, D. C.: Concern, Inc., 2233 Wisconsin Ave., N.W., Washington, D.C., 1978.

BUNKER, J., & WENNBERG, J. "Operation rates, mortality statistics and the quality of life." *New England Journal of Medicine,* 1973, *289,* 1249.

BUREAU OF RETIREMENT, INSURANCE, AND OCCUPATIONAL HEALTH. *Federal employees health benefits program report for fiscal year ended June 30, 1971.* Washington, D.C.: U.S. Civil Service Commission, 1971.

BURTON, B. T. *Human nutrition,* formerly *The Heinz handbook of nutrition, 3rd Edition.* New York: McGraw-Hill, 1976.

BUTLER, B. "The use of hypnosis in the care of the cancer patient." *Cancer,* 1954, *7,* 1–14.

CAFFREY, B. "Factors involving interpersonal and psychological characteristics: A review of empirical findings." II. *Milbank Memorial Fund Quarterly,* 1967, *45,* 119–139.

CAIRNS, R. J. "Opportunistic autoimmune disease and opportunistic malignancy from pimparied cell-mediated immunity." *British Journal of Dermatology,* 1974, *91,* 601.

CAMERON, E., & PAULING, L. "Supplemental ascorbate in the supportive treatment of cancer: Prolongation of survival times in terminal human cancer." *Proceedings of the National Academy of Science,* October 1976, *73*(1), 3685–3689.

CAMPBELL, A. "Subjective measures of well-being." *American Psychologist,* March 1976, 117–124.

CANNON, W. B. *Bodily changes in pain, hunger, fear and rage: An account of recent researches into the function of emotional excitement.* New York: D. Appleton & Co., 1929.

CANNON, W. B. *The wisdom of the body.* New York: Norton, 1942.

CAPLAN, R. D. "Organizational stress and individual strains: A social-psychological study of risk factors in coronary heart disease among administrators, engineers, and scientists." *Dissertation Abstracts International,* 1972, *32*(11-B), 6706–6707.

CAPLAN, R. D. *Job demands and worker health: Main effects and occupational differences.* Ann Arbor, MI: Institute for Social Research, Box 1248, Ann Arbor, Michigan 48106, 1970.

CAPLAN, R. D., & FRENCH, J. R., JR. *Physiological responses to work load: An exploratory study.* Unpublished manuscript, Institute for Social Research, Ann Arbor, Michigan, 1968.

CAPRA, F. "The new physics as a model for the new medicine." *Journal of Social and Biological Structures,* September 1977, *1*(1).

CAPRA, F. *The Tao of physics.* New York: Dell, 1977.

CARLEN, P. L., et al. "Reversible cerebral atrophy in recently abstinent chronic alcoholics measured by computed tomography scans." *Science,* June 2, 1978, *200,* 1076–1078.

CARLILE, F., & CARLILE, U. "T-wave changes in strenuous exercise." *Track Technique,* December 1960, *2,* 55–59.

CARLSON, R. J. *The end of medicine.* New York: Wiley, 1975.

CARN, S. M., & Clark, D. C. "Nutrition, growth, development and maturation: Findings from the ten-state nutrition survey of 1968–1970." *Pediatrics,* 1975, *56,* 306.

CASSELL, J. "Social science theory as a source of hypotheses in epidemiological research." *American Journal of Public Health,* 1964, *54,* 1482–1489.

CASTANEDA, C. *Tales of power.* New York: Simon & Schuster, 1974.

CHAMBERLAIN, D. "Spontaneous disappearance of carcinoma." *British Medical Journal,* 1938, *1,* 508–509.

"Changing health directions." *Behavior Today,* June 30, 1975.

CHAPMAN, J. S. "Health and medicine." *Archives of Environmental Health,* June 1974, *28,* 356–357.

CHARALAMBIDIS, P. H., & PATTERSON, W. B. "A clinical study of 250 patients with malignant melanoma." *Surgery, Gynecology and Obstetrics,* 1962, *115,* 333.

CHAUCHARD, P. *The brain.* Trans. by David Noakes. New York: Grove Press, 1962.

CHERASKIN, E., Ringsdorf, W. M., & BRECHER, A. *Psychodietetics.* New York: Bantam, 1976.

CHERASKIN, E., & RINGSDORF, W. M. *Predictive medicine.* Mountain View, CA: California Pacific Press, 1973.

CHOW, E. *Application to experimental health manpower project, State of California, Department of Health, for approval of pilot project: Training holistic and cultural health educators/practitioners.* San Francisco: East-West Academy of Healing Arts, 1977.

COCHRANE, A. L. "Effectiveness and efficacy: Random reflections on health services." *British Medical Journal,* 1974, *4,* 5.

COHEN, B. L. "Relative risks of saccharin and calorie ingestion." *Science,* March 3, 1978, *199,* 983.

COHEN, D. "Magnetic fields of the human body." *Physics Today,* August 1975, 34–43.

COHEN, L. "Immunity and resistance in clinical cancer." *South African Medical Journal,* 1956, *30,* 161–167.

COLBURN, H. N., & BAKER, P. M. "Health hazard appraisal—a possible tool in health protection and promotion." *Canadian Journal of Public Health,* September–October 1973, *64,* 490.

COLBURN, H. N., & BAKER, P. M. "The use of mortality data in setting priorities for disease prevention." *Canadian Medical Association Journal,* March 16, 1974, *11,* 679–681.

COLE, W. "Collective review. The mechanisms of the spread of cancer." *Surgery, Gynecology and Obstetrics,* 1973, *137,* 853–871.

Composition of foods: Raw, processed, prepared. Agriculture Handbook No. 8, U.S. Department of Agriculture. Washington, D.C.: Government Printing Office, 1963.

COMSTOCK, G. W., & PATRIDGE, K. B. "Church attendance and health." *Journal of Chronic Health,* 1972, *25,* 665–672.

"Controlling lead in the environment." *Science News,* December 24 and 31, 1977, *112,* 425.

COOPER, B., & RICE, D. *Social security bulletin.* Washington, D.C.: Social Security Administration, 1976.

COOPER, B., & WORTHINGTON, N. "Personal health care expenditures by state." *Public Funds 1966 and 1969, Vol. I.* Washington, D.C.: Government Printing Office, 1973.

COOPER, K. H. *The new aerobics.* New York: Bantam, 1975.

COOPER, K. H. *Aerobics.* New York: Bantam, 1976.

COOPER, K. H. *The aerobics way.* New York: M. Evans & Co., 1977.

COOPER, K. H., & COOPER, M. *Aerobics for women.* New York: Bantam, 1976.

CORBETT, M. D. *Help yourself to better sight.* North Hollywood, CA: Wilshire Book Co., 1972.

CORSON, S. A. "Psychological stress and target tissue." In E. M. Weyer and H. Hutchins, eds., *Psychophysiological aspects of cancer.* New York: New York Academy of Sciences, 890–915, 1966.

COULTER, H. L. *Divided legacy: A history of the schism in medical thought.* Vols. 1, 2, and 3. Washington, D.C.: Wehawken Book Co., 1977.

COUSINS, N. "Anatomy of an illness (as perceived by the patient)." *New England Journal of Medicine,* December 23, 1976, also *Saturday Review,* May 28, 1977, 4–51.

COUSINS, N. "The mysterious placebo: How mind helps medicine work." *Saturday Review,* October 1, 1977, 8–12.

COUSINS, N. "What I learned from 3,000 doctors." *Saturday Review,* February 18, 1978, 12–16.

COX, H. (An interview by Sherman Goldman.) *East West Journal,* May 1978, 22–33.

COX. H. *Turning east: The promise and peril of the new orientalism.* New York: Simon & Schuster, 1978.

CROSBY, W. H. "Can a vegetarian be well nourished?" *Journal of the American Medical Association,* August 25, 1975, *233*(8), 898.

CULLITON, B. J. "Health care economics: The high cost of getting well." *Science,* May 26, 1978, *200,* 883–885.

CURRIER, R. "Multiphasic examinations." *Public Health Reports,* 1977, *92,* 527.

CUTLER, M. "The nature of the cancer process in relation to a possible psychosomatic influence." In J. A. Generelli and F. J. Kirkner, eds., *The psychological variables in human cancer.* Berkeley, CA: University of California Press, 1954.

CUTLER, S., MYERS, M., & GREEN, S. "Trends in survival rates of patients with cancer." *New England Journal of Medicine,* 1975, *293,* 122.

CZACZKES, J. W., & DREYFUSS, F. "Blood cholesterol and uric acid of healthy medical students under stress of an examination." *Archives of Internal Medicine,* 1959, *103,* 708–711.

DANNER, S., & DUNNING, A. "Spared affluence, they've lived past 90." *Medical World News,* January 23, 1978, 42.

DAO, T. L. "Regression of pulmonary metastases of a breast cancer." *AMA Arch., Surg.,* 1962, *84,* 574.

DATEY, K. K., KESHMUKH, S. M., DAIVI, D. P., & VINEKAR, S. L. "Shavasan, a yogic exercise in the management of hypertension." *Angiology,* 1969, *20,* 325–333.

DAVIDSON, P. O. *Behavioral management of anxiety, depression and pain.* New York: Brunner-Mazel, 1976.

DAVIS, ADELLE. *Let's eat right to keep fit.* New York: Harcourt Brace, 1954.

DAVIS, C., & FESHBACH, M. "Life expectancy in the Soviet Union." *Wall Street Journal,* June 20, 1978.

DECOURCY, J. L. "Spontaneous regression of cancer." *Journal of Medicine,* 1933, *14,* 141.

DETRY, J. M. R. *Exercise testing and training in coronary heart disease.* Baltimore: Williams & Wilkins, 1973.

DHEW Publication No. (HRA) 74-1017, Series 2-No. 12. *Conceptual problems in developing an idea of health.*

DLIN, B. M. "Risk factors, lifestyle, and the emotions in coronary disease." *Psychosomatics,* October 1977, 28–31.

DODGE, D. L., & MARTIN, W. T. *Social stress and illness.* Notre Dame, IN: University of Notre Dame Press, 1970.

DOHERTY, K. J. "Relaxation in endurance running." *Track Technique,* June 1964, No. 16, 483–488.

DOHRENWEND, B. S., & DOHRENWEND, B. P., eds. *Stressful life events—their nature and effects.* New York: Wiley-Interscience, 1974.

DOMASH, L., FARROW, J., & ORME-JOHNSON, D. *Scientific research on transcendental meditation.* Los Angeles: Maharishi International University, 1976.

DORFMAN, W. "Closing the gap between medicine and psychiatry." Proceedings of the 1st International Congress of the Academy of Psychosomatic Medicine, E. Dunlop, ed. New York: Excerpta Medica Foundation, 1967, 11–14.

Dorland's illustrated medical dictionary. Philadelphia: W. B. Saunders, 1974.

DOWNING, G. *The massage book.* New York: Random House/Bookworks, 1973.

DREYER, P. "On Ludd, Illich and medicine." *The Nation,* August 28, 1976, 130.

DUBOS, R. *Mirage of health.* New York: Harper & Row, 1971.

DUBOS, R., MAYA PINES, AND EDITORS OF *LIFE. Health and disease.* New York: Time/Life, 1965.

DUBOS, R. *Man adapting.* New Haven: Yale University Press, 1965.

DUBOS, R. *Man, medicine and environment.* New York: Praeger, 1968.

DUBOS, R. "Medicine's living history." *Medical World News,* 1975, 77–85.

DUBOS, R. "The state of health and the quality of life." *Western Journal of Medicine,* July 1976, *125*(1), 8–9.

DUFTY, W. *Sugar blues.* New York: Warner Books, 1975.

DUHL, L. J. "Health, whole, hold, healing." *Cesar-Magazine,* Spring 1976, 4–16.

DUHL, L. J. *The definition of health: Or how complex can you get?* Unpublished manuscript, Department of Health and Medical Sciences, University of California, Berkeley, 1977.

DUNBAR, F. *Emotions and bodily changes.* New York: Columbia University Press, 1954.

DUNBAR, F. *Psychosomatic diagnosis.* New York: Harper & Row, 1954.

DUNN, H. L. "Points of attack for raising levels of wellness." *Journal of the American Medical Association,* July 1957, 225.

DUNN, H. L. *Development planning note* (N3-58-DAP). United States Public Health Service, May 1958.

DUNN, H. L. *High level wellness.* Mt. Vernon Publishing Co., 1961.

DUNPHY, J. E. "Some observations on the natural behavior of cancer in man." *New England Journal of Medicine,* 1950, *242,* 167.

EASSON, E. C. "False notion: Cancer—incurable." *UNESCO Courier,* 1970. *23,* 23–26.

ECCLES, J. C. *Facing reality—philosophical adventures by a brain scientist.* New York: Springer-Verlag, 1970.

EDSON, L. "Most things get better by themselves." *New York Times Magazine,* July 4, 1976, 105–111.

ELIASBERG, W. G. "Psychotherapy in cancer patients." *Journal of the American Medical Association,* 1951, *147,* 525–526.

ELLIS, A., & HARPER, R. *A guide to rational living.* North Hollywood, CA: Wilshire Book Co., 1973.

ELMADJIAN, F. "Adrenocortical function of combat infantrymen in Korea." *Ciba Foundation Colloquia in Endocrinology,* 1959, *8,* 627–642.

ENGEL, G. L. "Studies of ulcerative colitis: The nature of the psychologic process." *American Journal of Medicine,* 1955, *19,* 231.

ENGEL, G. L. "A unified concept of health and disease." *Perspectives in Biology and Medicine,* 1960, *3,* 459–485.

ENGEL, G. L. "A life setting conducive to illness—a psychological setting of somatic disease: The giving-up—given-up complex." *Bulletin of the Menninger Clinic,* 1968, *32,* 355–366.

ENGEL, G. L. "The psychosomatic approach to individual susceptibility to disease." *Gastroenterology,* 1974, *67,* 1085–1093.

ENGEL, G. L. "Psychologic factors in instantaneous cardiac death." *New England Journal of Medicine,* 1976, *294*(12), 664–665.

ENGEL, G. L. "The need for a new medical model: A challenge for biomedicine." *Science,* April 8, 1977, *196*(4286), 129–136.

ENGEL, G. L., & SCHMALE, A. "Conservation-withdrawal: A primary regulatory process for organismic homeostasis." *Physiology, Emotion and Psychosomatic illness.* Elsevier, NY: Ciba Foundation Symposium, *8,* 1972.

ENGLE, B. T., NIKOOMANESH, P., & SCHUSTER, M. M. "Operant conditioning of rectosphincteric responses in the treatment of fecal incontinence." *New England Journal of Medicine,* 1974, *290,* 646–649.

EVANS, E. *A psychological study of cancer.* New York: Langmans, 1928.

EVANS-WENTZ, W. Y. *The Tibetan book of the dead.* New York: Oxford University Press, 1960.

EVERSON, T. C. "Spontaneous regression of cancer." *Annals of the New York Academy of Sciences,* 1964, *114,* 721–735.

EVERSON, T. C. "Spontaneous regression of cancer." *Progr. Clin. Cancer,* 1967, *3,* 79–95.

EVERSON, T. C., & COLE, W. H. "Spontaneous regression of cancer: Preliminary report." *Ann. Surg.,* 1956, *144,* 366.

EVERSON, T. C., & COLE, W. H. "Spontaneous regression of malignant disease" (Guest editorial). *JAMA,* 1959, *169,* 758.

EVERSON, T. C., & COLE, W. H. *Spontaneous regression of cancer.* Philadelphia: W. B. Saunders, 1966.

EVERSULL, G. A. "Psycho-physiology training and the behavioral treatment of premature ejaculation: Preliminary findings." *Proceedings of the Biofeedback Research Society,* 1975.

FABREGA, H. "The need for an ethnomedical science." *Science,* 1975, *189,* 969.

FABREGA, H. "The position of psychiatry in the understanding of human disease." *Archives of General Psychiatry,* 1975, *32,* 1500.

FARQUHAR, J. W. *The American way of life need not be hazardous to your health.* New York: Norton, 1978.

FARQUHAR, J. W., et al. "Community education for cardiovascular health." *Lancet,* June 4, 1977, 1192–1195.

FARQUHAR, J. W., et al. "Heart disease prevention." *Lancet,* 1977-I, 1192.

FAVAZZA, A. R. "The days of our years." *MD,* October 1977, 19–101.

FEIN, R. "Some health policy issues: One economist's view." *Public Health Reports,* 1975, *90,* 387.

FELDENKRAIS, M. *Awareness through movement.* New York: Harper & Row, 1972.

FERGUSON, E. A. "The mind's eye: Nonverbal thought in technology." *Science,* August 26, 1977, *197,* 827–836.

FERGUSON, M. *Brain revolution.* New York: Bantam, 1973.

FERGUSON, T. "Your first marathon." *Medical Self-Care,* Winter 1977–78, 8–11.

FERNSTROM, J. D., & WURTMAN, R. J. "Nutrition and the brain." *Scientific American,* February 1974, 84–91.

FIER, B. "Recession is causing dire illness." *Moneysworth,* June 23, 1975.

FINCH, C. E., & HAYFLICK, L. *Handbook of the biology of aging.* New York: Van Nostrand Reinhold Co., 1977.

FINN, F., MULCAHY, R., & O'DOHERTY, E. F. "The psychological assessment of patients with coronary heart disease: A preliminary communication." *Irish Journal of Medical Science,* 1966, *6,* 399–404.

FISHER, S. *The female orgasm.* New York: Basic Books, 1973.

FISHER, S., & CLEVELAND, S. E. "Relationship of body image to site of cancer." *Psychosomatic Medicine,* 1956, *18,* 304–309.

FIXX, J. *The complete book of running.* New York: Random House, 1978.

FLINK, E. B. *Clinical manifestations of acute magnesium deficiency in man.* Second International Symposium on Magnesium, Montreal, Canada, 1976.

FOLKINS, C. H. "Temporal factors and the cognitive mediators of stress reactions." *Journal of Personality and Social Psychology,* 1970, *14,* 173–184.

FOOT, N. C., HUMPHREYS, G. A., & WHITMORE, W. F. "Renal tumors: Pathology and prognosis in 295 cases." *Journal of Urology,* 1951, *66,* 190.

FORKNER, C. E. "Spontaneous remission and reported cures of leukemia." *Chinese Medical Journal,* 1937, *52,* 1–8.

FOX, B. H. *Premorbid psychological factors as related to incidence of cancer: Background for prospective grant applicants.* National Cancer Institute, National Institutes of Health, 1976. Reprinted in *Journal of Behavioral Medicine,* March 1978.

FOX, H. M., MURAWSKI, B. J., BARTHOLOMAY, A. F., & GIFFORD, S. "Adrenal-steroid excretion patterns in 18 healthy subjects." *Psychosomatic Medicine,* 1961, *23*(1), 33–40.

FOX, S. M., NAUGHTON, J. P., & HASKELL, W. L. "Physical activity and the prevention of coronary heart disease." *Annals of Clinical Research,* 1971, *3,* 404.

Framingham Study, The: *An epidemiological investigation of cardiovascular disease.* Washington, D.C.: GPO, Section 10, September 1968.

FRANK, D. F. "Nature and functions of belief systems: Humanism and transcendental religion." *American Psychologist,* July 1977, 555–559.

FRANK, J. A., & DOUGHERTY, T. F. "The assessment of stress in human subjects by means of quantitative and qualitative changes on blood lymphocytes." *Journal of Laboratory and Clinical Medicine,* 1975, *42*(4), 538–549.

FRANK, J. D. "The faith that heals." *The Johns Hopkins Medical Journal,* 1975, *137,* 127–131.

FRANKENHAEUSER, M. "Looking at stress. Report to the Kittay Foundation on the psychopathology of human adaptation." Cited in *Behavior Today*, June 9, 1975, 6(23), 499.

FRANKENHAEUSER, M., & JOHANSSON, G. "Task demand as reflected in catecholamine excretion and heart rate." *Journal of Human Stress*, March 1976, 2(1)

FREIDSON, E. "Taking away the cake." *Behavior Today*, November 24, 1975, 625.

FRENCH, J. D. "The reticular formation." *Scientific American*, May 1957, 2–8.

FRENCH, J. D., LEEB, C. S., FAHRION, S. L., LAW, T., & JECHT, E. W. "Self-induced scrotal hyperthermia in man: A preliminary report." Paper presented at the Biofeedback Research Society Meeting, Boston MA, November 1972.

FRIEDMAN, M., & ROSENMAN, R. H. "Type A behavior pattern: Its association with coronary heart disease." *Annals of Clinical Research*, 1971, *3*, 300–312.

FRIEDMAN, M., & ROSENMAN, R. H. *Type A behavior and your heart.* New York: Knopf, 1974.

FRIEDMAN, M., ROSENMAN, R. H., & CARROLL, V. "Changes in the serum cholesterol and blood clotting time in men subjected to cyclic variation of occupational stress." *Circulation*, 1958, *18*, 852–861.

FRIEDMAN, S. B., & GLASGOW, L. A. "Psychologic factors and resistance to infectious disease." *Ped. Cl. N. Amer.*, 1966, *13*, 315–335.

FRIEDMAN, S. B., GLASGOW, L. A., & ADER, R. "Psychosocial factors modifying host resistance to experimental infections." *New York Academy of the Sciences*, 1969, *164*(2), 381–392.

FROST, J. W., DRYER, R. L., & KOHLSTAEDT, K. G. "Stress studies on auto race drivers." *Journals of Laboratory and Clinical Medicine*, 1951, *38*, 523–525.

FUCHS, V. *Who shall live?* New York: Basic Books, 1975.

FULLERTON, J. M., & HILL, R. D. "Spontaneous regression of cancer." *British Medical Journal*, 1963, *2*, 1589.

FUNKENSTEIN, D. H., KING, S. B., & DROLETTE, M. *Mastery of stress.* Cambridge: Harvard University Press, 1957.

GAARDER, K., & MONTGOMERY, P. S. *Clinical biofeedback: A procedural manual.* Baltimore: Williams & Wilkins, 1977.

GALIN, D. "Implications for psychiatry of left and right cerebral specialization." *Archives of General Psychiatry*, 1974, *31*, 572–583.

GALLAGHER, R. E., & GALLO, R. C. "Type C RNA tumor virus isolated from cultured human acute myelogenous leukemia cells." *Science,* 1975, *187,* 350–353.

GARB, S. "Neglected approaches to cancer." *Saturday Review,* June 1, 1968.

GARFIELD, S. R. "The delivery of medical care." *Scientific American,* April 1970, *222,* 42–58.

GATTOZZI, A. A. "Program reports on biofeedback." *NIMH Program Reports Number 5,* December 1971, 291–388.

GAUS, C., Cooper, B., & HIRSCHMAN, C. *Contrasts in HMO and fee-for-service performance.* Social Security Administration. Washington, D.C.: GPO, December 1975.

GAYLORD, H. R., & CLOWES, G. H. A. "On spontaneous cure of cancer." *Surgery, Gynecology, and Obstetrics,* 1903, *2,* 633–658.

GEBA, B. H. *Breathe away your tension.* New York: Random House/Bookworks, 1973.

GELLER, H., & STEELE, G. *The 1974 probability tables of dying in the next ten years from specific causes.* Indianapolis, IN: Methodist Hospital, 1979.

GELLER, I. "Ethanol preference in the rat as a function of photoperiod." *Science,* July 30, 1971, *173*(3995), 456–459.

GELLHORN, E. *Physiological foundations of neurology and psychiatry.* Minneapolis: University of Minnesota Press, 1953.

GELLHORN, E., & LOOFBOURROW, G. N. *Emotions and emotional disorders, a neurophysiological study.* Hoeber Medical Division. New York: Harper & Row, 1963.

GERRARD, D. *One bowl.* New York: Random House/Bookworks, 1973.

GLADMAN, A. E., & ESTRADA, N. "Biofeedback in clinical practice." In S. R. Dean, ed., *Psychiatry and mysticism.* New York: Nelson-Hall, 1975.

GLEMSER, B. *Man against cancer.* New York: Funk & Wagnalls, 1969.

GODFREY, F. "Spontaneous cure of cancer." *British Medical Journal,* 1910, *4,* 2027.

GOLDFARB, O., DRIESEN, J., & COLE, D. "Psychophysiologic aspects of malignancy." *American Journal of Psychiatry,* 1967, *123*(12), 1545–1551.

GOLDSMITH, S. "The status of health status indicator." *Health Service Reports,* 1972, *87*(3), 212–220.

GOLEMAN, D. "Meditation and consciousness: An Asian approach to mental health." *American Journal of Psychotherapy,* 1976, *30* (1), 41–54.

GOODFIELD, J. "Humanity in science: A perspective and a plea." *Science,* 1977, *198,* 580–585.

GORDON, T., et al. "Alcohol: A heart disease preventive." *Science News,* 1977, *112,* 102–103.

GORDON-TAYLOR, G. "The incomputable factor in cancer prognosis." *British Medical Journal,* 1959, *1,* 455–462.

GORMAN, P., & KAMIYA, J. "Voluntary control of stomach pH." Research note presented at the Biofeedback Research Society Meeting, Boston, November 1972.

GORTON, B. "Autogenic training." *American Journal of Clinical Hypnosis,* 1959, *2,* 31–41.

GOTTSCHALK, L. A. "Psychosmatic medicine today: An overview." *Psychosomatics,* February 1978, *19*(2), 89–93.

GOULD, A. P. Cancer. *Lancet,* 1910, *2,* 1665.

GOVINDA, L. A. *Way of the white clouds.* Berkeley CA: Shambhala, 1971.

GOVINDA, L. A. *Creative meditation and multi-dimensional consciousness.* Wheaton, IL: Theosophical Publishing House, 1976.

GRANICK, S., & PATTERSON, R. D. *Human aging II: An 11-year follow-up biomedical and behavioral study.* DHEW Publication No. (HSM) 71–9073, 1971.

GREAT BRITAIN GENERAL REGISTER OFFICE. *The survey of sickness of 1943–1952.* Studies of Medical Act Population Subjects, No. 12. London: H. M. Stationery Office, 1975.

GREDEN, J. F. "The caffeine crazies." *Human Behavior,* April 1975.

GREEN, E. E., GREEN, A. M., & WALTERS, E. D. "Voluntary control of internal states: Psychological and physiological." *Journal of Transpersonal Psychology,* 1970, *1,* 1–26.

GREEN, E., WALTERS, E. D., GREEN, A. M., & MURPHY, G. "Feedback technique for deep relaxation." *Psychophysiology,* 1969, *6,* 371–377.

GREEN, H. N. "An immunological concept of cancer: A preliminary report." *British Medical Journal,* 1954, *2,* 1374.

GREEN, J. "On how to live 90 to 100 health years (the syndrome of longevity . . . its seven great constants)." *Executive Health,* 1974, *6*(10).

GREENBERG, J. "The stress-illness link: Not if, but how." *Science News,* December 10, 1977, *112,* 394–398.

GREENE, W. A., JR. "The psychosocial setting of the development of leukemia and lymphoma." In E. M. Weyer and H. Hutchins, eds., *Psychophysiological aspects of cancer.* New York: New York Academy of Sciences, 1966, 294–801.

GREENE, W. A., JR., & MILLER, G. "Psychological factors and reticuloendothelial disease. Observations on a group of children and adolescents with leukemia. An interpretation of disease development in terms of the mother-child unit." *Psychosomatic Medicine*, 1958, *20*, 124–144.

GREENE,, W. A., JR., YOUNG, L., & SWISHER, S. N. "Psychological factors and reticuloendothelial disease. Observations on a group of women with lymphomas and leukemia." *Psychosomatic Medicine*, 1956, *18*, 284–303.

GREENLEIGH, L. "Timelessness and restitution in relation to creativity and the aging process." *Journal of American Geriatrics Society*, 1960, *8*, 353.

GRIMBY, G., NILSSON, G. N. J., & SALTIN, B. "Cardiac output during submaximal and maximal exercise in active middle-aged athletes." *Journal of Applied Psychology*, 1966, *21*(4).

GRUNDY, S. M., & GRIFFIN, A. C. "Effects of periodic mental stress on serum cholesterol levels." *Circulation*, 1959, *19*, 496–498.

GUNDERSON, E. K., & RAHE, R. H., eds. *Life stress and illness.* Springfield, IL: Charles C Thomas, 1974.

GUTSTEIN, W. H., HARRISON, F. P., KIU, G., & AVITABLE, M. "Neural factors contributing to atherogenesis." *Science*, 1978, *199*, 449–451.

GUYTON, A. C. *Textbook of medical physiology, 4th ed.* Philadelphia: W. B. Saunders, 1971.

HACKER, S., et al. "A humanistic view of measuring mental health." *Journal of Humanistic Psychology*, 1975, *12*(1) 94–106.

HAFNER, R. "Physiological change with stress in depression and obsessional neurosis." *Journal of Pyschological Research*, 1974, *17*, 175.

HAFNER, R. "Relationships between personality and autonomous nervous reactions to stress." *Journal of Psychosomatic Research*, 1974, *18*, 18–185.

HAGEN, D. Q. "The executive under stress." *Psychiatric Annals*, 1978, *8*(4), 49–51.

HALL, R. H. *Food for thought.* New York: McGraw-Hill, 1974.

HALSELL, G. *Los viejos—secrets of long life from the sacred valley.* Emmaus, PA: Rodale Press, 1976.

HAMBURG, D. A., & BROWN, S. S. "The science base and social context of health maintenance: An overview." *Science*, 1978, *200*, 847–849.

HAMPTON, J., STOUT, C., BRANDT, E., & WOLF, S. "Prevalence of myocardial infarction and reinfarction and related diseases in an Italian-American community." *Journal of Laboratory and Clinical Medicine,* 1964, *61,* 866.

HANDLEY, W. S. "The natural cure of cancer." *British Medical Journal,* 1909, *1,* 582–588.

HARDINGE, M. G., & STARE, F. J. "Nutritional studies of vegetarians: Nutritional, physical, and laboratory findings." *American Journal of Clinical Nutrition,* 1954, *2,* 73.

HARDYCK, C. D., PETRINOVICH, L. F., & ELLSWORTH, D. W. "Feedback of speech muscle activity during silent reading: Rapid extinction." *Science,* 1966, *154,* 1467–1468.

HARMAN, D. "Vitamin E and aging." *Science News,* March 18, 1972, 188.

HARNETT, W. L. "The relation between delay in treatment of cancer and survival rate." *British Journal of Cancer,* 1953, *7,* 19.

HARPER, A. E. "Official dietary allowances: Those pesky RDA's." *Nutrition Today,* March-April 1974, *9,* 15–25.

HARRINGTON, R. L., KORENEFF, C., NASSER, S., WRIGHT, C., & ENGELHARD, C. *Systems approach to mental health care in a HMO model.* Project MH 24109. Washington, D.C.: NIMH, 1977.

HARRIS, M. G., & HALLBARER, E. S. "Self-directed weight control through eating and exercise." *Behavioral Research and Therapy,* November 1973, *11*(4), 523–529.

HARRIS, M. J. "How to make it to 100." *New West,* January 3, 1977, 16–24.

HAUSER, P. M., et al. "Health statistics today and tomorrow." *American Journal of Public Health,* 1973, *63*(10), 890–910.

HAVENS, W. P., JR., & MARCK, R. E. "The leukocyte response of patients with experimentally induced infectious hepatitis." *American Journal of Science,* 1946, *212,* 129.

HAYES-BAUTISTA, D., & HARVESTON, D. S. "Holistic health care." *Social Policy,* March-April 1977, 7–13.

HAYFLICK, L. "The biology of aging." *Natural History,* August-September 1977, 22–25.

HAYFLICK, L. "On the facts of life: How old would you be if you didn't know how old you were?" *Executive Health,* 1978, *14*(9).

HEISENBERG, W. *Physics and philosophy.* New York: Harper Torchbooks, 1958.

HERRIGEL, E. *Zen and the art of archery.* New York: Random House, 1971.

HERSHKOWITZ, M. "Disappearance of metastases." *JAMA,* 1959, *170,* 996.

HIBBS, J. B., JR., TAINTOR, R. R., CHAPMAN, H. A., JR. & WEINBERG, J. B. "Macrophage tumor killing: Influence of the local environment." *Science,* 1977, *197,* 279–282.

HIGDON, H. *Fitness after forty.* Mountain View, CA: Runner's World, P.O. Box 366, 94042, 1977.

HIGDON, H. "Can running cure mental illness?" *Runner's World,* 1978, 36–43. (a)

HIGDON, H. "Running and the mind." *Runner's World,* 1978, 36–43. (b)

HILL, S. R., JR., GOETZ, F. C., FOX, H. M., MURAWSKI, B. J., KRAKAUER, L. J., REIFENSTEIN, R. W., GRAY, S. J., REDDY, W. J., HEDBERG, S. E., ST. MARK, J. R., & THORN, G. W. "Studies on adrenocortical and psychological response to stress in man." *Archives of International Medicine,* 1956, *97,* 269–298.

HINKLE, L. E., JR. *Beyond the germ theory: The roles of deprivation and stress in health and disease. Normal stress in normal experience.* New York: Health Education Council, 1954, 132–145.

HOAGLAND, H. "Studies of brain metabolism and electrical activity in relation to adrenocortical physiology." *Recent Progress in Hormone Research,* 1954, *10,* 29–63.

HOAGLAND, H., ELMADJIAN, F., & PINCUS, G. "Stressful psychomotor performance and adrenocortical functions as indicated by the lymphocyte response." *Journal of Clinical Endocrinology,* 1946, *6,* 301–311.

HOFFMAN, F. C. *The mortality from cancer throughout the world.* Newark, NJ: Prudential Press, 1915.

HOLDEN, C. "Cancer and the mind: How are they connected?" *Science,* 1978, *200*(23), 1363–1369.

HOLMAN, H. R. "The excellence deception in medicine." *Hospital Practice,* April 1976.

HOMBURGER, F. *The biological basis of cancer management.* New York: Harper & Row (Hoeber Medical Division), 1957.

HONSBERGER, R., & WILSON, A. F. "Transcendental meditation in treating asthma." *Respiratory Therapy: The Journal of Inhalation Technology,* 1973, *3,* 79–81.

HOROWITZ, M. "Life event questionnaires for measuring presumptive stress." *Psychosomatic Medicine,* 1977, *39*(6), 413–431.

HOUSE, J. "Occupational stress and coronary heart disease: A review and theoretical orientation." In O'Toole, ed., *Work and the quality of life.* Cambridge, MA: MIT Press, 1974.

HOUSE OF REPRESENTATIVES, COMMITTEE ON INTERSTATE AND FOREIGN COMMERCE. *Cost and quality of health care: Unneces-*

sary surgery. Washington, D.C.: Government Printing Office, 1976.

HOWARD, B. *Dance of the self.* New York: Simon & Schuster, 1974.

HOWE, G. R., BURCH, J. D., & MILLER, A. B. "Saccharin and bladder cancer in human subjects." *Lancet,* September 17, 1977.

HOXWORTH, P. I., & HAMBLETI, J. B. "Unexplained twelve-year survival after metastatic carcinoma of the colon." *American Journal of Surgery,* 1963, *105,* 126.

HOYMAN, H. S. "Rethinking an ecological systems model of man's health, disease, aging and death." *Journal of the School of Health,* 1975, *45*(9), 509–518.

HUGGINS, C. "Endocrine-induced regression of cancer." Address, December 13, 1966. *Science,* 1967, *156,* 1050–1054.

HUGHES, C. H. "The relations of nervous depression toward the development of cancer." *St. Louis Medical and Surgical Journal,* 1885.

HUGHES, X. J. *Cost and Quality of Health Care: Unecessary Surgery.* Report of U.S. House of Representatives Committee on Interstate and Foreign Commerce. Washington, D.C.: GPO, 1976.

HUMPHREYS, C. *Concentration and meditation.* Baltimore: Penguin, 1971.

HUTSCHNECKER, A. *The will to live.* New York: Crowell, 1953, New York: Cornerstone Library, 1974.

ILLICH, I. "Medicine is a major threat to health." An interview by Sam Keen. *Psychology Today,* May 1976, 66–77.

ILLICH, I. *Medical nemesis—the expropriation of health.* New York: Pantheon, 1976.

INGELFINGER, F. J. "Health: A matter of statistics or feeling." *NEJM,* February 24, 1977, 448–449.

INGELFINGER, F. J. "Medicine: Meritorious or meretricious?" *Science,* May 26, 1978, *200,* 942–946.

ISMAIL, A. H., & TRACHTMAN, L. E. "Jogging the imagination." *Psychology Today,* March 1973, 79–82.

ISSELBACHER, K. J. "Physicians must go public." *Focus* (Newsletter of Harvard Medical Community), May 4, 1978, 1–3.

JACKSON, I. *Yoga and the athlete.* Mountain View, CA: World Publications, Box 366, 1975.

JACOBSEN, O. *Heredity in breast cancer.* London: H. K. Lewis & Co., 1948.

JACOBSON, E. *Progressive relaxation.* Chicago: University of Chicago Press, 1938.

JACOBSON, E. *You must relax.* New York: McGraw-Hill, 1962.

JACOBSON, E. *Anxiety and tension control.* Philadelphia: J. B. Lippincott, 1964.

JACOBSON, E. "The two methods of tension control and certain basic techniques in anxiety tension control." *Modern treatment of tense patients.* Springfield, IL: Charles C Thomas, 1970. (a)

JACOBSON, E. *Modern treatment of tense patients.* Springfield, IL: Charles C Thomas, 1970. (b)

JAMES, M. *Born to win.* Reading, MA: Addison-Wesley, 1973.

JAMES, W. "The gospel of relaxation." *Talks to teachers on psychology; and to students on some of life's ideals.* New York: Henry Holt and Company, 1899.

JARVIK, L. F. "Thoughts on the psychobiology of aging." *American Psychologist,* May 1975, 576–592.

JENKINS, C. D. "Social and epidemiologic factors in psychosomatic disease." *Psychiatric Annals,* 1972, *2,* 8–21.

JENKINS, G. D. "Regression of pulmonary metastasis following nephrectomy for hypernephroma: Eight-year follow-up." *Journal of Urology,* 1959, *82,* 37.

JENKINS, G. D. "Final report—regression of pulmonary metastases following nephrectomy for hypernephroma: 13-year follow-up." *Journal of Urology,* 1965, *94,* 99–100.

JÖBSIS, F. F. "Nonivasive, infrared monitoring of cerebral and myocardial oxygen sufficiency and circulatory parameters." *Science,* 1977, *198,* 1264–1267.

JOHN LAME DEER, & ERDOES, R. *Lame Deer: Seeker of visions.* New York: Pocket Books, 1976.

JOHNSON, H. E., & GARTON, W. H. *A practical method of muscle reeducation in hemiplegia: Electromyographic facilitation and conditioning.* Pomona, CA: Casa Colina Hospital for Rehabilitative Medicine, 1973. Unpublished manuscript.

JONES, F. N. "Birth defects linked to airport noise." *Medical World News,* April 3, 1978, 84.

JONES, F. P. *Body awareness in action.* New York: Schocken, 1976.

JONES, T. *The incredible voyage.* Kansas City: Universal Press Syndicate, 1977.

KAMIYA, J. "Conscious control of brain waves." *Psychology Today,* 1968, *1*(11), 56–60.

KAMIYA, J. "Operant control of the EEG alpha rhythm and some of its reported effects on consciousness." In C. T. Tart, ed., *Altered states of consciousness.* New York: Wiley, 1969.

KAPLAN, H. S. *The new sex therapy.* New York: Brunner/Mazel, 1974.

KAPLAN, J. "Exercise: The new high." *Glamour,* May 1978, 248–250.

KARLINS, M., & ANDREWS, L. *Biofeedback: Turning on the power of your mind.* Philadelphia: J. B. Lippincott, 1972.

KARTZMAN, J., & GORDON, P. *No more dying: The conquest of aging and extension of human life.* New York: Dell, 1977.

KARVONEN, M. J. "Effects of vigorous exercise on the heart." In F. F. Rosenbaum, and E. L. BELKNAP, eds., *Work and the heart.* New York: Paul B. Hoeber Publishing, 1959.

KATZ, D., & KAHN, R. L. *The social psychology of organizations.* New York: Wiley, 1966.

KECK, L. R. *The spirit of synergy.* Nashville: Abingdon Press, 1978.

KEITH, R. A., LOWN, B., & STARE, F. J. "Coronary heart disease and behavior patterns: An examination of method." *Psychosomatic Medicine,* 1965, *27,* 424–433.

KENNETT, J. (RŌSHI). *How to grow a lotus blossom.* Shasta Abbey of the Reformed Sōtō Zen Church, Mt. Shasta, CA 96067, 1977.

KENT, S. "Technology in medicine." *Modern Medicine,* February 1, 1976, 54–63.

KESSEL, L. "Spontaneous disappearance of bilateral pulmonary metastases." *JAMA,* 1959, *169,* 1737.

KETY, S. S. "Psychoendocrine systems and emotion: Biological aspects." In D. C. Glass, ed., *Neurophysiology and emotion.* New York: Rockefeller University Press and Russell Sage Foundation, 1967, 103–108.

KETY, S. S. "From rationalization to reason." *American Journal of Psychiatry,* 1974, *131*(9), 957–963.

KEYS, A. "Coronary heart disease in seven countries." *Circulation,* 1970, Supplement 1:1-1-1-211, 41.

KIEV, A. *Magic, faith and healing.* New York: Free Press, 1969.

KILLEEN, R. N. F. "A review of Illich's *Medical Nemesis.*" *Western Journal of Medicine,* 1976, *125*(1), 67–69.

KIMBALL, R. W. "Studies on the pathogenesis of migraine." In J. Wortis, ed., *Recent advances in biological psychiatry, Vol. 3.* New York: Grune & Stratton, 1961, 200.

KINSEY, A.C., POMEROY, W., MARTIN, C., and GEBHARD, P. *Sexual behavior in the human female.* Philadelphia: W.B. Saunders, 1953.

KISCH, A. I. "Health care system and health." *Inquiry,* 1974, *11*(4), 269–274.

KISCH, A., & TORRENS, P. "Health status assessment in the health insurance study." *Inquiry,* 1974, *11,* 272.

KISSEN, D. M. "The significance of personality in lung cancer in men." In E. M. Weyer and H. Hutchins, eds., *Psychophysiological Aspects of Cancer.* New York: New York Academy of Sciences, 1966, 933–945.

KISSEN, D., & EYSENCK, H. J. "Personality in male lung cancer patients." *Journal of Psychosomatic Research,* 1962, *6,* 123–127.

KISSEN, D. M., BROWN, R. I. F., & KISSEN, M. "A further report on personality and psychosocial factors in lung cancer." *Annals of the New York Academy of Sciences,* 1969, *164,* 535–545.

KISSEN, D. M., & RAO, L. G. S. "Steroid excretion patterns and personality in lung cancer." *Annals of New York Academy of Sciences,* 1969, *164,* 476–479.

KIVETSKY, R. E., TURKEVICH, W. M., & BALITSKY, K. P. "On the psychophysiological mechanism of the organism's resistance to tumor growth." In E. M. Weyer and H. Hutchins, eds., *Psychophysiological Aspects of Cancer.* New York: New York Academy of Sciences, 1966, 933–945.

KLOPFER, B. "Psychological variables in human cancer." *Journal of Projective Techniques,* 1957, *21,* 331–340.

KNOWLES, J. H. "Editorial." *Science,* December 16, 1977.

KNOWLES, J. H. "The hospital." *Scientific American,* 1973, *229*(3), 128–138.

KNOWLES, J. H., ed. *Doing better and feeling worse.* New York: Norton, 1977. (a)

KNOWLES, J. H. "The responsibility of the individual." *Daedalus,* Winter 1977. Also *Proceedings of the American Academy of Arts and Sciences,* 1977, *106*(1). (b)

KOERNER, D. R. "Cardiovascular benefits from an industrial physical fitness program." *Journal of Occupational Medicine,* 1973, *15*(9), 700.

KOLATA, G. B. "Brain biochemistry: Effects of diet." *Science,* April 2, 1976, *192,* 41–42.

KOLATA, G. B., & MARX, J. L. "Epidemiology of heart disease: Searches for causes." *Science,* October 29, 1976, 509–512.

KONOWALCHUK, J., & SPEIRS, J. I. "Drinkers rejoice: A little wine may kill your virus." *Science,* June 3, 1977, *196,* 1074.

KORNEVA, E. A., & KHAI, L. M. "Effect of destruction of hypothalamic areas on immunogenesis." *Fizio. Zh. SRR. Sechenov,* 1963, *49,* 42.

KOSTRUBALA, T. *The joy of running.* New York: J. B. Lippincott, 1976.

KOWAL, S. J. "Emotions as a cause of cancer: Eighteenth and nineteenth century contributions." *Psychoanalytic Review,* 1955, *42,* 217–227.

KRAUT, A. I. *A study of role conflicts and their relationships to job satisfaction, tension and performance.* Doctoral dissertation. University of Michigan, Ann Arbor. University Microfilms, No. 67-8312, 1965.

KRINGLEN, E. "Heart disease and life stress." *Science News,* 1977, *112,* 166.

KRISTEIN, M. M., ARNOLD, C. B., & WYNDER, E. L. "Health economics and preventive care." *Science,* 1977, *195,* 457–462.

KRISTT, D. A., & ENGEL, B. T. "Learned control of blood pressure in patients with high blood pressure." *Circulation,* 1975, *51,* 370–378.

KUHN, T. S. *The structure of scientific revolutions.* Chicago: University of Chicago Press, 1962.

KURTZMAN, J. & GORDON, P. *No more dying.* Los Angeles: J. P. Tarcher, 1976, New York: Dell, 1977.

LACEY, J. I. "Differential emphasis in somatic response to stress." *Psychosomatic Medicine,* 1952, *14,* 71.

LACEY, J. I. "Individual differences in somatic response patterns." *Journal of Comparative Physiological Psychology,* 1952, *43,* 338.

LACEY, J. I. "Somatic response patterning and stress: Some revisions of activation theory." In M. Appley and R. Trumbull, eds., *Psychological stress.* New York: Appleton-Century-Crofts, 1967.

LACEY, J. I., BATEMAN, O. E., & VAN LEHAN, R. "Autonomic response specificity." *Psychosomatic Medicine,* 1958, *15,* 8.

LACEY, L. *Lunaception.* New York: Coward, McCann & Geoghegan, 1975.

LADER, M., & WING, L. "Habituation of the psycho-galvanic reflex in patients with anxiety states and in normal subjects." *Journal of Neurology, Neurosurgery, and Psychiatry,* 1964, *27,* 210–218.

LAFRAMBOISE, H. L. "Health policy: Breaking the problem down to more manageable segments." *Canadian Medical Association Journal,* 1973, *108,* 888.

LAING, R. D. *The politics of experience.* New York: Ballantine Books, 1969.

LALANDE, M. *A new perspective on the health of Canadians.* Ottawa,

Canada: Minister of National Health and Welfare Information, 1975.

LaMETTRIE, J. D. *L'Homme Machine.* Aram Vartanian, ed. Princeton: Princeton University Press, 1960.

LANG, J. S. "The fitness mania." *U.S. News and World Report,* February 27, 1978, 37–40.

LANGNER, T. S., & MICHAEL, S. T. *Life stress and mental health.* New York: Free Press, 1963.

LANGONE, J. *Long life.* Boston: Little, Brown, 1978.

LANSKY, S., GOGGIN, E., & HASSANEIN, K. "Male child with cancer the more anxious? Yes and no. . . ." Roche Pharmaceuticals: *Psychiatric News,* 1975.

LAPPÉ, F. M. *Diet for a small planet, rev. ed.* New York: Ballantine Books, 1975.

LARSEN, O. A., & MALMBORG, R. O., eds. *Coronary heart disease and physical fitness.* Copenhagen, Denmark: Munksgaard, 1971.

LATTIME, E. C., & STRAUSSER, H. R. "Arteriosclerosis: Is stress-induced immune suppression a risk factor?" *Science,* 1977, *198,* 302–303.

LAUCK, D. "Winning through imagination." *Mainliner,* March 1978, 48.

LAUREL, G. "General warmup exercise program." *Track Technique,* June 1963, No. 12, 377–378.

LAZARUS, A. A. "Broad-spectrum behavior therapy." *Newsletter of the Association for the Advancement of Behavior Therapy,* 1969, *4,* 5–6.

LAZARUS, R. *Patterns of adjustment.* New York: McGraw-Hill, 1976.

LAZARUS, R. S. *Psychological stress and the coping process.* New York: McGraw-Hill, 1966.

LAZARUS, R., OPTON, E. M., NOMIKOS, M. S., & RANKIN, N. O. "The principle of short-circuiting of threat: Further evidence." *Journal of Personality,* 1965, *33,* 622–635.

LAZARUS, R. S., SPEISMAN, J. C., MORDKOFF, A. M., & DAVIDSON, L. A. "A laboratory study of psychological stress produced by a motion picture film." *Psychological Monographs,* 1962, *76,* No. 553.

LEAF, A. "Every day is a gift when you are over 100." *National Geographic,* 1973, *143*(1), 93–118. (a)

LEAF, A. "Getting old." *Scientific American,* September 1973, 45–52.

LEAF, A. "On the physical fitness of men who live to a great age." *Executive Health,* August 1977, *13*(11).

LEAF, A. Personal communication, 1978.

LEBOVITS, B. Z., et al. "Prospective and retrospective psychological studies of coronary heart disease." *Psychosomatic Medicine*, 1967, *29*, 265–272.

LEBOYER, F. *Birth without violence.* New York: Knopf, 1975.

LEGIER, J. F. "Spontaneous regression of primary bile duct carcinoma." *Cancer*, 1964, *17*, 730.

LEIGH, H., & REISER, M. F. "Major trends in psychosomatic medicine —the psychiatrist's evolving role in medicine." *Annals of Internal Medicine*, 1977, *87*, 233–239.

LEIGHTON, A. Informal paper prepared for the 25th Anniversary Meeting, Department of Psychology and Behavioral Science, University of Washington, Seattle, 1974.

LEIZON, K. "Spontaneous disappearance of bilateral pulmonary metastases: Report of case of adrenocarcinoma of kidney after nephrectomy." *JAMA*, 1959, *169*, 1737–1919.

LEONARD, G. *The ultimate athlete.* New York: Viking, 1975.

LEONARD, G. "The holistic health revolution." *New West*, May 10, 1976, 40–49.

LEONARD, J. N., HOVER, J. L., & PRITIKIN, N. *Live longer now.* New York: Grosset & Dunlap, 1976.

LeSHAN, L. "A basic psychological orientation apparently associated with malignant disease." *The Psychiatric Quarterly*, 1961, *35*, 314–330.

LeSHAN, L. "A psychosomatic hypothesis concerning the etiology of Hodgkin's disease." *Psychological Reports*, 1957, *3*, 565–575.

LeSHAN, L. "Psychological states as factors in the development of malignant disease: A critical review." *National Cancer Institute Journal*, 1959, *22*(1), 1–18.

LeSHAN, L. "An emotional life-history pattern associated with neoplastic disease." *Annals of New York Academy of Sciences*, 1966, *125*(3), 780–793.

LeSHAN, L. *How to meditate.* New York: Bantam, 1974. (a)

LeSHAN, L. *The medium, the mystic, and the physicist.* New York: Viking, 1974. (b)

LeSHAN, L., & GASSMAN, M. "Some observations on psychotherapy with patients with neoplastic disease." *American Journal of Psychotherapy*, 1958, *12*, 723–734.

LeSHAN, L., & WORTHINGTON, R. E. "Some psychologic correlates of neoplastic disease: Preliminary report." *J. Clin. and Exper. Psychol.*, 1955, *16*, 281–288.

LeSHAN, L., & WORTHINGTON, R. E. "Loss of cathexes as a common psychodynamic characteristic of cancer patients: An attempt at statistical validation of a clinical hypothesis." *Psychol. Rep.*, 1956, *2*, 183–193. (a)

LeSHAN, L., & WORTHINGTON, R. E. "Personality as a factor in the pathogenesis of cancer. A review of the literature." *British J. M. Psychol.*, 1956, *29*, 49–56. (b)

LeSHAN, L., & WORTHINGTON, R. E. "Some recurrent life history patterns observed in patients with malignant disease." *J. Nerv. Ment. Dis.*, 1956, *124*, 460–465. (c)

LEVI, L. *Stress: Sources, management and prevention; medical and psychological aspects of the stress of everyday life.* New York: Liveright Publishing, 1967.

LEVI, L. "Sympatho-adrenomedullary and related reactions during experimentally induced emotional stress." In R. P. Michael, ed., *Endocrinology and Human Behavior.* London: Oxford University Press, 1968, 200–219.

LEVI, L. *Society, stress and disease.* New York: Oxford University Press, 1971.

LEVIN, A. S. *Protocol for immunologic assessment of cancer patients undergoing psychotherapy.* Grant proposal. Oakland, CA: Western Laboratories Medical Group, 1979.

LEVIN, E. J. "Spontaneous regression (cure?) of a malignant tumor of bone." *Cancer*, 1957, *10*, 377.

LEVINE, J. D., GORDON, N. C., and FIELDS, H. L. "The mechanism of placebo analgesia." *Lancet*, September 23, 1978, 654–657.

LEVINE, S., GOLDMAN, L., & COOVER, G. D. "Expectancy and the pituitary-adrenal system." *Physiology, Emotion, and Psychosomatic Illness.* Elsevier, NY: Ciba Foundation Symposium 8, Excerpta Medica, 1972.

LEWIS, J. M., BEAVERS, W. R., GOSSETT, J. T., & PHILLIPS, V. A. "The family system and physical illness." In *No single thread, psychological health in family systems.* New York: Brunner/Mazel, 1976.

LEWIS, R. *The way of silence: The prose and poetry of Basho.* New York: Dial Press, 1970.

LIBOW, L. S. "Interaction of medical, biological and behavioral factors on aging, adaption and survival: An 11-year longitudinal study." *Geriatrics*, 1974, *29*(11), 75–88.

LIEF, A., ed. *The commonsense psychiatry of Dr. Adolf Meyer.* New York: McGraw-Hill, 1948.

"Life and death and medicine." *Scientific American* (special issue), 1973, *229*(3).

LINDEMANN, E. "Symptomatology and management of acute grief." *American Journal of Psychiatry*, 1944, *101*, 141–148.

LINDEMANN, H. *Relieve tension the autogenic way.* New York: Peter H. Wyden, 1973.

LINDEN, W. "Practicing of meditation by school children and their levels of field independence-dependence, test anxiety, and reading achievement." *Journal of Consulting and Clinical Psychology,* 1973, *41,* 139–143.

LINDER, F. E. "The health of the American people." *Scientific American,* June 1966, *214*(6), 21–29.

LIPOWSKI, Z. J. "Psychosomatic medicine in the seventies: An overview." (102 references). *American Journal of Psychiatry,* 1977, *134*(3), 233–244.

LLOYD, O. C. "Regression of malignant melanoma as a manifestation of a cellular immunity response." *Proc. Roy. Soc. Med.,* 1969, *62,* 543–545.

LOGAN, R. F. L. "Assessment of sickness and health in the community." Parts I and II. *Medical Care,* 1964, *2*(3), 173–190; *2*(4), 218, 225.

LOMBARD, W. P. "Some of the influences which affect the power of voluntary muscle contractions." *Journal of Physiology,* 1892, *13,* 1–58.

LONGGOOD, W. *The poisons in your food.* New York: Simon & Schuster, 1960.

LOVE, W. A. "Problems in therapeutic application of EMG feedback." *Proceedings of the Biofeedback Research Society,* 1972.

LOVE, W. A., MONTGOMERY, D. D., & MOELLER, T. A. "A post hoc analysis of correlates of blood pressure reduction." *Proceedings of the Biofeedback Research Society,* 1974.

LOWEN, A. *The language of the body.* New York: Collier, 1971.

LOWEN, A. *Bioenergetics.* New York: Coward, McCann & Geoghegan, 1975.

LOWN, B., et al. "Basis for recurring ventricular fibrillation in the absence of coronary heart disease and its management." *NEJM,* 1976, *294*(12), 623–629.

LUBLIN, J. S. "Seeking a cure: Companies fight back against soaring cost of medical coverage." *Wall Street Journal,* May 10, 1978, 1.

LUCE, G. G. *Body time.* New York: Bantam, 1973.

LUCE, G. "Muscle and EEG feedback." In J. Segal, ed., *Mental health program reports,* 1973, 20852, 109–121. 6, National Institute of Mental Health, Rockville, Maryland.

LUTHE, W. "Method, research and application of autogenic training." *American Journal of Clinical Hypnosis,* 1962, *5*(1), 17–23.

LUTHE, W. *Autogenic training.* New York: Grune & Stratton, 1965.

LUTHE, W., ed. *Autogenic therapy,* Vol. I. New York: Grune & Stratton, 1969. (a)

LUTHE, W., ed. *Autogenic therapy: Applications in psychotherapy,* Vol. III. New York: Grune & Stratton, 1969. (b)

LUTHE, W. *Creativity mobilization techniques.* New York: Grune & Stratton, 1976.

LUTHE, W. *A training workshop for professionals: Introduction to the methods of autogenic therapy.* Orlando, FL: Biofeedback Society of America, 1977.

LUTYENS, M. *Krishnamurti: The years of awakening.* New York: Avon, 1975.

LYNN, R. *Attention, arousal and the orienting response.* Oxford: Pergamon Press, 1966.

MACKWORTH, J. F. *Vigilance and habituation.* Baltimore: Penguin, 1970.

MACMILLAN, M. B. "A note on LeShan and Worthington's 'Personality as a factor in the pathogenesis of cancer.'" *British J. M. Psychol.* 1957, *30,* 49.

McCAIN, G., PAULUS, P. B., & COX. V. C. "Crowding, death rates linked in humans." *Science News,* November 19, 1977, *112,* 341.

McCARTHY, E., & WIDNER, G. "Effects of screening by consultants on recommended elective surgical procedures." *New England Journal of Medicine,* 1974, *291,* 1331.

McCORD, J. "Thirty-year follow up: Counseling fails." *Science News,* November 26, 1977, *112,* 357.

McGOVERN, G. *Dietary goals for the United States—supplemental views.* Select Committee on Nutrition and Human Needs. U.S. Senate. Washington, D.C.: GPO. Price: $5.75. No stock number given.

McGOVERN, G. *Dietary goals for the United States.* A report of the Select Committee on Nutrition and Human Needs, U.S. Senate, February 1977. Washington, D.C.: GPO. Stock No. 052-070-04376-8. Price: $2.50. and the "Second Edition" of the above document in expanded form, December 1977. Stock No. 052-070-04376-8 ($2.50).

McKEOWN, T. "A historical appraisal of the medical task." In *Medical history and medical care.* New York: Oxford University Press, 1971.

McKEOWN, T. "The major influences on man's health." Unpublished paper. England: University of Birmingham, 1973.

McKEOWN, T. *The modern rise of population.* London: Blackwell Scientific Publications, 1976.

McKEOWN, T. *The role of medicine: Dream, mirage, or nemesis.* London: Nuffield Provincial Hospital Trust, 1976.

McKEOWN, T. "Determinants of health." *Human Nature,* April 1978, 60–67.

McQUADE, W., & AIKMAN, A. *Stress.* New York: Dutton, 1974.

MALININ, G. I., et al. "Evidence of morphological and physiological transformation of mammalian cells by strong magnetic fields." *Science,* 1976, *194,* 844–846.

MALMO, R. B. "Studies of anxiety: Some clinical origins of the activation concept." In C. D. Speilberger, Ed., *Anxiety and behavior.* New York: Academic Press, 1966.

MALMO, R. B., & SHAGASS, C. "Physiologic study of symptom mechanisms in psychiatric patients under stress." *Psychosomatic Medicine,* 1949, *11,* 27–29.

MANHOLD, J. H. "Extension of a hypothesis: Psychosomatic factors in wound healing." *Psychosomatics,* 1978, *19*(3), 143–147.

MANN, G. V. "Diet-heart: End of an era." *NEJM,* 1977, 297(12), 644–650.

MANN, G. V., et al. "Atherosclerosis in the Masai." *American Journal of Epidemiology,* 1972, *95,* 26–37.

MANNHEIMER, D. I., DAVIDSON, S. T., BALTER, B. B., MELLINGER, G. D., CISIN, I. H., & PARRY, H. J. "Popular attitudes and beliefs about tranquilizers." *American Journal of Psychiatry,* 1973, *130,* 1246.

MARGOLIS, J., & WEST, D. "Spontaneous regression of malignant disease: Report of three cases." *J. Amer. Geriatrics Society,* 1967, *15,* 251–253.

MARINACCI, A. A. *Applied electromyography.* Philadelphia: Lea & Febiger, 1968.

MARTIN, B. *Anxiety and neurotic disorders.* New York: Wiley, 1971.

MARTIN, E. A. "Organic disease as the cause of admission to a psychiatric hospital." *Journal of the Irish Medical Association,* 1962, *50,* 117–122.

MASLOW, A. *Farther reaches of human nature.* New York: Viking, 1971.

MASLOW, A. H. *Toward a psychology of being.* New York: Nostrand, 1968.

MASON, J. W. "A review of psychoendocrine research on the pituitary-adrenal cortical system." *Psychosomatic Medicine,* 1968, *30,* 576–607.

MASON, J. W. "The scope of psychoendocrine research." II. *Psychosomatic Medicine,* 1968, *30*(5), 565–575.

MASON, J. W. "A historical view of the stress field." I and II. *Journal of Human Stress,* June 1975, 22036; March 1975, 6–12.

MASON, J. W. "Psychologic stress and endocrine function." In E. J. Sachar, ed., *Topics in psychoendocrinology.* New York: Grune & Stratton, 1975.

MEARES, R. "A model of psychosomatic illness." *The Medical Journal of Australia,* July 19, 1975, *2,* 97–100.

MECHANIC, D. "Stress, illness and illness behavior." *Journal of Human Stress,* 1976, *2*(2).

"Medicine in the 2000's." *The Western Journal of Medicine,* July 1976, 64–66.

MEERLOO, J. "Psychological implications of malignant growth: survey of hypotheses." *Brit. J. M. Psychol.* 1954, *27,* 210–215.

MELLORS, R. C. "Prospects for the biological control of cancer." *Bull. N. Y. Acad. Med.,* 1962, *38,* 75.

MELZACK, R. "How acupuncture works: A sophisticated western theory takes the mystery out." *Psychology Today,* June 1973, 28–38.

MENNINGER, R.W. "Psychiatry 1976: Time for a holistic medicine." *Annals of Internal Medicine,* May 1976, *84,*(5), 603–604.

MERCK, SHARP & DOHME. *The hypertension handbook.* "Presented as a service to medicine." West Point, PA: Merck, Sharp & Dohme, 1974.

MILLER, E. E., & LUETH, D. *Feeling good: How to stay healthy.* Englewood Cliffs, NJ: Prentice-Hall, 1978.

MILLER, F. R., & JONES, H. W. "The possibility of precipitating the leukemic state by emotional factors." *Blood,* 1948, *3*(2) 880–884.

MILLER, J. A. "Are rats relevant?" *Science News,* July 2, 1977, *112,* 12–13.

MILLER, J. Z., et al. "Therapeutic effect of vitamin C." *JAMA,* January 17, 1977, *237*(3), 248–251.

MILLER, M. K., & STOKES, C. S. *Health status, health resources, and consolidated structural parameters: Implications for public health care policy.* Reprint, Department of Rural Sociology, Cornell University, 1978. (a)

MILLER, M. K., & STOKES, C. S. "Cornell study suggests that physicians are killing their patients." *Behavior Today,* March 20, 1978, *9*(10). (b)

MILLER, N. E. "Learning of visceral and glandular responses." *Science,* 1969, *163,* 434–445.

MILLER, N. E., DICARA, L. V., SOLOMON, H., WEISS, J. M., & DWOR-

KIN, B. "Learned modification of autonomic functions: A review and some new data." In T. X. Barber, et al, eds., *Biofeedback and self-control.* Chicago: Aldine-Atherton, 1970.

MILLER, N. E., et al. "The Troms heart study: High density lipo-protein and coronary heart-disease: A prospective case-control study." *Lancet,* 1977, *1,* 965–967.

MILLER, S., REMEN, N., BARBOUR, A., NAKLES, M. A., MILLER, S., & GARELL, D. *Dimensions of humanistic medicine.* San Francisco: Institute for the Study of Humanistic Medicine, 1975.

MILLMAN, M. *The unkindest cut.* New York: Morrow, 1977.

MINC, S. "Psychological factors in coronary heart disease." *Geriatrics,* 1965, *20,* 747–755.

MINTER, R. E., & KIMBALL, C. P. "Life events and illness onset: A review." *Psychosomatics,* 1978, *19*(6), 334–339.

MOELLER, T. A., & LOVE, W. A., JR. "A method to reduce arterial hypertension through muscular relaxation." Paper presented at the Biofeedback Research Society Meeting, Boston, 1972.

MOORMAN, L. T. "Tuberculosis on the Navajo reservation." *American Review of Tuberculosis,* 1950, *61,* 586.

MOOS, R. H., & SOLOMON, G. F. "Psychologic comparisons between women with rheumatoid arthritis and their nonarthritic sisters." *Psychosomatic Medicine,* 1965, *2,* 150.

MOREHOUSE, L., & GROSS, L. *Total fitness.* New York: Simon & Schuster, 1975.

MOREHOUSE, L., & GROSS, L. *Maximum performance.* New York: Simon & Schuster, 1977.

MORGAN, J., et al. "Psychological effects of chronic physical activity." *Medicine and Science in Sports,* Winter 1970, *2*(4), 213–217.

MORRIS, J. N., et al. "Incidence and prediction of ischaemic heart disease in London busmen." *Lancet,* 1966, *2,* 553–559.

MORTIMER, E. A. "Immunization against infectious disease." *Science,* May 26, 1978, *200,* 902–906.

MOSER, R. H. "Ruminations—Host factors: An overview." *JAMA,* 1975, *232*(5), 516–519.

MOSER, R. H. "Knowledge is not enough." *NEJM,* April 21, 1977.

MOSS, G. E. *Illness, immunity, and social interaction: The dynamics of biosocial resonation.* New York: Wiley, 1973.

MURPHY, M. *Golf in the kingdom.* New York: Delta, 1972.

MURPHY, M. "Sport as yoga." Appendix in M. Spino's *Beyond Jogging.* Millbrae, CA: Celestial Arts, 1976.

MUSES, C. M., & YOUNG, A. M. *Consciousness and reality.* New York: Outerbridge and Lazard, 1972.

NAISMITH, D. J., STOCK, A. L., & YUDKIN, J. "Effect of changes in the proportions of the dietary carbohydrates and energy intake on the plasma lipid concentrations in healthy young men." *Nutrition and Metabolism,* 1974, *16*(5), 295–304.

NARANJO, C., & ORNSTEIN, R. E. *On the psychology of meditation.* New York: Viking, 1971.

NATIONAL ADVISORY COMMISSION ON HEALTH MANPOWER. *Report of the National Advisory Commission on Health Manpower,* Vol. 2. Washington, D.C.: GPO, 1967.

National Health Federation Bulletin (published monthly). P. O. Box 688, Monrovia, California 91016.

NELSON, D. "Spontaneous regression of cancer." *British Medical Journal,* 1960, *2,* 670.

NELSON, D. H. "Spontaneous regression of cancer." *Clinical Radiology,* 1962, *13,* 138.

NEMIAH, J. C., & SIFNEOS, P. E. "Affect and fantasy in patients with psychosomatic disorders." In O. W. Hill, ed., *Modern trends in psychosomatic medicine.* New York: Appleton-Century-Crofts, 1970, 26–34.

"Nervous factor in the production of cancer." *British Medical Journal,* 1925, *20,* 1139.

NEWELL, K. W., ed. *Health by the people.* Geneva: World Health Organization, 1975.

NIDICH, S., SEEMAN, W., & DRESKIN, T. "Influence of transcendental meditation: A replication." *Journal of Counseling Psychology,* 1973, *20,* 565–566.

NOLAN, G. H. "Key to reducing risks of teenage pregnancy is psychosocial, physician declares." *Behavior Today,* October 24, 1977, *8*(41), 2–3.

NOLEN, W. A. *Surgeon under the knife.* New York: Dell, 1977.

NOSSAL, G. J. V. "The body's immune defense system in health and disease." In E. H. Kone and H. J. Jordan, eds., *The greatest adventure—basic research that shapes our lives.* New York: Harper & Row, Perennial Library, 1974.

NOVOSTI PRESS AGENCY. "Very old people in the USSR." *Gerontologist,* 1970, *10*(2), 151–152.

NUNN, C. Z. "Is there a crisis of confidence in science?" *Science,* December 9, 1977, *198*(4321), 1.

OBRIST, P. A., et al., eds. *Cardiovascular psychophysiology.* Chicago: Aldine, 1974.

OCHSNER, A. "On the role of vitamins C and E in medicine." *Executive Health,* 1970, *10*(5).

OLGAS, M. "Relationship between parents' health status and body image of children." *Nursing Research,* July-August 1974, *23*(4), 319–324.

"On walking—nature's own amazing "anti-age antibiotic!" " *Executive Health,* July 1978, *14*(10),

OOKA, H., SEGALL, P. E., & TIMIRAS, P. S. "Neural and endocrine development after chronic trytophan deficiency in rats: Pituitary-thyroid axis." *Mechanisms of Aging and Development,* 1978, (7), 19–24.

OREM-JOHNSON, D. W. "Autonomic stability and transcendental meditation." *Psychosomatic Medicine,* 1973, *35,* 341–349.

ORR, M. L., & WATT, B. K. *Amino acid content of foods.* U. S. Department of Agriculture, Home Economics Research Report No. 4, Washington, D.C.: GPO, 1968.

OSLER, W. *Aequanimitas.* New York: McGraw-Hill, 1906.

OSLER, W. Quoted in R. Dubos, *Mirage of health.* New York: Harper & Row, 1971.

OTIS, L. S. "The facts on transcendental meditation: If well-integrated but anxious, try TM." *Psychology Today,* 1974, 7, 45–46.

OTTO, H. A., & MANN, J. *Ways of growth.* New York: Viking, 1968.

PACIFIC RESEARCH SYSTEMS. *Nutrition, health and activity profile.* Los Angeles, 2222 Corinth Avenue, Los Angeles, CA 90064.

PAFFENBARGER, R., et al. "Exercise and heart disease: An abstract." *Circulation,* October 1977.

PAFFENBARGER, R. S., et al. "Work energy level: Personal characteristics and fatal heart attack: A birth cohort effect." *American Journal of Epidemiology,* 1977, *105,* 200–213.

PAGE, I. H. "Preventive medicine." *Science,* September 3, 1976, *193* (4256), 1.

PAGE, I. H. *The cholesterol fallacy.* Cleveland: Coronary Club, 1977.

PAGE, T., HARRIS, R. H., & EPSTEIN, S. S. "Drinking water and cancer mortality in Louisiana." *Science,* July 2, 1976, *193,* 55–57.

"Paradise Lost," A staff report in *Nutrition Today,* May-June 1978, 6–9.

PARKER, W. *Cancer, a study of ninety-seven cases of cancer of the female breast.* New York: 1885.

PARKES, C. M. *Bereavement: Studies of grief in adult life.* New York: International Universities Press, 1972.

PARSONS, T. *The social system.* New York: Free Press, 1951.

PARSONS, T. "Definitions of health and illness." In Jaco, ed., *Patients, physicians, and illness.* New York: Free Press, 1972, 97–117.

PASSMORE, R., & DURNIN, J. V. G. A. "Human energy expenditure." *Physiology Review,* 1955, *35,* 801.

PASSWATER, RICHARD A. *Supernutrition for Healthy Hearts.* New York: Dial Press, 1977.

PATEL, C. H. Yoga and biofeedback in the management of hypertension." *Lancet,* November 10, 1973.

PATEL, C. H., & DATEY, K. K. "Yoga and biofeedback in the management of hypertension: Two control studies." Proceedings of The Biofeedback Research Society, Monterey, California, 1975.

PAUL, G. L. "Physiological effects of relaxation training and hypnotic suggestion." *Journal of Abnormal Psychology,* 1969, *74*(4), 425–437.

PAULING, L. *Vitamin C and the common cold.* San Francisco: W. H. Freeman and Co., 1970.

PAULING, L. "On vitamin C and cancer." *Executive Health,* January 1977, *13*(4).

PAULING, L. *Linus Pauling before Congress.* Stanford, CA: Linus Pauling Institute, 1978. (a)

PAULING, L. "Vitamin C and heart disease." *Executive Health,* January 1978, *14*(4). (b)

PAYKEL, E. S., MYERS, J. K., DIENELT, M. N., KLERMAN, G. L., LINDENTHAL, J. J., & PEPPER, M. P. "Life events and depression." *Archives of General Psychiatry,* 1969, *21,* 753–760.

PEARCE, J.C. *The crack in the cosmic egg.* New York: Julian, 1971.

PEARSE, I. H. *Is health a suitable study for academic consideration?* Scotland: University of St. Andrews, 1971.

PEARSE, I. H., & CROCKER, L. H. *The Peckham experiment: A study of the living structure of society, 6th ed.* Rushden, Great Britain: Northhamptonshire Printing and Publishing, 1947.

PEARSE, I. H., & WILLIAMSON, G. S. *The case for action, a survey of everyday life under modern industrial conditions with special reference to the question of health, 3rd ed.* London: Faber & Faber, 1938.

PEARSON, H. E. S., & JOSEPH, J. "Stress and occlusive coronary-artery disease." *Lancet,* 1963, *1,* 415–418.

Peckham Experiments. *Health of the individual, of the family, of society.* Sussex, England: The Pioneer Health Centre, 1971.

PELLETIER, K. R. "Influence of transcendental meditation upon autokinetic perception." *Journal of Perceptual and Motor Skills,* 1974, *39,* 1031–1034. Reprinted in Shapiro, D., ed., *Meditation:*

Self-Regulation Strategy and Altered States of Consciousness. Chicago: Aldine, 1979.

PELLETIER, K. R. "Neurological, psychophysiological, and clinical differentiation of the alpha and theta altered states of consciousness." *Dissertation Abstracts International,* 1974, *35*(1), 74–14, 806.

PELLETIER, K. R. "Psychophysiological parameters of the voluntary control of blood flow and pain." In D. Kanellakos and J. Lukas, eds., *The psychobiology of transcendental meditation.* Reading, MA: W. A. Benjamin, 1974, 34.

PELLETIER, K. R. "Diagnostic and treatment protocols for clinical biofeedback." *Journal of Biofeedback,* Fall-Winter 1975, *2*(4).

PELLETIER, K. R. "Neurological substates of consciousness." *Journal of Altered States of Consciousness,* 1975, *2*(1).

PELLETIER, K. R. "Theory and applications of clinical biofeedback." *Journal of Contemporary Psychotherapy,* 1975, *7*(1).

PELLETIER, K. R. "Holistic applications of clinical biofeedback and meditation." *Journal of Holistic Health,* 1976, *1.*

PELLETIER, K. R. "Neurophysiological parameters of the voluntary control of blood flow and pain." *Journal of Altered States of Consciousness,* 1976.

PELLETIER, K. R. *Mind as healer, mind as slayer.* New York: Delacorte Press/Seymour Lawrence, 1977.

PELLETIER, K. R. "Biofeedback." In *Collier's Encyclopedia.* New York: MacMillan, 1977.

PELLETIER, K. R. "Mind as Healer, Mind as Slayer," *Psychology Today,* February 1977.

PELLETIER, K. R. *Toward a science of consciousness.* New York: Delacorte Press, 1978.

PELLETIER, K. R. "Stress: Managing and overcoming it." In "Tools for Transformation," *New Realities,* August 1978, 43–45.

PELLETIER, K. R. "Adjunctive biofeedback with cancer patients: A case presentation." Proceedings of the Biofeedback Society of America. Denver: Biofeedback Society of America, 1977. Reprinted in *Biofeedback and Self-Regulation,* September 1977, *2* (3), 317. Reprinted in C. Garfield, ed., *Stress and Survival: The emotional realities of life-threatening illness.* St. Louis: The C. V. Mosby Company, 1979.

PELLETIER, K. R., & GARFIELD, C. *Consciousness: East and West.* New York: Harper & Row, 1976.

PELLETIER, K. R., & GARFIELD, C. "Meditative states of consciousness." In P. Zimbardo and C. Maslach, eds., *Psychology for our times: Readings.* 2nd Edition. Glenview, IL.: Scott, Foresman & Company, 1977.

PELLETIER, K. R. "Holistic Medicine: From pathology to prevention." *Western Journal of Medicine,* September 1979.

PELLETIER, K. R. "A Preventive approach to psychosomatic medicine," in D. Bresler, J. Gordon, and D. Jaffe, eds., *Body, Mind, and Health: Toward an Integral Medicine.* Washington, D.C.: National Institute of Mental Health, 1979.

PELLETIER, K. R., GLADMAN, A. E., & MIKURIYA, T. H. "Clinical protocols—professional group specializing in psychosomatic medicine." *Handbook of Physiological Feedback.* Berkeley: Autogenic Systems, Inc., 1976.

PELLETIER, K. R., & PEPER, E. " The chuzpah factor in altered states of consciousness." *Jounal of humanistic psychology,* 1977, *17*(1). Reprinted in G. Hendricks and J. Fadiman, eds., *Transpersonal Education,* Englewood Cliffs, N.J.: Prentice-Hall, 1976

PELLETIER, K. R., & PEPER, E. "Alpha EEG feedback as a means for pain control." *Journal of Clinical and Experimental Hypnosis,* 1977, 25(4), 361–371.

PELLETIER, K. R., & PEPER, E. "Clinical biofeedback: A holistic approach to psychosomatic medicine." In C. Garfield and J. Garfield, eds., *Rediscovery of the body: An inquiry into mind-body processes.* Manuscript in preparation.

PELLETIER, K. R., & PEPER, E. "Developing a biofeedback model: Alpha EEG feedback as a means for pain control." *Biofeedback and Self-Regulation,* 1977. In press.

PELNER, L. "Host-turn antagonism. III. Prolonged survival of certain patients with cancer. Fortuitous occurrence or immunity mechanism." *Journal of American Geriatric Society,* 1956, *4,* 1126.

PENDERGRASS, E. *Presidential address to the American Cancer Society.* Meeting, 1959.

PENFIELD, W. *The mystery of the mind.* Princeton, NJ: Princeton University Press, 1975.

PEPER, E. *Biofeedback as a core technique in clinical therapies.* Paper presented at the Biofeedback Research Society Meeting, Boston, 1972.

PEPER, E. *Applications of biofeedback to reduce stress and for preventive health.* Paper presented at the 82nd Annual Convention of the American Psychological Association, New Orleans, 1974.

PEPER, E. "Problems in biofeedback training: An experiential analogy—urination." *Perspectives in Biology and Medicine,* Spring 1976.

PEPER, E., PELLETIER, K.R., and TANDY, B. "Biofeedback training: Holistic and transpersonal frontiers." In Peper, E., Ancoli, S., and Quinn, M., eds., *Mind/body integrations: Essential readings in biofeedback.* New York: Plenum Press, 1979.

PERLS, F. S. *Gestalt therapy verbatim.* Lafayette, IN: Real People Press, 1969.

PERRY, J. W. "Reconstitutive process in the psychopathology of the self." *Annals of the New York Academy of Sciences,* 1962, *96,* 853–876.

PERSKY, H. "Adrenocortical function in anxious human subjects: The disappearance of hydrocortisone from plasma and its metabolic fate." *Journal of Clinical Endocrinological Metabolism,* 1957, *17,* 760–765.

PERSKY, H. "Adrenocortical function and anxiety." *Psychoneuroendocrinology,* 1975, *1,* 37–44.

PERSKY, H., GROSZ, H. J., NORTON, H. A., & McMURTRY, M. "Effect of hypnotically-induced anxiety on the plasma hydrocortisone level of normal subjects." *Journal of Clinical Endocrinological Metabolics,* 1959, *19,* 700–710.

PERSKY, H., HAMBURG, D. A., BASOWITZ, H., GRINKLER, R. R., SABSHIN, M., KORCHIN, S. J., HERZ, M., BOARD, F. A., & HEATH, H. A. "Relation of emotional responses and changes in plasma hydrocortisone level after stressful interview." *AMA Archives of Neurology and Psychiatry,* April 1958, *79,* 434–447.

PERSKY, H., KORCHIN, S. J., BASOWITZ, H., BOARD, F. A., BABSHIN, M., HAMBURG, D. A., & GRINKLER, R. "Effect of two psychological stresses on adrenocortical function." *AMA Archives of Neurology and Psychiatry,* 1959, *81.*

PETERS, M. "Hypertension and the nature of stress." *Science,* October 7, 1977, *198,* 80.

PICKERING, T. "Yoga and biofeedback in hypertension." *Lancet,* December 22, 1973.

PIRSIG, R. M. *Zen and the art of motorcycle maintenance.* New York: Bantam, 1974.

PITTS, F. N., JR., & McCLURE, J. N., JR. "Lactate metabolism in anxiety neurosis." *New England Journal of Medicine,* 1967, *277,* 1329–1334.

PLAG, J. "U.S. fliers held by Viets healthier." *Omaha World-Herald,* November 12, 1977, No. 49, 1.

POLEDNAK, A. P. "College athletics, body size, and cancer mortality." *Cancer,* July 1976, 382–387.

POPENOE, C. *Wellness.* New York: Random House, 1977.

"Pound of prevention ounce of cure?" *Medical World News,* May 15, 1978, 46–62.

POWLES, J. "On the limitations of modern medicine." *Science, Medicine, and Man,* 1973, *1,* 1–30.

PRAUL, D. "Ailing boy who preferred to die." *San Francisco Chronicle,* February 1978, 1.

Prevention Magazine (monthly). 33 East Minor Street, Emmaus, PA 18049.

PRIBRAM, K. H. "Emotions: Steps toward a neuropsychological theory." In D. Glass, ed., *Neurophysiology and Emotion.* New York: Rockefeller University Press and Russell Sage Foundation, 1967.

PRICE, D. B., TAHLER, M., MASON, J. W. "Preoperative emotional states and adrenal cortical activity." *AMA Archives of Neurology and Psychiatry,* 1957, *77,* 646–656.

PRIOR, I. "The onslaught of a western diet." *Behavior Today,* April 25, 1977, 5.

PUBLIC HEALTH SERVICE. *Federal employees health benefit program utilization study.* Washington, D.C.: Public Health Service, January 1955.

QUINT, J. V., & CODY, J. "Preeminence and mortality." *American Journal of Public Health,* 1970, *60*(6), 1118–1124.

RAHE, R. H. "Subjects' recent life changes and their near-future illness reports." *Annals of Clinical Research,* 1973, *4,* 1–16.

RAHE, R. H., MAHAN, J. L., & ARTHUR, R. J. "Prediction of near-future health change from subject's preceding life changes." *Journal of Psychosomatic Research,* 1970, *14,* 401–406.

RAHE, R. H., MEYER, M., SMITH, M., KJAER, G., & HOLMES, T. H. "Social Stress and Illness Onset." *Journal of Psychosomatic Research,* 1964, *8,* 35–44.

RAHE, R. H., & RANSOM, J. A. "Life change and illness studies: Past history and future directions." *Journal of Human Stress,* March 1978, 3–15.

RAHE, R. H., & ROMO, M. "Recent life changes and the onset of myocardial infarction and coronary death in Helsinki." In E. K. E. Gunderson and R. H. Rahe, eds., *Life stress and illness.* Springfield, IL: Charles C Thomas, 1974, 105–120.

RASMUSSEN, H. "Medical education—revolution or reaction?" *Pharos,* 1975, *53,* 38–45.

RAY, B. S. "Discussion of T. C. Everson and W. H. Cole: Spontaneous regression of cancer." *Ann. Surg.,* 1956, *144*(1) 366–383.

REES, W. D., & LUTKINS, S. G. "Mortality of bereavement." *British Medical Journal,* 1967, *4,* 13.

REICHARD, S. E. *Letter of HHA instructions.* Baltimore, MD: U. S. Public Health Service Hospital, 1975.

REMEN, N. *The masculine principle, the feminine principle, and humanistic medicine.* San Francisco: Institute for the Study of Humanistic Medicine, 1975.

Report of the Committee to evaluate the National Center for Health Statistics. *American Journal of Public Health,* 1973, *63*(10), 890–910.

REUBEN, D. *The save-your-life diet.* New York: Random House, 1975.

RICHARDS, M. C. *Centering.* Middletown: Wesleyan University Press, 1962.

RICHARDS, V. "On the nature of cancer. An analysis from concepts in current research." *Oncology,* 1967, *21,* 161–188.

RILEY, V. "Mouse mammary tumors: Alteration of incidence as apparent function of stress." *Science,* 1975, *189,* 465–467.

ROBBINS, L. C. *How to practice prospective medicine.* Indianapolis: Methodist Hospital, 1970.

ROBERTSON, L., FLINDER, C., & GODFREY, B. *Laurel's kitchen.* Berkeley, CA: Nilgiri Press, 1976.

ROCHE LABORATORIES. *Medical considerations for psychiatrists: Cardiovascular considerations.* Nutley, NJ: Hoffman-La Roche, 1979.

RODALE, J. I. *The complete book of vitamins.* Emmaus, PA: Rodale Press, 1977.

RODIN, J., & LANGER, E. J. *Journal of Personality and Social Psychology,* 1977, *35*(12), 903–911.

ROELANTS, G. E. "Biochemical evidence against a physiologic role for macrophage RNA-antigen complexes in the immune induction." In D. C. Dumonde, ed., *The role of lymphocytes and macrophages in the immunological response.* Munich, New York: International Congress of Haematology, Spring-Verlag, 1971.

ROSA, K. R. *You and AT.* New York: Dutton, 1976.

ROSE, S. *The conscious brain.* New York: Knopf, 1973.

ROSENBERG, J. L. *Total orgasm.* New York: Random House/Bookworks, 1973.

ROSENMAN, R. H., et al. "Coronary heart disease in the western collaborative group study: A follow-up experience of 4½ years." *Journal of Chronic Diseases,* 1970, *23,* 173–190.

ROSENMAN, R. H., BRAND, R. J., JENKINS, C. D., FRIEDMAN, M.,

STRAUSS, R., & WORM, M. "Coronary heart disease in the western collaborative group study: Final follow-up experience of 8½ years." *Journal of the American Medical Association,* 1975, *233*(8).

ROSENSTOCK, I. M. "What research in motivation suggests for public health." *American Journal of Public Health,* March 1960, *50*(3), 295–301.

ROTH, W. T. "Some motivational aspects of exercise." *Journal of Sports Medicine,* March 1974, *14*(1), 40–47.

"Roughage in the diet." *Medical World News,* September 6, 1974, 35–42.

ROXBURGH, D. "Spontaneous regression of cancer." *British Medical Journal,* 1935, *1,* 39.

Royal Norwegian Ministry of Agriculture Report No. 32. *Norwegian nutrition and food policy.* Oslo, Norway: Storting, 1975–1976.

Runner's World Magazine. Mountain View, CA: World Publications.

RUSH, A. K. *Getting clear: Body work for women.* New York: Random House/Bookworks, 1973.

RUSSEK, H. I. "Stress, tobacco, and coronary heart disease in North American professional groups." *Journal of the American Medical Association,* 1965, *192,* 189–194.

RUSSEK, H. I., & RUSSEK, L. G. "Is emotional stress an etiologic factor in coronary heart disease?" *Psychosomatics,* 1976, *17*(2), 63.

RYAN, A. J. "Sports medicine today." *Science,* May 26, 1978, *200,* 919–924.

SACHAR, E. J. "Corticosteroid in depressive illness: A review of control issues and the literature." *Archives of General Psychiatry,* 1967, *17,* 544.

SACHAR, E. J. "Psychological factors relating to activation and inhibition of the adrenocortical stress response in man: A review." In D. WeWied and J. Weijnen, eds., *Progress in brain research, Vol. 32,* New York: Elsevier, 1970.

SACKS, O. W. *Migraine.* Berkeley: University of California Press, 1970.

SALES, S. M. *Differences among individuals in affective, behavioral, biochemical and physiological responses to variations in workload.* Doctoral dissertation, University of Michigan, Ann Arbor, Michigan. University Microfilms No. 69-18098, 1969.

SALES, S. M., & HOUSE, J. "Job dissatisfaction as a possible risk factor in coronary heart disease." *Journal of Chronic Diseases,* 1971, *23,* 867–873.

SALK, J. *Man unfolding* (R. N. Anshen, ed.). New York: Harper & Row, 1972.

SALK, J. *Survival of the wisest.* New York: Harper & Row, 1973.

SAMUELS, MIKE, & BENNETT, HAL. *The well body book.* New York: Random House, 1973.

SAMUELS, M., & SAMUELS, N. *Seeing with the mind's eye.* New York: Random House/Bookworks, 1975.

SANCHEZ, A., et al. "Role of sugars in human neutrophilic phagocytosis." *American Journal of Clinical Nutrition,* 1973, *26*(11), 1180–1184.

SARGENT, J. D., GREEN, E. E., & WALTERS, E. D. "The use of autogenic feedback training in a pilot study of migraine and tension headaches." *Headache,* 1972, *12,* 120–124.

SATIR, V. *Peoplemaking.* Palo Alto, CA: Science and Behavior Books, 1972.

SATO, KOJI. "Death of Zen masters." *Psychologia,* 1964, *7,* 143–147.

SARAVAY, S. M., & KORAN, L. M. "Organic disease mistakenly diagnosed as psychiatric." *Psychosomatics,* June 1977, 6–11.

SAWARD, E. W. "The effect on future physician requirements of an HMO policy after national health insurance." *Journal of Community Health,* 1975, *1*(1), 53–71.

SAWARD, E. W. "Medicare, medical practice, and the medical profession." *Public Health Reports,* July–August 1976, *91*(4), 317–321.

SAWARD, E., BLANK, J., & LAMB, H. *Some information descriptive of a successfully operating HMO.* Washington, D.C.: Department of HEW, 1972.

SAWARD, E., & SORENSEN, A. "The current emphasis on preventive medicine." *Science,* May 26, 1978, *200,* 889–894.

SAYERS, G. "Factors influencing the level of ACTH in the blood." *Ciba Foundation Colloquia on Endocrinology,* 1957, *11,* 138–149.

SAYERS, G., & SAYERS, M. A. "Regulation of pituitary or adrenocorticotrophin activity during response of rate to acute stress." *Endocrinology,* 1947, *40,* 265–273.

SCHEFLEN, A. E. "Malignant tumors in the institutionalized psychotic population." *Arch. Neurol. Psychiat.,* 1951, *64,* 145–155.

SCHILDKRAUT, J. J., & KETY, S. S. "Biogenic amines and emotion." *Science,* 1967, *156,* 21–30.

SCHLESS, G. L., & VON LAUERAN-STIEVAR, R. "Recurrent episodes of diabetic acidosis precipitated by emotional stress." *Diabetes,* 1964, *13,* 419–420.

SCHMALE, A. H., JR., & ENGEL, G. L. "The giving up-given up complex illustrated on film." *Arch. Gen. Psychiat.,* 1967, *17,* 135–145.

SCHMALE, A. H. "Giving up as a final common pathway to changes in health." In Z. J. Lipowski, ed., *Psychosocial aspects of physical illness, Vol. 8.* New York: Basel S. Karger, 1972, 20–40.

SCHOFIELD, J. E. "Teratoma of testis; spontaneous disappearance of lung metastases." *British Medical Journal,* 1947, *1,* 411.

SCHOOLMAN, H. M., & BERNSTEIN, L. M. "Computer use in diagnosis, prognosis, and therapy." *Science,* May 26, 1978, *200,* 926–931.

SCHULMAN, S., & SMITH, A. M. "The concept of health among Spanish-speaking villagers of New Mexico and Colorado." *Journal of Health and Human Behavior,* 1963, *4,* 226.

SCHULTZ, J., & LUTHE, W. *Autogenic training: A psychophysiologic approach in psychotherapy.* New York: Grune & Stratton, 1959.

SCHWARTZ, G. E. *Biofeedback as therapy: Some theoretical and practical issues.* Paper delivered to the Third Annual Brockton Symposium on Behavior Therapy, April 1972.

SCHWARTZ, G. E. *Pros and cons of meditation: Current findings on physiology and anxiety, self-control, drug abuse, and creativity.* Paper delivered at the 81st annual convention of the American Psychological Association, Montreal, Canada, 1973.

SCHWARTZ, G., ed. *Biofeedback: Theory and research.* New York: Academic Press, 1978.

SCHWARTZ, G. E., & GOLEMAN, D. J. *Meditation as an alternative to drug use: Accompanying personality changes.* Submitted for publication, 1974.

SCHWARTZ, G., & SHAPIRO, D. *Consciousness and self-regulation: Advances in research.* New York: Plenum Press, 1976.

SCHWARTZ, G. E., SHAPIRO, D., & TURSKY, B. "Learned control of cardiovascular integration in man through operant conditioning." *Psychosomatic Medicine,* 1971, *33,* 57–62.

SCHWARZENEGGER, A. "The powers of the mind: An interview with Arnold Schwarzenegger." *New Age,* March 1978, 38–43.

SCOTT, J. B. "Spontaneous regression of cancer." *British Medical Journal,* 1935, *1,* 230.

SEELEY, J. *The Americanization of the unconscious.* New York: International Science Press, 1967.

SEGAL, J. "Biofeedback as medical treatment." *JAMA,* 1975, *232*(2), 179–180.

SEGALL, P. E. "Long-term tryptophan restriction and aging in the rat." *Aktuelle Gerontologie,* Band 7, Heft 10, Stuttgart, Germany, October 1977, 535–538.

SEGALL, P. E., OOKA, H., ROSE, K., & TIMIRAS, P. S. "Neural and endocrine development after chronic tryptophan deficiency in rats: Brain monoamine and pituitary responses." *Mechanisms of Ageing and Development*, 1978, No. 7, 1–17.

SEGALL, P. E., & TIMIRAS, P. S. "Age-related changes in thermoregulatory capacity of tryptophan-deficient rats." *Federation Proceedings*, January 1975, *34*(1), 83–85.

SEGALL, P. E., & TIMIRAS, P. S. "Patho-physiologic findings after chronic tryptophan deficiency in rats: A model for delayed growth and aging." *Mechanisms of Ageing and Development*, 1976, No. 5, 109–124.

SEGUIN, C. A. "Migration and psychosomatic disadaptation." *Journal of Psychosomatic Medicine*, 1956, *18*, 404–409.

SELIGMAN, A. M. *Helplessness.* San Francisco: W. H. Freeman, 1975.

SELIGMAN, A. M. A review of Everson, Tilden, Cole, Waner: "Spontaneous regression of cancer: A study and abstracts of reports in the world medical literature and of personal communications concerning spontaneous regression of malignant disease." *JAMA*, 1966, *198*(6), 680.

SELYE, H. *Stress without distress.* New York: Dutton, 1974.

SELYE, H. *From dream to discovery.* Montreal, Canada: International Institute of Stress. Also New York: Arno Press, 1975.

SELYE, H. "Secret of coping with stress." An interview in *U.S. News and World Report*, March 21, 1977, 51–53. (a)

SELYE, H. "Stress can be good for you." *Behavior Today*, October 31, 1977. (b)

SHAPIRO, D., & SCHWARTZ, G. E. "Biofeedback and visceral learning: Clinical applications." *Seminars in Psychiatry*, 1972, *4*, 171–184.

SHAPIRO, D., TURSKY, B., GERSON, E., & STERN, M. "Effects of feedback and reinforcement on the control of human systolic blood pressure." *Science*, 1969, *163*, 588.

SHAPIRO, S. L. "Spontaneous regression of cancer." *Eye, Ear, Nose, Throat Monthly*, October 1967, *46*, 1306–1310.

SHEALY, N. *Ninety days to self-health.* New York: Dial, 1977.

SHEDRIN, H. "Brain wave correlates of subliminal stimulation, unconscious attention, primary and secondary process thinking, and repressiveness." *Psychological Issues*, 1973, *8*(2), 56–87.

SHIMKIN, M. B., GRISWOLD, M. H., & CUTLER, S. J. "Survival in untreated and treated cancer." *Ann. Intern. Med.*, 1956, *45*, 255–267.

SHRIFTE, M. "Toward identification of a positive variable in host resistance to cancer." *Psychosomatic Medicine*, 1962, *24*, 390.

SILVERMAN, S. *Psychologic cues in forecasting physical illness.* New York: Appleton-Century-Crofts, 1970.

SIMEONS, A. T. W. *Man's presumptuous brain.* New York: Dutton, 1960.

SIMMONS, L. W. "The relation between the decline of anxiety-reducing and anxiety-resolving factors in a deteriorating culture, and its relevance to bodily disease." *Proc. Ass. Res. Neurol. Ment. Disease,* 1950, *29,* 127.

SIMONTON, O.C., & MATTHEWS-SIMONTON, S. "Belief systems and management of the emotional aspects of malignancy." *Journal of Transpersonal Psychology,* 1975, 7 (1), 29–47.

SIMONTON, O.C., MATTHEWS-SIMONTON, S., & CREIGHTON, J. *Getting well again.* Los Angeles: J.P. Tarcher, 1978.

"Skyrocketing costs of health care, The." *Business Week,* May 17, 1976, 144–147.

SLATER, P. *Survey of sickness, October 1943 to December 1945.* London: Ministry of Health, August 1946.

SLOANE, R. B. "Some behavioral and other correlates of cholesterol metabolism." *Journal of Psychosomatic Research,* 1961, *5,* 183–190.

SMITH, M. *When I say no, I feel guilty.* New York: Bantam, 1975.

SOBEL, D. S., & HORNBACHER, F. L. *An everyday guide to your health.* New York: Grossman, 1973.

SOLOFF, L. A. "Sexual activity in the heart patient." *Psychosomatics,* October 1977, 23–28.

SOLOMON, G. F. "Emotions, stress, the central nervous system, and immunity." *New York Academy of Science Annals,* 1969, 164(2), 335–343.

SOLOMON, G. F., AMKRAUT, A. A., & KASPER, P. "Immunity, emotions and stresses (with special reference to the mechanisms of stress effects on the immune system)." *Psychotherapy and Psychosomatics,* 23, 1974, 209–217.

SONTAG, SUSAN. *Illness as metaphor.* New York: Farrar, Straus & Giroux, 1978.

SOROCHAN, W. "Health concepts as a basis for orthobiosis." *Journal of the School of Health,* 1968, *38*(10), 673–682.

SPINO, M. *Beyond jogging.* Millbrae, CA: Celestial Arts, 1976.

SPITZER, W. O., FEINSTEIN, A. R., & SACKETT, D. L. "What is a health care trial?" *JAMA,* July 14, 1975, *233*(2), 161–163.

"Spontaneous regression of cancer." *British Medical Journal,* 1962, *2,* 1245.

STALLONES, R. A. *Environment, ecology, and epidemiology.* Washington, D.C.: Pan-American Health Organization Scientific Publication No. 231, 1971.

STAMLER, J. Paper presented at a meeting of the American Heart Association, New York, 1975; and to the Second Science Writers Forum, Marro Island, Florida, January 1975.

STANYAN, M. "Secrets of long life from the Andes." *San Francisco Examiner & Chronicle,* September 26, 1976, *3.*

STAPLETON, R. C. *The gift of inner healing.* New York: Word, Inc., 1975.

STAPLETON, R. C. *The experience of inner healing.* New York: Word, Inc., 1976.

STATE OF CALIFORNIA, BOARD OF MEDICAL EXAMINERS. Compilation of laws relating to the practice of medicine and surgery, physical therapy, physician's assistants, podiatry, psychology, dispensing opticians, hearing aid dispensers, speech pathologists, and audiologists with rules and regulations and directory. Sacramento, 1972–1973.

STEIN, J. *Meditation, habituation, and distractability.* Unpublished undergraduate honors thesis, Harvard University, 1973.

STEIN, M. "Some psychophysiological considerations of the relationship between the autonomic nervous system and behavior." In D. C. Glass, ed., *Neurophysiology and emotion.* New York: Rockefeller University Press and Russell Sage Foundation, 1967, 145–154.

STEPHENSON, H., & GRACE, W. J. "Life stress and cancer of the cervix." *Psychosomatic Medicine,* 1954, *16,* 287–294.

STERMAN, M. B., & FRIAR, L. "Suppression of seizures in the epileptic following sensorimotor EEG feedback training." *EEG Journal,* 1972, *33,* 89–95.

STERMAN, M. B., MACDONALD, L. R., & STONE, R. K. "Biofeedback training of the sensori-motorelectroencephalogram rhythm in man: Effects of epilepsy." *Epilepcia,* 1974, *15,* 395–416.

STERN, J. A., SURPHLIS, W., & KOFF, E. "Electrodermal responsiveness as related to psychiatric diagnosis and prognosis." *Psychophysiology,* 1965, *2,* 61–66.

STERNBACH, R. A. *Principles of psychophysiology.* New York: Academic Press, 1966.

STEVENS, C. M. "Physician supply and national health care goals." *Industrial Relations,* 1971, *10,* 119–144.

STEWART, C. T., JR. "Allocation of resources to health." *Journal of Human Resources,* 1971, *6*(1), 103–121.

STEWART, F. W. "Experiences in spontaneous regression of neoplastic disease in man." *Texas Rep. Biol. Med.,* 1952, *10,* 239.

STOKES, J. F., NABARRO, J. D. N., & ROSENHEIM, M. L. "Physical disease in a mental observation unit." *Lancet,* 1954, *2,* 862–863.

STONE, H. B., CURTIS, R. M., & BREWER, J. H. "Can resistance to cancer be induced?" *Ann. Surg.,* 1951, *134,* 519–528.

STONE, H. B., & SCHNAUFER, L. "Attempts to induce resistance to cancer." *Ann. Surg.,* 1955, *141,* 329.

STOUT, C., MORROW, J., BRANDT, E., & WOLF, S. "Unusually low incidence of death from myocardial infarction: Study of an Italian-American community in Pennsylvania." *Journal of the American Medical Association,* 1964, *188,* 845–849.

STOYVA, J., & BUDZYNSKI, T. "Cultivated low arousal—an antistress response?" In L. V. DiCara, ed., *Recent advances in limbic and autonomic nervous system research.* New York: Plenum Press, 1973.

STRAUSS, S. "Abkhazia." *Harper's,* June 1973, 6.

STREISGUTH, A. P., et al. "Caffeine, nicotine, and alcohol effects with pregnant women." *Medical World News,* September 19, 1977, 12–14.

STROEBEL, C. *Personal communication.* Hartford, CT: Institute of Living, 1975.

STUART, R. B., & DAVIS, B. *Slim chance in a fat world.* Champaign, IL: Research Press, 1972.

SUINN, R. M. "Body thinking: Psychology for Olympic champs." *Psychology Today,* July 1976, 38–43.

SUMNER, W. C., & FORAKER, A. G. "Spontaneous regression of human melanoma: Clinical and experimental studies." *Cancer,* 1960, *13,* 79–81.

SWAMI RAMA. *A practical guide to holistic health.* Honesdale, PA: Himalayan Institute, 1978.

SYME, L. S. "Social and psychological risk factors in coronary disease." *Modern Concepts of Cardiovascular Disease,* 1975, 44, *17.*

SZENT-GYÖRGY, A. *Electronic biology and cancer: A new theory of cancer.* New York: Marcel Dekker, 1976. (a)

SZENT-GYÖRGI, A. "On a substance that can make us sick (if we do not eat it!)" *Executive Health,* June 1977, *13*(9), 1–6. (b)

SZENT-GYÖRGI, A. "How new understandings about the biological functions of ascorbic acid may profoundly affect our lives." *Executive Health,* May 1978, *14*(8). (c)

Tape cassettes: Psychology Today Cassettes, 11116 Cashmere Street, Los Angeles, CA 90049.

TARLAU, M., & SMALHEISER, I. "Personality patterns in patients with

malignant tumors of the breast and cervix; exploratory study."
Psychosomatic Medicine, 1951, *13,* 117–121.

TART, C. T. *Altered states of consciousness.* New York: Wiley, 1969.

TART, C. T. *States of consciousness.* New York: Dutton, 1975.

TAUB, E. "Self-regulation of human tissue temperature." In G. E.
Schwartz and J. Beatty, eds., *Biofeedback: Theory and research.*
New York: Academic Press, 1976.

TAYLOR, G. J. "The mind-body dichotomy." *Psychosomatics,* May
1978, *19*(5), 264–267.

TAYLOR, G. R. "People pollution." *Ladies' Home Journal,* October
1970, 74–79.

TAYLOR, R. *Hunza health secrets for long life and happiness.* Engel-
wood Cliffs, NJ: Prentice-Hall, 1964.

Teaching asaras: An Ananda Marga manual for teachers. Los Altos
Hills, CA: 1973.

THEORELL, T., & RAHE, R. H. Behavior prior to myocardial infarction. In T. Theorell, ed., *Psychosocial factors in relation to the
onset of myocardial infarction and to some metabolic variables: A
pilot study.* Stockholm: Karolinska Institute, 1970.

THOMAS, C. B. "What becomes of medical students, the dark side."
Johns Hopkins Medical Journal, 1976, *138*(5), 185–189.

THOMAS, C. B., & DUSZYNSKI, K. R. "Closeness to parents and the
family constellation in a prospective study of five disease states:
Suicide, mental illness, malignant tumor, hypertension and coronary heart disease." *Johns Hopkins Medical Journal,* 1974, *134*(5),
251–270.

THOMAS, C. B., & MURPHY, E. A. "Further studies on cholesterol
levels in the Johns Hopkins medical students: The effect of stress
at examinations." *Journal of Chronic Diseases,* 1958, *8,* 661–668.

THOMAS, L. *The lives of a cell.* New York: Bantam, 1975.

THOMAS, L. "The future place of science in the art of healing."
Journal of Medical Education, 1976, *51,* 23.

THOMAS, L. "On the science and technology of medicine." In J. H.
Knowles, ed., *Doing better and feeling worse.* New York: Norton,
1977, 35–46.

THURLOW, H. J. "Illness in relation to life situation and sick-role
tendency." *Journal of Psychosomatic Research,* 1971, *15,* 73–88.

TILLICH, P. "The meaning of health." *Perspectives in Biology and
Medicine,* 1961, *5,* 92–100.

TINBERGEN, N. "Ethology and stress diseases." *Science,* 1974, *185,*
20–27.

TOOMIN, M. K., & TOOMIN, H. "GSR biofeedback response patterns in psychotherapy." *Psychotherapy: Theory, research and practice,* December 1975.

TOP, F. H. "Environment in relation to infectious diseases." *Archives of Environmental Health,* December 1964.

TORNSTAM, L. "Health and self-perception: A systems theoretical approach." *Gerontologist,* June 1975, *15*(3), 264–270.

TRAVIS, J. W. *Wellness inventory.* Mill Valley, CA: Wellness Center, 1975.

TRAVIS, J. W. *Wellness workbook.* Mill Valley, CA: Wellness Center, 1979.

TRAVIS, J. W., & REICHARD, S. E. *Health hazard appraisal: User's guide to P.H.S. computerized health hazard appraisal.* Baltimore: USPHS Hospital, 1978.

TRUNGPA, C. *Meditation in action.* Berkeley, CA: Shambhala, 1969.

TRUNGPA, C. *Cutting through spiritual materialism.* Berkeley, CA: Shambhala, 1973.

TSUJI, K., ASHIZAWA, S., SASA, H., et al. "Clinical and statistical observations on spontaneous regression of cancer." *Jap. J. Cancer Clin.,* 1969, *15,* 729–733.

TUKE, D. H. *Illustrations of the influence of the mind on the body in health and disease designed to elucidate the action of the imagination. . . . , 2nd ed.* London: J. & A. Churchill, 1884.

TULKU, T. *Reflections of the mind.* Berkeley: Dharma Press, 1975.

TWADDLE, A. D. *The concept of health status.* Presented at the 2nd International Conference on Social Science and Medicine, Aberdeen, Scotland, 1970.

ULLYOT, J. *Women's Running.* Mountain View, CA: World Publications, 1976.

UNITED STATES DEPARTMENT OF HEW. *Forward plan for health.* FY 1977–1981. Washington, D.C.: GPO, 631-613/489, 1975.

VACHON, L. Cited in "Biofeedback in action." *Medical World News,* March 9, 1973.

VAN, J. "Dr. Knowles has a prescription for health care." *Boston Globe,* August 5, 1977, 2.

VAN DER VALK, J. M. & GROEN, J. J. "Personality structure and conflict situation in patients with myocardial infarction." *Journal of Psychosomatic Research,* 1967, *11,* 41–46.

VARTANIAN, A., ed. *La Mettrie's l'homme machine: A study in the origins of an idea.* Princeton, NJ: Princeton University Press, 1960.

VAYDA, E. "Keeping people well: A new approach to medicine." *Human Nature,* July 1978, 64–71.

VEATCH, R. M. "The medical model: Its nature and problems." *The Hastings Center Studies,* 1973, *1*(3), 58–76.

VICKERY, D. M., & FRIES, J. F. *Take care of yourself: A consumer's guide to medical care.* Reading, MA: Addison-Wesley, 1977.

VIRCHOW, R. *Cellular pathology.* Translated by Frank Chance. Ann Arbor, MI: Edwards Brothers, 1940.

VIRCHOW, R. *Disease, life and man.* Stanford, CA: Stanford University Press, 1958.

VITHOULKAS, G. *Homeopathy: Medicine of the new man.* New York: Avon, 1972.

VOLEN, M., & BRESLER, D. *A guide to good nutrition.* Los Angeles: Center for Integral Medicine, 1979.

WADE, N. "Thomas S. Kuhn: Revolutionary theorist of science." *Science,* July 8, 1977, *197,* 143–145.

WALLACE, R. K. "Physiological effects of transcendental meditation." *Science,* 1970, *167,* 1751–1754.

WALLACE, R. K., BENSON, H., WILSON, A. F., & GARRETT, M. D. "Decreased blood lactate during transcendental meditation." *Federation Proceedings,* 1971, *30,* 376.

WALLACE, R. K., BENSON, H., & WILSON, A. F. "A wakeful hypometabolic state." *American Journal of Physiology,* 1971, *221,* 795–799.

WALLACE, R. K., & BENSON, H. "The physiology of meditation." *Scientific American,* 1972, *226,* 84–90.

WATSON, G. *Nutrition and your mind.* New York: Harper & Row, 1972.

WATT, E. W., PLOTNICKI, B. A., & BUSKIRK, E. R. "The physiology of single and multiple daily training programs." *Track Technique,* 1972, No. 49, 1554–1555.

WEED, L. L. *Medical records, medical education, and patient care.* Chicago: Case Western Reserve University Press, 1970.

WEIL, A. *The natural mind.* Boston: Houghton Mifflin, 1972.

WEISS, E., et al. "Emotional factors in coronary occlusion." *Archives of Internal Medicine,* 1957, *99,* 628–641.

WEISS, R., & ENGEL, B. "Operant conditioning of heart rate in patients with premature ventricular contractions." *Psychosomatic Medicine,* 1971, *33*(4), 301–321.

WELBORN, S. N. "Are you eating right?" *U.S. News and World Report,* November 28, 1977, 39–43.

WERTLAKE, P. T., et al. "Relationship of mental and emotional stress to serum cholesterol levels." *Proceedings of the Society for Experimental Biology and Medicine*, 1958, *97*, 163–165.

WESHOW, H. J., & REINHART, G. "Life change and hospitalization— a heretical view." *Journal of Psychosomatic Research*, 1974, *18*, 393–401.

WEST, P. M. "Origin and development of the psychological approach to the cancer problem." In J. A. Gengerelli and F. J. Kirkner, eds., *The psychological variables in human cancer*. Berkeley, CA: University of California Press, 1954.

WEYER, E. M., & HUTCHINS, H., eds. *Psychophysiological aspects of cancer*. New York: New York Academy of Sciences, 1966.

WHATMORE, G. B., & KOHLI, D. R. "Dysponesis: A neurophysiologic factor in functional disorders." *Behavioral Science*, 1968, *13*(2), 102–104.

WHATMORE, G. B., & KOHLI, D. R. *The Psychopathology and treatment of functional disorders*. New York: Grune & Stratton, 1974.

WHEATLEY, D. "Evaluation of psychotropic drugs in general practice." *Proceedings of the Royal Society of Medicine*, 1962, *65*, 317.

WHEELER, J. I., JR., & CALDWELL, B. M. "Psychological evaluation of women with cancer of the breast and of the cervix." *Psychosomatic Medicine*, 1955, *17*, 256–268.

WHEELIS, A. *How people change*. New York: Harper & Row, 1973.

WHITE, J. *The highest state of consciousness*. New York: Doubleday, 1972.

WHITE, J. *Relax*. New York: Dell, 1976.

WHITE, L. S. "Sounding board: How to improve the public's health." *New England Journal of Medicine*, 1975, *293*(15), 773–774.

WICKRAMASKERA, I. "Effects of EMG feedback training on susceptibility to hypnosis: Preliminary observations." *Proceedings of the American Psychological Association*, 1971, 783–784.

WICKRAMASKERA, I., ed. *Biofeedback, behavior therapy and hypnosis*. Chicago: Nelson Hall, 1976.

WILLIAMS, G. "Biological and analytic components of variation in long-term studies of serum constituents in normal subjects." *Clinical Chemistry*, 1970, *16*(12), 1016–1032.

WILLIAMS, G. "Comparison of estimates of long-term analytical variation derived from subject samples and control serum." *Clinical Chemistry*, 1977, *23*(1).

WILLIAMS, J. F. *Personal hygiene applied*. Philadelphia: W. B. Saunders, 1934.

WILLIAMS, R. J. *Biochemical individuality.* New York: Wiley, 1956.

WILLIAMS, R. J. *Nutrition in a nutshell.* New York: Dolphin Books, 1962.

WILLIAMS, R. J. *Nutrition against disease.* New York: Bantam, 1973.

WILLIAMS, R. J. *The wonderful world within you.* New York: Bantam, 1977.

WILLIAMS, R. J., & DWIGHT, K. *A physician's handbook on orthomolecular medicine.* New York: Pergamon Press, 1977.

WILLIAMSON, G. S., & PEARSE, I. H. *Biologists in search of material: An interim report on the work of the Pioneer Health Centre, Peckham, 2nd ed.* London: Faber & Faber, 1947.

WILLIAMSON, G. S., & PEARSE, I. H. *Science, synthesis and sanity.* London: Collins, 1965.

WILSON, W. "Correlates of avowed happiness." *Psychological Bulletin,* 1967, *67*(4), 294–306.

WINGFIELD, R. T. "Psychiatric symptoms that signal organic disease." *Virginia Medical Monthly,* 1967, *94,* 153–157.

WOLF, S. "Disease as a way of life: Neural integration in systemic pathology." *Perspectives in Biology and Medicine, Vol. IV.* Chicago: University of Chicago Press, 1969–1961, 288–305.

WOLF, S. *The stomach.* New York: Oxford University Press, 1965.

WOLF, S. "A bell for Roseto: Town loses immunity to stress." *Brain/Mind Bulletin,* July 17, 1978, *3*(17), 2.

WOLFF, H. G. *Stress and disease.* Springfield, IL: Charles C Thomas, 1953.

WOLFF, H. G. *Headache and other head pain.* New York: Oxford University Press, 1963.

WOLFGANG, O. "Is immortality real?" *Modern Maturity,* April-May 1978, 25–26.

WOLPE, J. *Psychotherapy by reciprocal inhibition.* Stanford, CA: Stanford University Press, 1958.

WOLPE, J., & LAZARUS, A. A. *Behavior therapy techniques.* New York: Pergamon Press, 1966.

WOOD, L. L. *Medical records, medical education, and patient care.* Chicago: Case Western University Press, 1971.

WOODWARD, K. L., et al. "Sister Ruth: Healer Ruth Carter Stapleton." *Newsweek,* July 17, 1978, 58–66.

World Health Organization. "Constitution of the World Health Organization, Annex I." In the *First ten years of the World Health Organization.* Geneva: World Health Organization, 1958.

WRIGHT, I. S. "Can your family history tell you anything about your chances for a long life?" *Executive Health,* February, 1978, 14(5).

WRIGHT, L. "Conceptualizing and defining psychosomatic disorders." *American Psychologist,* August 1977, 625–628.

WYNDER, E. L., & BROSS, L. I. "Factors in human cancer development." *Cancer,* 1959, *12,* 1016.

YANDELL, R. J. "The imitation of Jung—an exploration of the meaning of 'Jungian.' " Spring 1978.

YOUNG, A. M. *The reflexive universe.* New York: Delacorte, 1976.

YOUNG, J. B., & LANDSBERG, L. "Suppression of sympathetic nervous system during fasting." *Science,* 1977, *196,* 1473–1475.

ZIMBARDO, P. G. *The cognitive control of motivation.* Glenview, IL: Scott, Foresman, 1969. (a)

ZIMBARDO, P. G. "The human choice: Reason and order versus impulse and chaos." *Nebraska Symposium on Motivation,* March 1969. (b)

INDEX

A

Abelson, Philip H., 214
Abkhaz Republic (Caucasus), 189, 191, 200
Abraham, 188
Accidents, 57, 88. *See also* Auto accidents
Achterberg, Jeanne, 116, 117–19, 213–14
ACTH, 115
Acupuncture, 15
Additives, 133–42
Adenoidectomy, 89
Adolescence, 42–43, 193
Adrenals, 100, 105, 113. *See also* Stress
Aequanimitas, 208
Aerobics, 167–74ff., 195–96
Aerobics, 169–70, 174
Aerobics for Women, 171
Aerobics Way, The, 171
Age, 57, 143. *See also* Health Hazard Appraisal; Longevity

Alcohol (drinking), 9, 12, 39, 55ff., 62, 63, 66, 68, 155, 157, 160, 192
Ali, S. Magsood, 192
Alikishiyev, Ramazan, 188
American Dietetic Association, 147
American Heart Association, 147
American Medical Association, 147
American Way of Life Need Not Be Hazardous to Your Health, The, 217
Amino Acid Content of Foods, 153
Amino acids, 62, 130, 152, 153
Anemia, 153
Antibiotics, xv, 1
Antibodies, 203
Apple, Dorrian, 32
Archery, 187
Archives of Environmental Health, 5
Arteriosclerosis, 87, 88, 101, 107. *See also* Atherosclerosis
Arthritis, 1, 12
Ashley, Richard, 133
Astrand, Per-Olaf, 168, 174, 177, 182, 196
Atherosclerosis, 107, 150, 155, 194, 197

B

C

F

G

H

I

J

O

P

Q

U

T

Z

About the Author

KENNETH R. PELLETIER, PH.D., is an Assistant Clinical Professor in the Department of Psychiatry and the Langley Porter Neuropsychiatric Institute, University of California School of Medicine, San Francisco. He is Director of the Psychosomatic Medicine Clinic in Berkeley, California. During graduate school at the University of California at Berkeley, he was Phi Beta Kappa, a Woodrow Wilson Fellow, and studied at the C. G. Jung Institute in Zurich, Switzerland. He has published numerous articles on psychosomatic medicine, clinical biofeedback, and neurophysiology. Dr. Pelletier is co-author of *Consciousness: East and West* (New York: Harper and Row, 1976), author of the international best seller *Mind as Healer, Mind as Slayer: A Holistic Approach to Preventing Stress Disorders* (New York: Delacorte and Delta, 1977), *Toward a Science of Consciousness* (New York: Delacorte and Delta, 1978), and *Holistic Medicine* (New York: Delacorte and Delta, 1979).

MAILING ADDRESS:

Kenneth R. Pelletier, Ph.D.
The Psychosomatic Medicine Clinic
2510 Webster Street
Berkeley, CA 94705
(415) 548–1115